# SCHOOL PSYCHOLOGY
# FOR THE 21ST CENTURY

# SCHOOL PSYCHOLOGY FOR THE 21ST CENTURY

## Foundations and Practices

**Kenneth W. Merrell**
**Ruth A. Ervin**
**Gretchen A. Gimpel**

The Guilford Press
New York   London

© 2006 The Guilford Press
A Division of Guilford Publications, Inc.
72 Spring Street, New York, NY 10012
www.guilford.com

Printed in the United States of America

This book is printed on acid-free paper.

Last digit is print number:  9  8  7  6  5  4  3  2  1

**Library of Congress Cataloging-in-Publication Data**

Merrell, Kenneth W.
  School psychology for the 21st century : foundations and practices /
Kenneth W. Merrell, Ruth A. Ervin, Gretchen A. Gimpel.
     p. cm.
  Includes bibliographical references and index.
  ISBN 1-59385-250-9
 1.  School psychology—United States.  I. Ervin, Ruth A. II. Gimpel,
Gretchen A. III. Title.
  LB1027.55.M47 2006
  371.4—dc22                        2005021693

# About the Authors

**Kenneth W. Merrell, PhD,** is Professor and Director of the School Psychology Program at the University of Oregon, where he teaches courses in school psychology and leads the Oregon Resiliency Project. Earlier in his career he worked for 3 years full-time as a school psychologist, and he has worked as a consulting school psychologist in three states while working as a university educator. Dr. Merrell's teaching and research interests are focused on social–emotional assessment and intervention for at-risk children and adolescents, as well as social–emotional learning in schools. He has a long list of publications, including five books and five nationally normed assessment instruments related to these areas. He is a Fellow in both the Division of School Psychology (Division 16) and the Society for Clinical Child and Adolescent Psychology (Division 53) of the American Psychological Association. Having previously served as an editorial board member or consulting editor for several professional and scientific journals, Dr. Merrell currently serves as an editorial board member for *School Psychology Review*, and is the series editor for The Guilford Practical Intervention in the Schools Series.

**Ruth A. Ervin, PhD,** is Associate Professor of School Psychology and Special Education at the University of British Columbia, Vancouver, Canada. Her professional teaching and research interests lie within the domains of promoting systems-level change to address research-to-practice gaps in school settings; collaborative consultation with school personnel, parents, and other service providers for the prevention and treatment of emotional and/or behavioral disorders such as attention-deficit/hyperactivity disorder and oppositional defiant disorder via a data-driven, solution-oriented problem-solving approach; and linking assessment to intervention to promote academic performance and socially significant outcomes for school-age children. Emphasis in Dr. Ervin's work has been placed on systems-level change and the merging of research and practice agendas to support school personnel in the timely provision of primary, secondary, and tertiary prevention efforts to address student needs.

**Gretchen A. Gimpel, PhD,** is Associate Professor of Psychology at Utah State University, where she coordinates the National Association of School Psychologists-approved master's degree program in school psychology and is on the program faculty of the combined (school/clinical/counseling) American Psychological Association-accredited PhD program. Dr. Gimpel is a licensed psychologist and certified school psychologist. She teaches core child therapy and behavioral assessment courses for psychology graduate students and is the faculty internship supervisor for school psychology students. Dr. Gimpel also coordinates child therapy services within the Psychology Department's Community Clinic and supervises graduate students who provide services in this clinic. Her publications and professional presentations are in the area of child behavior problems and family issues as related to child behaviors. Dr. Gimpel currently serves on the editorial advisory boards of several school psychology-related journals.

# Acknowledgments

We have enjoyed the support of many colleagues as we have developed this volume, and we wish to acknowledge their contributions. We are particularly indebted to our editor at The Guilford Press, Chris Jennison. He is a gentleman, a supportive and patient editor, a colleague, and a friend. It was Chris's persistent encouragement (and occasional nudging) of one of us (KWM) over a period of 2 years to write an introductory book on the field of school psychology that led to this book becoming a reality. We were fortunate to have three excellent reviewers for the first draft of the manuscript: Ed Daly (University of Nebraska at Lincoln), Dan Olympia (University of Utah), and Tammy Gilligan (James Madison University). Their insightful and astute comments led to several important changes in the final manuscript, and this book is better because of their efforts. We are indebted to our colleagues and students at our respective institutions (University of Oregon, University of British Columbia, and Utah State University) for helping to create intellectual environments in which we could conceptualize and articulate what we think is a progressive view of school psychology. We are also grateful to our own mentors and past colleagues in the field. Finally, we are indebted to the many scholars, practitioners, and leaders in the field of school psychology over the past several decades who, through their life's work, have helped bring the field to the critical and promising point where it is at the present time. As we wrote this book we truly stood on the shoulders of giants.

# Preface

The field of school psychology is at a critical juncture. Until recently considered to be a young field, school psychology is now showing signs of maturity. It is moving into a new era in which it is beginning to fulfill its potential to significantly affect the education and mental health needs of children, adolescents, and their families in a positive way and to become a key player in the advancement of American education. But let's face it: Growing up is hard. Arriving at a point at which maturity exists almost inevitably involves at least some of these four C's: confusion, chaos, compromises, and changes. The arrival of school psychology at this crossroads has coincided to a great extent with the move from the 20th to 21st centuries. Two of the seminal occurrences of this transition have been a special issue of *School Psychology Review* (vol. 29, no. 4, 2000) titled "School Psychology in the 21st Century" and the 2002 Future of School Psychology Conference, which was held in Indianapolis and simultaneously webcast on the Internet. A quick perusal of the content of these two projects indicates an emerging consensus regarding the maturation of school psychology from a philosophically based to a scientifically based profession and the need for maps or an overall vision to help it make the successful transition beyond the crossroads. The common understanding that emerged from these efforts is that school psychology is moving out of its decades-long struggle for identity. It is now beginning to marshal its vast resources into a rich vision for helping to solve the enormous challenges of promoting the education and mental health of young people in our complex society and troubled times. In a twist on the 19th-century German philosopher Friedrich Nietzsche's famous statement "out of chaos comes order," one of the presentations at the 2002 Futures conference was a panel discussion entitled "Out of Chaos Comes Resolutions." This presentation (and its great title) summarized much of our view about where school psychology is as a field and what needs to happen for the field to successfully get past the crossroads:

1. Our focus should be increasingly on *context and systems*, and not just individuals.
2. We should focus primarily on diagnosing competence and the conditions that enable and support it, not solely on the description and categorization of pathology.

3. School psychologists should direct their efforts toward helping *all* students, not just those who have been referred because of serious problems.
4. Our practices and decision-making processes must be *outcome focused* and *data based*.

Not coincidentally, the title of this volume, *School Psychology for the 21st Century: Foundations and Practices*, invokes the temporal element of change and references the current development and crossroads of the field. Early in the first decade of this new century, we as authors began a discussion that led to the conception and creation of this volume. As we discussed the feasibility of writing an introduction to school psychology, we quickly found that we shared a viewpoint and vision for our professional field and that we were all enthusiastic about the possibilities that exist at this important juncture. We embarked on this work not only to provide a solid introduction to school psychology but also to help shape the further development and progress of the field.

This volume is designed to provide an introduction and orientation to the field of school psychology. We especially intend for it to be of interest and use to graduate students who are beginning to prepare for careers in the field. Almost all of the hundreds of graduate programs in school psychology in the United States and Canada offer an introductory class on the field and its professional issues. Students typically take this class during their first year of graduate study, often during their first semester or term. We believe that it is ideally suited for use in such introductory graduate classes, where we hope that it will help to shape the views and practices of the emerging generation of school psychologists. We believe that it will also be of interest to undergraduate students in psychology and education who are considering graduate studies and careers in these fields and who desire to learn more about the possibilities that school psychology may hold for them. We also intend this book to be of use to individuals who are considering a career change into school psychology and need a resource to help them explore the field. Individuals who currently work as school psychology practitioners, trainers, administrators, and researchers will find this volume to be a fresh introduction and guide to our dynamic and exciting field.

The first two chapters present a foundation and context for understanding school psychology. Chapter 1 provides an introduction to the field, and Chapter 2 gives an overview of the history of school psychology, as well as the historical context of its place in psychology and American education. Chapter 3 provides a foundation for effective school psychology practices in an increasingly diverse cultural context. Chapters 4 through 6 provide a foundation for the professional practice of school psychology, focusing on training and credentialing, employment trends and issues, and legal and ethical aspects of practice in this field. Chapters 7 through 12 provide the details of our vision of best practice in school psychology and focus on the wide range of roles that we believe school psychologists should pursue, including a data-oriented problem-solving approach to practice; assessment; prevention and intervention; facilitating systems-level change via implementing a public health perspective on school psychology services; and being involved as a consumer and producer of research and evaluation. Chapter 13 provides some concluding comments regarding moving the field of school psychology forward and mapping our own future as professionals. Together, the 13 chapters in this book provide a comprehensive and, in our view, state-of-the-art introduction to the field of school psychology.

This volume was written deliberately to reflect the shared points of view of the authors, as well as a shared vision of what school psychology can become. As we began to discuss the possibility of writing an introductory volume to school psychology, none of us was interested in simply providing another overview of the history, current status, and issues of the field. Rather, we wrote this book because we were interested in promoting a forward-thinking vision of the exciting and dynamic possibilities within the field of school psychology. We believe that school psychology has much to offer and that its potential is just beginning to emerge. The possibilities for this field to make a strong positive impact in schools and other settings and in the lives of children, adolescents, and their families are simply enormous. We also believe that there are still several barriers to achieving this vision, foremost of which are the low expectations of many professionals and institutions for school psychology, some of which have unfortunately been perpetuated by the narrow vision of school psychology that is held by some of its own practitioners and trainers. We are not naive about the challenges, obstacles, and barriers that many school psychologists face in using their professional skills and interests to achieve the maximum good. Rather, we believe that through a concerted effort over time, school psychologists can individually and collectively advance the field at all levels, and that in doing so, school psychology will make an enormous positive impact.

Although each chapter within this book is unique, these chapters were developed through a collective vision for the book. Some of the "big ideas" on which this book and our vision for the field of school psychology are based include the following:

• North American society has become increasingly diverse and pluralistic with respect to the cultural background, race, ethnicity, and language of its citizens, and it will continue to become increasingly diverse during the 21st century. School psychologists should develop cultural competence so that they can work appropriately and effectively with individuals and groups from a variety of backgrounds (see Chapter 3).

• School psychology practice has been and should continue to be primarily focused in school or other educational settings. The educational setting is a primary focus of our vision and of this book. However, school psychologists have much to offer outside of the context of school settings, and we encourage the practice of school psychology in a variety of settings and contexts (see Chapter 5).

• School psychology practice should be outcome focused and data driven. School psychologists should base their decisions on valid data and use effective data collection techniques to inform, monitor, and modify intervention activities (see Chapter 7).

• Individual psychoeducational assessment of children and adolescents has been and will continue to be a mainstay activity of school psychologists. However, individual assessment activities should do more than simply describe or diagnose problems. Rather, the most useful assessment strategies are those that provide a foundation for implementing and monitoring effective interventions (see Chapter 8).

• School psychologists have historically worked with a limited segment of student populations, primarily those who have or are suspected of having disabilities and those who are otherwise at high risk for negative outcomes in life. We believe that there will always be a need for school psychologists to focus some of their effort on the small percentage of students who have serious learning, behavioral, and social–emotional problems. We also recognize that longitudinal research points to the chronic nature of such problems and the critical need for *early* intervention if negative long-term outcomes are to be curtailed. Thus we strongly contend that school psychologists should use their unique expertise to positively affect *all students in school settings*, not just those who currently exhibit serious learning, behavioral, or social–emotional problems.

- Although assessment activities have had and will continue to have an important place among the school psychologist's varied responsibilities, effective prevention and intervention activities should occupy a significant percentage of his or her time (see Chapters 9 and 10).

- Prevention and intervention activities can occur with individuals, within small groups, within classrooms, within entire schools, and within school district- or community-based contexts. School psychologists should engage in prevention and intervention activities at each of these levels, so that a larger number of individuals may be positively influenced (see Chapters 9 and 10).

- School psychologists do not typically function in isolation but work as part of a system. School psychologists should strive to use their expertise to develop a solid understanding of the systems in which they work and to help facilitate systems-level change as needed (see Chapter 11).

- School psychologists should be savvy consumers of research and should have the skills to engage in research and evaluation activities within their respective settings that will help to advance practice (see Chapter 12).

- School psychology is a field with incredible potential for helping to solve the "big" problems facing education. And yet this potential is still largely unrealized. We believe that school psychologists should play an active, important, and essential role in this regard. This book is built on the foundation of a progressive, forward-thinking vision of school psychology, and we are optimistic that collectively individual school psychologists can continue to move the field forward through their efforts (see Chapter 13).

We hope that this book will receive a broad audience and that it will meet the needs of those who use it, perhaps even inspire them to think about and practice school psychology in a new way. In sum, school psychology is a dynamic and exciting field that has incredible and still unrealized potential for positively affecting education, psychology, and the lives of children, adolescents, and their families. It is our hope that this book will provide a useful and engaging guide to the field of school psychology and will help the field continue to move forward.

# Contents

# Introduction to the Field of School Psychology

It is fitting for the first chapter of this introductory volume about school psychology to provide a general introduction to and overview of this exciting field. Individuals who are investigating this field or who are new to it often have some basic questions, and this chapter is an attempt to answer some of these basic questions and to provide a useful orientation to this book. The chapter begins with a discussion of the various definitions of school psychology and how these definitions inform and shape the field. General characteristics of school psychologists are described, including such aspects as number and location of individuals who work in the field, demographic characteristics of school psychologists, professional organizations, and level of training. To help provide a more direct and personal introduction to the field, we present vignettes about six individuals who work in school psychology. These vignettes show the diversity, strength, and creativity within the profession. Some aspects of entry into the field are described, including graduate training and credentialing of school psychologists. School psychology is differentiated from some of the more closely related fields in psychology and education. Finally, we include a guide to using this book and an overview of some of the "big ideas" on which the book was developed.

## DEFINING SCHOOL PSYCHOLOGY

At the beginning of a book introducing readers to the field of school psychology, it is reasonable to consider the questions "What is school psychology?" and "What is a school psychologist?" Individuals who have worked in this field for several years might assume that the meaning and definition of school psychology is self-evident. However, a closer look at the development of the field, the evolution of a professional identity, and some of the controversies regarding issues that might seem to outsiders to be straightforward show us that to define school psychology we must examine it closely and consider the importance of "what's in a definition."

## Previous Definitions

It is interesting to look through the literature from a few decades ago to see how the defining characteristics of school psychology have evolved over time. In their 1961 book *The School Psychologist*, White and Harris stated, "In our view school psychology is that branch of psychology which concerns itself with the personality of the pupil in interaction with the educational process," and argued that the field "encompasses not only the learning process, as part of education, but also the personality of the learner as a member of school society, as a member of a family unit, and as a member of the community" (p. 1). In her landmark book *The Psychologist in the Schools*, the original treatise on problem solving as the professional aspiration of school psychologists, Susan Gray (1963) posited that school psychologists had two primary roles: one as *data-oriented problem solvers* in schools, and the other as *transmitters of psychological knowledge and skills*. Bardon and Bennett, in their book *School Psychology* (1974), wrote "The specialty in psychology concerned with how schooling affects children in general and with the pupil in interaction with a specific school is called school psychology. The specialty includes knowledge about research and theory dealing with what happens between children and others when they are together in schools; more than that, school psychology deals with how school for a child in Jackson Junior High is different than school for a child in Wilson Junior High" (p. x).

## Current Definitions

In contrast to statements from notables in the 1960s and 1970s, which tended to define the field by focusing on what school psychologists do or should do rather than on what the specialty is, the most current definitions of school psychology tend to be more direct in defining the essential characteristics of school psychology. In the *What Is a School Psychologist?* area of the National Association of School Psychologists (NASP) website, the answer to "who are school psychologists?" is provided:

> School psychologists have specialized training in both psychology and education. They use their training and skills to team with educators, parents, and other mental health professionals to ensure that every child learns in a safe, healthy and supportive environment. School psychologists understand school systems, effective teaching and successful learning. Today's children face more challenges than ever before. School psychologists can provide solutions for tomorrow's problems through thoughtful and positive actions today.
>
> The training requirements to become a school psychologist are a minimum of 60 graduate semester hours including a year-long internship. This training emphasizes preparation in mental health, child development, school organization, learning, behavior and motivation. To work as a school psychologist, one must be certified and/or licensed by the state in which services are provided. School psychologists also may be nationally certified by the National School Psychology Certification Board. (National Association of School Psychologists, 2005, paragraphs 1 and 2)

Another definition or description of school psychology is provided by the Division of School Psychology (Division 16) of the American Psychological Association (APA). In the Goals and Objectives section of their website, the archival description of the specialty of school psychology reads:

School Psychology is a general practice and health service provider specialty of professional psychology that is concerned with the science and practice of psychology with children, youth, families; learners of all ages; and the schooling process. The basic education and training of school psychologists prepares them to provide a range of psychological assessment, intervention, prevention, health promotion, and program development and evaluation services with a special focus on the developmental processes of children and youth within the context of schools, families, and other systems.

School psychologists are prepared to intervene at the individual and system level, and develop, implement, and evaluate preventive programs. In these efforts, they conduct ecologically valid assessments and intervene to promote positive learning environments within which children and youth from diverse backgrounds have equal access to effective educational and psychological services to promote healthy development. (APA Division of School Psychology, 2005, paragraphs 1 and 2)

Because these definitions are from the two most influential entities representing the field of school psychology in the United States, they have particular importance. What do these definitions have in common? They indicate that school psychology is a profession concerned with the development, mental health, and education of children and youths. They indicate that school psychologists provide services to children, youths, and their families within the context of educational settings but are not limited to those settings. They indicate that school psychologists are concerned with supporting children, youths, their families, and other professionals who work with them in educational and other settings. Importantly, these definitions tell us that school psychology is part of the broader field of psychology and that it also is connected to the field of education and to other professional fields as well. Formulating definitions of school psychology and subsequent efforts to refine these definitions have been exceedingly difficult at times. These issues are not trivial. Professional identity and activities are shaped in great measure by how a specialty is defined. The short answer to "what's in a definition" is "more than you might think."

## CHARACTERISTICS OF SCHOOL PSYCHOLOGISTS

Definitions aside, another way to obtain a snapshot of the field of school psychology is to look at the characteristics of school psychologists. Like a good working definition of the field, it is surprisingly complex to provide a simple description of those who call themselves school psychologists. Because the practice of school psychology is governed by various credentialing bodies within the individual states and provinces, and because membership in professional organizations is voluntary, there is no unitary list or registry of school psychologists. This section provides some basic data regarding school psychologists, particularly the number of individuals who are estimated to work in the field, and some of their basic demographic characteristics, including gender and ethnicity. In Chapter 5, we provide more details regarding the characteristics of school psychologists, specifically in the context of employment.

Perhaps the most direct way to make inferences regarding basic characteristics of school psychologists is to look at available data from national organizations. However, even this method is fraught with challenges because the actual percentage of school psychologists who join professional organizations is unknown and because many school psychologists (like ourselves) belong to two or more professional organizations that represent the field.

Data provided to the authors by the NASP membership office indicated that as of May 31, 2003, there were 21,336 members of NASP. The majority of these NASP members resided in the United States, but nearly 300 lived in Canada, and a handful came from other nations. This figure is very close to the 21,408 members of NASP that Fagan and Wise (2000) reported from a June 1999 survey. Fagan and Wise made a conservative estimate that there were 25,000 school psychologists in the United States. More recently, Fagan (2002) has asserted that the best current estimates of the number of school psychologists in the United States range from 25,000 to 30,000. Based on our own experiences and conversation with school psychologists, we believe that Fagan and Wise's estimate that about 70% of all school psychologists in the United States are NASP members may be overly optimistic. We are more confident in an estimate that no more than 60% of school psychologists are NASP members. If we are correct, then a minimum of 30,000 school psychologists in the United States and Canada is probably a reasonable estimate. However, this number is nothing more than an educated guess. Not only do we not know the percentage of school psychologists who belong to NASP, but we must also recognize that there are some individuals who are NASP members who are not specifically trained as school psychologists or who are working in related fields. Using APA Division 16 data is less informative in terms of estimating the number of school psychologists. As of 2004 there were approximately 3,000 members of Division 16, but it is widely understood that far fewer school psychologists join APA than NASP, and it is unknown how many individuals are members of both organizations. One reason that APA Division 16 has far fewer members than NASP is that a doctoral degree is required for full APA membership, but the majority of practicing school psychologists do not have doctoral degrees.

Internationally, the number of school psychologists is also something of a puzzle, and it is even more difficult to ascertain than the number within the United States. Oakland and Cunningham (1992) conducted an international survey and estimated the number of individuals globally in the field of school psychology to be 87,000. If our own estimates and the Oakland and Cunningham figure are both reasonably correct, then about one out of three school psychologists in the world are within the United States. Although we are using the term "school psychologists" very generally to make these worldwide comparisons, it is worth noting that the role of school psychologists outside of the United States and Canada (who are also referred to in some nations as "educational psychologists") may differ considerably from the role of school psychologists in the United States and Canada. Particularly in the United States, the role of the school psychologist has been strongly linked to public law for education of students with disabilities. In most other nations, this situation is not the case. (For more information on the practice of school psychology worldwide, go to the International School Psychology Association website at www.ispaweb.org.)

With respect to gender of school psychologists, there is considerable evidence that the field has become a female-dominated profession in recent years and that the percentage of women in the field continues to increase. The most recent membership survey data available from NASP (December 2003 data from the 2002–2003 membership renewal survey) indicated that approximately 73% of NASP members were women. This figure indicates a 1% increase over the November 1999 estimate of 72% reported by Fagan and Wise (2000) and even more over the 67% female figure reported in the first edition of the Fagan and Wise (1994) book. In commenting on the fairly recent shift in gender composition of school psychologists since about the 1970s, Reschly (2000) stated that the increased proportion of women in the field during this time period constituted "the clearest changes in school psychology during the past two decades" (p. 508).

Future trends regarding the characteristics of school psychologists are difficult to predict. Because the field does not exist in isolation, future trends will inevitably be shaped by external forces, such as the economy, the development of public education, new federal laws and mandates, advocacy by national and state organizations, and national and worldwide social trends. However, it appears that in the immediate future several trends are very likely. The field of school psychology should continue to grow at least modestly, and school psychologists will continue to enjoy good employment prospects. Public school settings will almost certainly continue to be the primary place of employment for school psychologists, although expansion into nontraditional settings will continue. The large majority of school psychology practitioners will hold master's or specialist degrees as their highest academic degrees, although the percentage of school psychologists with doctoral degrees will continue to increase slightly, as it has in recent years. For the foreseeable future, the large majority of school psychologists will be women, and it is likely that the percentage of women in the field may even continue to increase. Fagan (2002) has asserted that "the proportion of women in school psychology may rise to as high as 80%" (p. 210). The available evidence indicates that NASP will continue to have substantially larger membership numbers than APA Division 16, but membership in both organizations is likely to evidence a modest increase.

# BEING THERE: SIX VIGNETTES

Although the general professional definitions of school psychology are extremely important and have broad impact on how the field is perceived both internally and externally, they give us only a small glimpse of what school psychologists do in their day-to-day work. Definitions cannot capture the diversity of roles that school psychologists fill, nor can they adequately convey how each practicing school psychologist is in a unique situation and setting and has a unique perspective on the field. In addition, general definitions cannot possibly convey the wealth of experience, passion, and personal commitment that individual school psychologists bring to their work. Perhaps a better way to illustrate what school psychology looks like at the point of actual practice is to catch a glimpse of what professional life is like for several school psychologists. The following six vignettes were developed through interviews with school psychologists who agreed to talk about their own professional experiences and views.

## Expanding the Role

When interviewed for this vignette, Deanna Sanders was a school psychologist with the Tacoma Public School District in Washington State. Her career has thus far taken her full circle, from west coast to east coast and back. Deanna was raised in Seattle and attended the public schools there. She entered the field of school psychology in 1988, when she enrolled in a master's degree training program in school psychology at Central Washington University, where she had recently completed her undergraduate education. During the third year of her graduate program, she completed a year-long internship in the Tacoma schools. After graduating in 1991, she went on a road trip with a friend and stopped in Las Vegas, Nevada. While there, she inquired regarding opportunities for school psychologists in the Clark County School District. She was quickly hired into her first professional position.

Deanna spent 3 years working as a school psychologist in Las Vegas. Reflecting back on this first job, she notes, "I was prepared for the basic evaluation role, but quickly encountered many other situations, like dealing with crises, helping families find resources, and repairing relationships between schools and the school psychology staff." Her assignment included serving as a school psychologist for three different schools of widely varying circumstances. One was located in a high poverty area and had many homeless children, including those from "families who lived in their cars in the desert." Another was in a lower-middle-class area and had a very diverse student population. The third school was in an upper-middle-class area of the city, with a relatively high-achieving student population. "There was a huge difference between the three schools, and my roles in them," she reflects. Overall, her basic responsibilities included assessment and evaluation, processing referrals, communicating assessment results to parents and teachers, and some direct intervention work (counseling) with students. However, as she defined her role through 3 years of experience, she found herself focusing increasingly on helping students and their families in poverty situations locate and access services, "sort of a social work role," she says. "Overall, I was very happy with my initial role there, but I learned quickly that you can develop your role to be broader than just assessment."

In 1994, Deanna left Las Vegas to pursue a doctoral degree in a program that had recently been started at James Madison University (JMU) in Harrisonburg, Virginia. The JMU program was a combined program in clinical, counseling, and school psychology, and it focused on recruiting students who already had earned master's or specialist degrees and who had prior professional experience. She found the transition to being a full-time student once again to be "intimidating at first, but it got better as the first year went on. It was great to study more about school psychology now that I had experience in the field and a reference for it." After completing the on-campus portion of her course work, she left Harrisonburg for Richmond, Virginia, where she completed her predoctoral internship and worked for 3 additional years as a school psychologist. She completed her doctoral degree in 1997. The transition to Richmond was challenging for her initially. In Washington and Nevada, she had been used to a low-key, laid-back "west coast" professional culture, but she found the school district in Richmond, a southern city, "to have a much more formal culture with respect to professional dress, distinctions between students and professionals, and more formality in general." An additional adjustment was the ethnic or racial makeup of the student population. As an African American woman who was raised in the Pacific Northwest, Deanna was used to being a minority. However, she recalls that the schools to which she was assigned "were 97% to 98% African American, and it was a different culture than I grew up with in the northwest." The crushing poverty of many of the students and families she served in Richmond proved to be an impetus to expand her role further. "My role was pretty much traditional assessment, evaluation, and consultation, but it grew into varied other roles, like linking community resources to families, helping families deal with basic needs like getting their electricity turned on and getting clothes for their children." She worked closely with social workers and ended up "taking on a social work type of role."

In 1998, Deanna returned to her home state of Washington, accepting a position as a school psychologist in the Tacoma Public Schools, where she had completed her master's program internship and where she continues to work. Once again, she experienced the adjustments that come with moving into a new assignment and a new system. She notes that it was important to quickly "learn the culture of the individual schools" to which she was assigned so she could be more effective within each system. Although her current job description has a "heavier emphasis on assessment than all other areas," she once more has learned to expand her professional role. For example, she has developed new interests and skills in working with teachers regarding interventions for student reading problems, and she has found that she needs to develop effective behavior supports for many students with behavioral and emotional problems. "As many as a third of the families in the schools I serve are involved in the drug culture, so I have had to move into working with student behavior problems related to this issue. Some of these kids are being raised by grandparents, who need lots of support. Many of the kids have not had effective and stable home situations. I now do heavy consultation focused in this area."

Among the greatest challenges she experiences in her current role include having increased expectations along with diminishing resources, the burden of excessive paperwork, and not being able to enact enough change with students who do not have supportive families. "It's very frustrating to know that a child is hurting and that the family is not willing to make changes" she says. What she likes most about her current work is "working with teachers through consultation, where I have seen an attitude shift, with more willingness to enact change and try new things." Overall, Deanna's advice to future school psychologists is to try to follow a maxim that has guided her throughout her career for nearly two decades now: "Try to maintain a focus on students as individuals, and not as numbers or results."

## Surviving the Assessment Marathon

Bob Green has worked in the fields of special education and school psychology since the late 1970s. A native of Michigan, Bob went into the military immediately after high school, serving in the U.S. Air Force from 1968 to 1972 during the Vietnam War. After his military service, he began attending college on the G.I. Bill, first at the University of Michigan at Flint and then at Brigham Young University in Utah, where he earned a bachelor's degree in special education and a master's degree in educational psychology and fulfilled the requirements for several teaching certificates.

Bob's first professional position was in Coos Bay, Oregon, in 1977, where he was a special education teacher with specific responsibilities for student assessment and diagnosis. After one year in Oregon, he returned to Utah and soon began a certification program in school psychology at the University of Utah. He completed the program over a 2-year period while he worked full time. He worked briefly as a special education teacher for the Weber County, Utah, School District and was then hired as a school psychologist in the Ogden, Utah, City School District, where he worked from 1980 to 2002. In 2002 Bob retired from the Ogden School District and then was immediately hired by Davis School District in Utah.

Bob's professional role as a school psychologist for more than 25 years has been focused heavily on the traditional activities of assessment, evaluation, and diagnosis of students; writing reports; and consulting with parents and teachers. By most standards, his work in this area has had a marathon-like quality. During his years in Ogden, he was one of three school psychologists in a district with a student population ranging from 10,000 to 15,000, with an average school psychologist-to-student ratio over the years of about 1:4,000. In this role, he specialized in assessment of students with severe disabilities and "did an average of one complete assessment per work day, or about 150 to 200 complete assessments per school year." Most of his assessment activities involved the use of standardized norm-referenced tests, but in the late 1980s, he was trained in the use of curriculum-based measurement (CBM), which he continues to use and which he views as a very important tool. Bob is fluent in both Spanish and Russian, and during his years in Ogden he was able to use his Spanish-language skills frequently in working with the district's growing population of Spanish-speaking families. Since his move to Davis County, with a school psychologist-to-student ratio of 1:1,500, he has been able to expand his role beyond assessment, and he now enjoys being able to provide direct services to students and to engage in more consultation with parents, teachers, and colleagues.

One of the noteworthy aspects of Bob Green's career has been his commitment to professional development and service. He has been a member of NASP and of the Utah Association of School Psychologists (UASP) for many years. At the state level, he has been active in supporting the organization and in providing leadership. He developed the Utah Association of School Psychologists website and continues to manage it. More recently, he has served as president of UASP. He strongly encourages new school psychologists to become involved in their professional organizations at the state and national levels. "They provide a great opportunity for professional development, networking, and keeping your skills sharp."

## Systems-Level Intervention and Leadership

Margaret McGlinchey has been a school psychologist for more than two decades. A Michigan native, she was raised in Detroit and has spent her professional career working in Michigan public schools. She completed her undergraduate studies in secondary education, with a major in psychology. She was attracted to what she learned about teaching and learning in her psychology major, and she decided to pursue school psychology graduate studies because she wanted to make a broad impact on schools and to focus on prevention. She received her Ed.S. in school psychology at Western Michigan University (WMU) and immediately began working full time as a school psychologist. She also earned a PhD in school psychology from WMU in 1988 while she was working in the field full time. She was attracted to WMU's program because of its focus on function-based assessment, applied behavior analysis, and prevention/intervention.

She currently works for the Kalamazoo, Michigan, Public School District, where she has been since 1984. She notes that she is fortunate to have always had a good school psychologist-to-student ratio in Kalamazoo, which has averaged about 1:1,000 over the years she has been there. "These numbers have allowed us to focus on prevention and intervention. Our psychologists conduct an average of 40 to 50 evaluations per year, working within a building team structure. These numbers and the structure have allowed us to focus on pre-referral interventions, and to emphasize appropriateness of referrals." Since 2001, Margaret's role has expanded to include leadership and program development responsibilities. The local intermediate service district (ISD) has purchased half of her time to work on grants to develop systems capacity and to implement data-based decision making, using curriculum-based measurement and the DIBELS assessment system for evaluation of early literacy skills.

An important part of Margaret's professional role for the past two decades has been training and mentoring school psychology graduate students as they prepare to enter the profession. She estimates that she has served as field supervisor for 20–30 practicum students and at least 20 interns over the years, mostly students from Western

Michigan University. "Working with graduate students and being affiliated with the university in this capacity has been an important part of my own ongoing professional development over the years." She also teaches courses in norm-referenced and curriculum-based measurement and in corrective-remedial intervention strategies as an adjunct faculty member at WMU.

Having worked in the field for several years, Margaret has seen various professional trends (and sometimes fads) come and go and has seen the field develop and mature. She notes that "the original prereferral intervention systems we used were a good idea, but had flaws . . . by the time kids became a focus of concern, it was too late to impact them in a meaningful way." She has also been frustrated at times with the separation of general and special education, which she considers to be "an artificial separation that can create confusion and problems in service delivery. We need to shift our thinking toward a collective and collaborative responsibility for all students in a building." Her perspective on the field over more than two decades of professional work has allowed her to appreciate the current direction the field is taking. "This is definitely the most exciting time in my career and in school psychology. I am thrilled to see the positive changes in the field—the increasing emphasis on prevention, intervention, function-based assessment, building-wide systems of service delivery, and the move to a problem-solving role."

## Let the Data Be Your Guide

For Marty Ikeda, the path from Hawaii to Iowa has been both long and circuitous. Marty was raised in Honolulu. As he completed his high school education, he desired to leave the islands to experience other parts of the nation. His search took him to Marquette University in Wisconsin, where he completed his undergraduate education in psychology. Wanting to pursue graduate study in psychology, he started a doctoral program in industrial/organizational psychology in Colorado but soon realized it was not the right field for him. He quit graduate school and took a job as a family liaison at a boarding school in South Dakota, where he worked under the supervision of a school psychologist. His experience in this setting helped him to realize what he wanted to do, and he ended up in the doctoral program in school psychology at the University of Oregon, where he received his PhD in 1994. While there, he worked extensively on projects related to severe disabilities and single-subject research design and was trained in data-oriented problem solving.

Following his predoctoral internship at the Meyer Rehabilitation Institute in Omaha, Nebraska (now the Munroe–Meyer Institute), Marty worked for a year as a school psychologist at the Heartland Area Education Agency in Iowa. He then left for a year to pursue a postdoctoral training experience at the Seashore House, affiliated with Children's Hospital of Philadelphia, and returned to the Heartland Agency in Iowa the next year. His first positions at Heartland involved a combination of practice and research assignments. In addition to providing direct services for students with attention-deficit/hyperactivity disorder (ADHD), autism, and other conditions, he conducted research on the effectiveness of Heartland's emerging problem-solving model. He participated in a federally funded grant on early intervention services for students with autism, and he was often asked to problem solve with students who had other types of severe disabilities.

In 2001, Marty became coordinator of research and special projects in an administrative and supervisory position. In this capacity, he has used his school psychology training and experience to improve student outcomes through research. Some of the research projects he has conducted or supervised include implementing universal screening through curriculum-based measurement, effective interventions for students with autism, measuring the effectiveness of school-based problem-solving teams, and responding to federal education initiatives such as the No Child Left Behind (NCLB) act.

Marty's perspective on school psychology is that the current time is one of the most exciting times in the history of the field. "In the past, we have gotten involved with a lot of individual assessment and intervention, but with tightening budgets and more accountability, we need to move into impacting larger groups and systems, to impact all students." Marty contends that school psychologists have always had much to offer the field of education but that the timing has never been better than now. "Schools are screaming for help, and we now have the opportunity to do it." He views the most important roles of school psychologists as "selecting and implementing universal screening tools, developing data management plans, and using single subject research data to help inform practice." His advice to future psychologists is to "be visible, be in classrooms, work with kids, try different approaches, and let the data be your guide."

## Behavioral School Psychologist in a Nontraditional Setting

When we interviewed her for this vignette, Trina Spencer was a parent education coordinator and school psychologist working for the Hawthorne Country Day School (HCDS). This school is part of the Hawthorne Foundation, a private, nonprofit organization based in Westchester County, New York, a few miles north of New York City. The school provides comprehensive services to individuals with autism and other developmental disabilities and has several programs, including an early intervention program, preschool and school-age programs, a Manhattan Annex, and a parent education program. Most of the students at HCDS are referred there by public school districts in the New York City metropolitan area. These districts are seeking out-of-district placements for students with moderate to severe disabilities and intense educational and life skills needs. Funding for these services comes from tuition from the school districts, private fund-raising, and grants. HCDS focuses its educational program on the principles of applied behavior analysis.

Trina's path to New York started in Logan, Utah, where she was raised and where she attended Utah State University (USU). As an undergraduate psychology major, she developed a strong interest in behavioral psychology and applied behavior analysis. She took all of the courses and supplemental experiences in this area that she could, and she was encouraged to continue her studies in USU's specialist-level master's program in school psychology, where she started as a graduate student in 1998. Trina knew from the onset of her graduate training that she wanted to receive all of the applied behavior analysis training that she could and to ultimately pursue the Board Certified Behavior Analyst credential (BCBA), along with her school psychology license. She took graduate courses and practica from instructors who were knowledgeable in behavioral school psychology and applied behavior analysis, but her specialized career goals required her to do her internship year at a site where she could be supervised by someone who held the BCBA credential, as well as a school psychology license/certificate. She found such a site at the Fred S. Keller School in Yonkers, New York, and her internship there ultimately led her to her current position.

Within only 2 years of accepting this position, Trina saw her role evolve considerably. "When I started here, I was mainly doing functional behavioral assessments (FBAs), but it consumed all of my time. I was working with one student and teacher at a time, and I was not able to make the kind of impact I wanted," she notes. As a response to this situation, she decided to train the teachers at the school to conduct FBAs, which proved to be a highly successful approach that allowed her to increase her time as a consultant and trainer. "Now, I mainly train and consult with our teachers, and run our parent education program, which includes conducting workshops two times a month for parents of children with disabilities from across the New York City area. We are now much further along in the problem-solving process than we were two years ago." The parent workshops cover such varied topics as principles of applied behavior analysis, play skills, using a token economy, toilet training, and self-management. She also holds biweekly meetings with individual parents, visiting them in their homes and coaching them through the implementation of procedures they learn about in the workshops. She also spends a smaller percentage of her time working in some traditional school psychology roles, including conducting direct behavioral observations in classrooms, developing behavior intervention plans, conducting special education reevaluations, and counseling. Of her current role Trina says, "It is interesting and varied, which is why I love my job so much."

What Trina likes most about her professional role is seeing behavior change and being appreciated. "I know I'm doing the right thing when I hear a student say 'mama' for the first time, or when a parent says 'thank you.' " Unlike students in public schools, the students and families at HCDS are self-selected, and they specifically want to be there for what the program can offer them. "They want to be here, and we have developed a very close community, helping families to build networks." What she finds most frustrating about her role can be summed up simply, and it is a challenge that can be appreciated by many school psychologists and educators: insufficient resources. Despite the positive impact she is able to accomplish in her position, she says "there is not enough money available to purchase the materials we need, to provide all the services that are needed, and we are stretched too thin to serve the intense needs of so many parents." The limited resources create a situation in which "I can't do all that I want to do and what they need." Still, Trina values her work and role and says that "school psychology is a good fit for me. It allows me to pursue my goals and make a difference."

## University Professor and Trainer

Heather Sterling-Turner is an associate professor of school psychology in the psychology department at the University of Southern Mississippi (USM), in Hattiesburg, Mississippi, where she has worked since 1998. In her current professional role Heather trains and mentors the next generation of school psychologists, students who are in USM's doctoral program in school psychology. She also has an active program of research and scholarly work centering on her interests in applied behavior analysis, functional assessment and analysis, behavioral consultation, and pediatric psychology.

Heather was raised in Alexandria, Louisiana, "literally on the grounds of a state mental institution," as she likes to say. Her father was a clinical psychologist and staff member at this hospital. He was trained in behavior modification and analysis during the 1960s, when this emphasis was a common focus in clinical psychology training programs. In retrospect, the unique environment and family connection greatly influenced Heather's own career choice. She was an undergraduate at the University of the South in Sewanee, Tennessee, where she earned a bachelor's degree in psychology and where the curriculum emphasized behavioral models and animal research; the department chair was a former student of the legendary B. F. Skinner. Despite her strong exposure to the field of psychology, Heather "didn't know anything about school psychology" early in her undergraduate education. She knew that she wanted to work with children, but she struggled to define a clear path to doing that. "I figured I could either hang out a shingle and do the 50-minute hour, put on a white coat and work with rats, or work for a state institution."

During her senior year Heather learned about the field of school psychology and found out that there were a small number of doctoral programs that had strong behavioral orientations. This focus became her goal, and she ultimately enrolled in the graduate program in school psychology at Mississippi State University, where she received strong training in applied behavior analysis, functional assessment, consultation, single-subject research design, and academic assessment. Of her graduate school experience, Heather says, "I wasn't at first interested in pursuing an academic position, but got excited about research by working with the faculty at MSU." By her 3rd of 4 years full time in graduate school, she was focused on working as a university faculty member. Heather's predoctoral internship was at Children's Hospital of Philadelphia, where she received additional training in developmental disabilities, pediatric psychology, and functional assessment. She joined the faculty at the University of Southern Mississippi immediately after the conclusion of her internship. She accepted her current position because of several aspects that were appealing to her. "I liked the behavioral school psychology orientation, the program's focus on a data-based problem-solving model, and I liked the idea of returning to Mississippi. I was very interested in going somewhere where I could have an opportunity to make change, and this environment was very appealing in that way."

Regarding her work as a university faculty member, Heather says, "I love working with students who are not yet in the field, those who have a strong interest in our training model." She particularly enjoys seeing students develop and grow in their professional expertise and identity during their graduate training, and she likes that she is still able to maintain a focus on school psychology practice through her work in consulting on cases and supervising practica. In terms of the role and demands of a faculty member, Heather finds the flexibility of the job very appealing: "I don't punch a clock, and I can to some extent arrange my schedule around my needs, which helps to balance work and family." Among the challenges she finds in working at a public research university is the continual cutting of state appropriations for higher education, resulting in pressure to obtain external funding for research and in having to make difficult choices regarding balancing her time well to blend the research, teaching, and service aspects of the job.

Heather is very encouraged by some of the opportunities and recent developments in the field of school psychology. She is particularly encouraged by some of the changes that resulted from the December 2004 reauthorization of the Individuals with Disabilities Education Act (IDEA). "I'm very excited about the inclusion of the 'response to intervention' model for learning disabilities identification, and am so glad that the law is changing to no longer mandate the use of the ability-achievement discrepancy model for LD services. . . . I don't think that the discrepancy model helps to inform intervention, and I think that in so many cases our systems have set up low performing kids to fail if we cannot diagnose them." Her advice to current school psychology students is to "synthesize what you learn . . . don't forget what you learn from one course or from one setting to another." She also advocates that students and practitioners "stick to a research to practice model where you can evaluate what you do, using data to make decisions and select empirically supported interventions."

## Tying It Together

The variety, personal investment, and impact reflected in the professional lives of the six school psychologists featured in these vignettes could easily be duplicated by conducting similar interviews with any six randomly selected school psychologists. It is also noteworthy that professional lives evolve over time. Those school psychologists profiled in this section who have been in the field for several years have seen their career paths develop and change, sometimes in ways they never anticipated. The same could be said for any school psychologist who is committed to making in impact in the field. Although tied together by a collective professional identity and associations, every school psychologist has a unique story, makes unique contributions, and follows a unique path. And yet, there is a commonality among them that ties them together and that reflects the shared vision and unique identity that defines school psychology. We believe that this vision and identity stem from a focus on affecting the academic, behavioral, and social-emotional problems of children and youths in educational settings through the effective use of psychological principles and procedures and through the medium of "school psychology." This vision is also clearly tied to the personal commitment and idealism of those individuals who choose to join the field of school psychology. Although school psychologists have differing backgrounds, job descriptions, expectations, and professional ambitions, as a group they share a collective desire to positively influence the lives of children, adolescents, and their families. It is the incredible power of this collective individual idealism that fuels the impact and potential of the field.

# HOW DOES ONE BECOME A SCHOOL PSYCHOLOGIST?

Having established a definition of school psychology and some of the characteristics of school psychologists, the next question that might be asked by someone who is exploring the field is "How does one become a school psychologist?" This question is dealt with in extensive detail in Chapter 4, which covers training and credentialing issues in the field. To help us establish our basic introduction to school psychology, a few of the more elemental details regarding the paths that must be traveled to become a school psychologist are covered in this section.

To become a school psychologist, one must have completed a graduate-level program in school psychology and have received a credential (i.e., a certificate or license) to practice in the field. The specialist-degree level of training has become the standard of minimum preparation for entering the field. This level of training typically (but not always) requires approximately 2 years of full-time graduate study beyond the bachelor's degree and includes a field experience component (practicum and internship). NASP has advocated for a specialist standard of preparation requiring a minimum of 60 semester credits of graduate study and including a full-time academic-year internship. Because these standards are integrated into NASP's Nationally Certified School Psychologist credential (the NCSP, which is promoted and offered by NASP's National School Psychology Certification Board), the 60 credit/1,200 internship hours specialist level of training has become the de facto standard in the field. It is worth noting that many graduate programs do not offer a specialist degree by that name but provide an equivalent level of training through a master's degree (MS, MA, or MEd) or certificate of advanced graduate study (CAGS) program.

Although the efforts of NASP to advocate for minimum training at the 60/1,200 specialist level have created a general standard, it is important to recognize that neither NASP nor any other professional organization actually credentials school psychologists for work in the field. There is no national-level licensing body that provides clearance to work as a school psychologist anywhere. Rather, credentialing of school psychologists is the responsibility of individual states and provinces. For school psychologists to work in public school settings, they must usually obtain a credential, which may be called a certificate or a license, from the educational licensing agency of the particular state or province where they intend to work. Usually, these agencies are part of the state or provincial department of education. Each state sets its own standards for entry into the field in that state, and some states have lower entry-level requirements than others. However, the NASP-advocated specialist level of training is almost always sufficient for credentialing in any state or province.

As if the differentiation between NASP professional standards and various state education department standards is not confusing enough, newcomers to the field are frequently surprised to find that there is another level of credentialing that is usually necessary to practice as a school psychologist outside of school settings. To become licensed as a psychologist to practice independently or to practice in settings such as hospitals, clinics, and community mental health agencies with the use of the title "psychologist," one must hold a doctoral degree in psychology (school psychology, counseling psychology, or clinical psychology) and be licensed by the professional psychology licensing board of a particular state or province. The doctoral level of professional psychology training, which usually requires 1 year of supervised predoctoral internship and 1 year of supervised postdoctoral residency (as well as passing written and oral competency examinations that are required by many states) before the license is granted, is what is advocated by APA and its various state affiliates. However, the APA position, as well as most state psychology licensing laws, include provisions for the use of the title "school psychologist" (as opposed to "psychologist" or "licensed professional psychologist") with less than the doctoral level of training and without a psychology license, providing that the work is limited to school settings and is conducted under the banner of a school psychology credential from a state department of education.

There are currently more than 200 institutions of higher education in the United States and Canada that provide graduate-level training in school psychology at some level, and approximately 300 different training programs exist at these institutions (Fagan & Wise, 2000; Thomas, 1998). Although the specialist level of graduate training has become the standard and typical mode of entry into the field for most school psychologists, a substantial percentage of school psychologists have earned doctoral degrees. The most recent estimate was that 26% of school psychologists have doctoral degrees (Fagan & Wise, 2000). It is likely that the current percentage is slightly higher, because this has been the trend for the past 30 years.

Individuals who enroll in school psychology graduate training programs have a variety of undergraduate backgrounds, the most common of which are psychology and education. A generation ago, it was not uncommon for individuals entering the field of school psychology to have had backgrounds in education, perhaps some experience as teachers, and in many cases to be midcareer (i.e., in their 30s or 40s); but these background characteristics appear to be less common than they were two or three decades ago. We are not aware of any studies or data that have tracked the age, undergraduate preparation, and background of students entering school psychology programs over the years, but it has been our experience that the trend has been toward students entering graduate school in their early to mid-20s, more often than not with an undergraduate degree in psychology, and often with little or no full-time professional experience in psychology or education. We anticipate that as education and mental health fields become increasingly professionalized and that as higher levels of educational attainment become more common, these trends in school psychology training will continue and become even more noticeable.

# DIFFERENTIATING SCHOOL PSYCHOLOGY FROM RELATED PROFESSIONS

In addition to understanding what school psychology is all about and how one becomes a school psychologist, prospective graduate students who are beginning to explore the possibility of a career in this field must also decide whether to pursue school psychology or some closely related field. As school psychology faculty members, we visit with prospective graduate students on an ongoing basis. Although many prospective school psychologists have a very clear idea what being a school psychologist involves and how school psychology differs from some of its sister fields, many do not. We have all sat through meetings with prospective students who assumed that they were considering entering a school counseling training program, for example. Because there are important differences not only in the entry-level requirements but also in the typical role and function of various fields, it is very important for prospective graduate students to get a clear picture of how school psychology is both similar to and different from its sister fields in psychology and education.

## Related Fields in Psychology

At the doctoral level of training, there are other areas of professional psychology that overlap considerable with school psychology and that may prepare professional psychologists to work with children, adolescents, and their families. Historically, school psychology has been included with two other fields, *clinical psychology* and *counseling psychology*, as one of the three health care areas of professional psychology. Completing a doctoral program in any one of these three fields will prepare one to become a board-licensed professional psychologist and to work in a variety of clinic, private practice, community, and medical settings. Clinical and counseling psychology have not traditionally focused on schools and educational issues as school psychology has, and they do not typically prepare students to work primarily in school settings. However, many clinical and counseling psychology programs focus on working with children, adolescents, and their families and provide a path toward a predoctoral internship and postdoctoral residency year in a child-focused setting, providing assessment, intervention, and consultation services. Historically, there have been some important differences between clinical and counseling psychology, with the former field focusing more on abnormal behavior and psychopathology and the latter focusing more on normal developmental and adjustment issues of life. However, these distinctions have become increasingly blurred in recent years, and today it is not uncommon to find clinical psychologists working in college counseling centers and to find counseling psychologists working in hospitals and clinics.

Within clinical, counseling, and school psychology, some subspecialties focusing on children, youths, and their families have emerged in recent years, and these subspecialties are usually not specific to one field of psychology. For example, just as APA has a division devoted to school psychology (Division 16), it now has separate divisions devoted to child, family, and youth services (Division 37), clinical child and adolescent psychology (Division 53), and pediatric psychology (Division 54). Child and adolescent neuropsychology has also emerged as a strong subspecialty within the division of neuropsychology (Division 40). These specialty areas include doctoral-level psychologists who are graduates of school, clinical, or counseling psychology programs, who have received specific specialty training, and who have developed particular expertise and interests in the respective specialty area.

With these related psychology fields and specialty areas, school psychology shares a focus on children, youths, and their families. What makes school psychology unique among these related areas within psychology is the specific focus on schools as practice settings and on educational and learning issues as primary concerns. Although some overlap exists among these areas, they all have a unique identity.

## Related Fields in Education

Because school psychology is rooted in education, as well as psychology, there are some professions that are specific to education with which we share some common concerns and some professional overlap. *School counseling* is perhaps the best known of these related educational professions. This field grew out of the mental hygiene and child guidance movements of the early 20th century, and it has evolved from a field focused on vocational guidance and college placement to a field that strives to promote a comprehensive model of student development, adjustment, and growth at all grade levels. The American School Counselor Association has been in existence since 1952 and currently has more than 14,000 members. Many more school counselors than school psychologists are employed in schools. Within the United States, the national average ratio of school counselors to students is about 1:500 (American School Counselor Association, 2003, paragraph 7), whereas the national average for school psychologists is slightly less than 1:2,000 (Fagan, 2002). In terms of differences in training and job focus between the two fields, school psychologists tend to receive more training in individual assessment methods and intervention techniques than do school counselors and have historically focused more on students with disabilities. School counselors are more likely to be assigned to work at a single school, whereas school psychologists are often itinerant and may have responsibility for two to four schools or may work on a districtwide basis. Much of this difference in site-based versus itinerant service models is related to the large differences in professional to student ratios, which are much smaller for school counselors.

In addition to school psychologists and school counselors, *school social workers* are also employed in public and private schools. This profession is part of the larger field of social work, and it began in the early 1900s in the large urban areas of the northeast United States out of a concern for underprivileged students. The first school social workers often were part of psychological clinics in the schools and had the title of "visiting teachers." Their role was often focused on home visits and advocacy for children and their families who were living in tenements in industrial areas. Today, school social workers maintain some of the same historical emphasis on advocacy and working with at-risk students, but they tend to work on multidisciplinary teams with psychologists, counselors, teachers, and nurses and to focus on a broad array of mental health and social-behavioral adjustment issues. It is difficult to estimate the number of school social workers nationwide. It is widely understood that there are far fewer school social workers than school psychologists, although an exact professional-to-student ratio for this field is not known.

Although school counseling and school social work are the two best known professions within education that are closely related to school psychology, there are other professional roles in schools that have much in common with our field. These other roles are not necessarily defined as separate professions but have evolved as specialty positions in education in many school systems. Special education consultants, service coordinators, or consulting teachers are often employed in larger school districts and have the responsibility of working with teachers, other educators, and parents in developing appropriate educational programs for students, especially those who are at risk for negative outcomes or who are otherwise having difficulty in school. Such consultant or coordinator positions are often filled from the ranks of experienced and talented teachers, but sometimes they are filled by individuals with school psychology backgrounds. These roles usually involve extensive indirect intervention through consultation, and they may have a problem-solving or training focus as well. In addition, some schools hire teachers or counselors to serve as educational diagnosticians or educational assessment specialists. These types of positions include an exclusive focus on individual assessment of students with learning and behavior problems, and on the surface they seem quite similar to the role of school psychologists who are in very traditional "test-and-place" assessment roles.

Although most school psychologists remain employed with that title, those who have the aptitude and interest to pursue other roles within schools often find that there are opportunities for career shifts within school systems. Some school psychologists move into educational leadership positions, such as pupil personnel directors, special education administrators, and school principals. Typically, career moves of this type require the individual to obtain additional graduate-level education in order to receive an administrative credential. School psychologists who have particular expertise in research methods, statistics, and psychometrics sometimes move into district-level positions as directors of research services, directors of testing, and so forth.

## USING THIS BOOK: A VISION FOR SCHOOL PSYCHOLOGY

As is stated in the preface, this book is designed to provide an introduction and orientation to the field of school psychology. We especially intend for this book to be of special interest and use to graduate students who are beginning to prepare for careers in the field of school psychology. We also intend for this book to be of use to individuals who are considering careers in school psychology and need a resource to help them explore the field, as well as by individuals who are currently working as school psychologists and who are interested in an introduction and guide to this dynamic and exciting field.

Following this introductory chapter, Chapter 2 provides brief overviews of the historical context of the field, as well as of history and trends in American education. Chapters 3 through 6 provide a foundation for the professional practice of school psychology, focusing on cultural and linguistic diversity, training and credentialing issues, employment trends and challenges, and legal and ethical aspects of practice in this field. Chapters 7 through 12 detail our vision of best practice in school psychology and focus on the wide range of roles that we believe school psychologists should pursue, including a data-oriented problem-solving approach to practice; assessment; prevention and intervention; facilitating systems-level change; and being involved as a consumer and producer of research and evaluation. Chapter 13 provides some concluding comments regarding moving the field of school psychology forward and mapping our own future as professionals. Together, the 13 chapters in this book provide a comprehensive and, in our view, state-of-the-art introduction to the field of school psychology.

You may have noted that we use the phrase "school psychology for the 21st century" in the title of this book. Our focus on the 21st century was a very deliberate choice on our part. In deciding to write this book, we were not interested in simply providing an overview of the history and current status of the field, which have been well documented in other sources. Rather, we wrote this book because we were interested in promoting a forward-thinking vision of the exciting and dynamic possibilities within the field of school psychology. We believe that the field of school psychology has much to offer and that its potential is just beginning to emerge. The possibilities of this field making a strong positive impact in schools and other settings and in the lives of children, adolescents, and their families are simply enormous. We also believe that there are still several barriers to achieving this vision, foremost of which are the low expectations of other professionals for school psychology, which have unfortunately often been perpetuated by the narrow vision that some school psychologists and school psychology trainers have had. We are not naive about the institutional challenges, obstacles, and barriers that many school psychologists face in using their professional skills and interests to achieve the maximum good. Rather, we believe that through a concerted effort over time, school psychologists can individually and collectively advance the field at all levels, and that in doing so, school psychology will make an enormous positive impact.

Although each chapter within this book is unique, these chapters were developed through a collective vision for the book. Some of the "big ideas" on which this book and our vision for the field of school psychology are based include the following:

• The general fields of psychology and education, as well as the specific field of school psychology, have given us rich and sometimes challenging historical precedents for the present practice of school psychology. Although it is important to have a strong understanding of these historical elements and how they have shaped the present, we agree with the premise that *the past is not necessarily the future*, and we advocate that the time has come for the field of school psychology to move forward from some of the historical challenges that have limited it in realizing its full potential.

• American society has become increasingly diverse and pluralistic with respect to cultural background, race, ethnicity, and language of its citizens, and it will continue to become increasingly diverse during the 21st century. School psychologists should develop cultural competence so that they can work appropriately and effectively with individuals and groups from a variety of backgrounds (see Chapter 3).

• School psychology has been and should continue to be primarily focused in school or other educational settings. The educational setting is a primary focus of our vision and of this book. However, school psychologists have much to offer outside of the context of school settings, and we encourage the practice of school psychology in a variety of settings and contexts (see Chapters 4 and 5).

• Individual psychoeducational assessment of children and adolescents has been and will continue to be a mainstay activity of school psychologists. However, individual assessment activities should do more than simply describe or diagnose problems. Rather, the most useful assessment strategies are those that provide a foundation for effective interventions (see Chapter 8).

• School psychology practice should be data oriented or data driven. School psychologists should base their decisions on valid data and use effective data collection techniques to inform, monitor, and modify intervention activities (see Chapter 7).

• School psychologists should be savvy consumers of research and should have the skills to engage in research and evaluation activities within their respective settings that will help to advance practice (see Chapter 12).

• School psychologists have historically worked with a limited segment of student populations, primarily those who have or are suspected of having disabilities and those who are otherwise at high risk for negative outcomes in life. We believe that there will always be a need for school psychologists to focus some of their effort on the small percentage of students who have serious learning, behavioral, and social-emotional problems. We also recognize that longitudinal research points to the chronic nature of such problems and the critical need for *early* intervention if negative long-term outcomes are to be curtailed. Thus we strongly contend that school psychologists should use their unique expertise to positively affect *all students in school settings*, not just those who have severe needs.

• Although assessment activities have had and will continue to have an important place among the school psychologist's varied responsibilities, effective prevention and intervention activities should occupy a significant percentage of his or her time (see Chapters 9 and 10).

• Prevention and intervention activities can occur with individuals, within small groups, within classrooms, within entire schools, and within school district or community-based contexts. School psychologists should engage in prevention and intervention activities at each of these levels, so that a larger number of individuals may be positively influenced (see Chapters 9 and 10).

• School psychologists do not typically function in isolation but work as part of a system. School psychologists should strive to use their expertise to develop a solid understanding of the systems in which they work and to help facilitate systems-level change as needed (see Chapter 11).

• School psychology is a field with incredible potential for helping to solve the "big" problems facing education. And yet this potential is still largely unrealized. We believe that school psychologists should play an active, important, and essential role in this regard. This book is built on the foundation of a progressive, forward-thinking vision of school psychology, and we are optimistic that collectively individual school psychologists can continue to move the field forward through their efforts (see Chapter 13).

In sum, school psychology is a young, dynamic, and exciting field that has incredible and still unrealized potential for positively affecting education, psychology, and the lives of children, adolescents, and their families. It is our hope that this book will provide a useful and engaging guide to the field of school psychology and will help serve to continue to move the field forward.

## DISCUSSION QUESTIONS AND ACTIVITIES

1. Individuals who are being introduced to the field of school psychology are often surprised to find that the definition of school psychology is not necessarily clear-cut and that at times it has been a point of controversy. Discuss the power of definitions and how they can shape the field of school psychology and how it is perceived.

2. During the past several decades, the characteristics of school psychologists have changed somewhat. Characterize some of these changes, and describe the current characteristics of those who work in the field of school psychology.

3. Interview one or more school psychologists in your area. Find out how they entered the field, what their career trajectory has been, what their responsibilities and roles are, and how they spend a typical day, week, and month in their workplace. Ask them what they like most or find most rewarding about their work as school psychologists, as well as what they find to be the most frustrating or difficult.

4. One of the first decisions that new graduate students in school psychology make is whether to pursue a master's/specialist degree or a doctoral degree. How do the two levels of training differ, and what are the costs and benefits, pros and cons, to each?

5. At the doctoral level of training, differentiate between the training and roles of school psychologists from the two other primary areas of professional psychology: clinical psychology and counseling psychology. At the specialist or master's level, differentiate between the training and roles of school psychologists from the fields of school counseling and school social work.

# 2

# The Historical Context
# of School Psychology

In relation to most other scientific and academic fields, school psychology is quite young. It has been in existence for barely a century and has been a formidable organized professional entity for only a few decades. To fully understand the field of school psychology in the 21st century, it is essential to understand its roots. We agree with Reschly and Ysselydyke's (2002) observation that the past is not necessarily the future with respect to the field of school psychology, but we also believe that a basic understanding of the past is essential if we are to move the field forward. This chapter provides a brief excursion into the historical context of school psychology. First, we explore its philosophical and intellectual foundations, ranging from classical Greek to modern European influences. Some of the major events, movements, and individuals in the emergence of the field of psychology in general, and then the field of school psychology in particular, examined. We then detail some aspects of the historical context of American education as they relate to the development of school psychology. We provide an overview of major events and issues in the development and professionalization of the field of school psychology and link them to the recent history of the field, with a particular emphasis on legal developments and training and credentialing issues that have had a strong impact on the recent history of school psychology. Ongoing tensions or "culture wars" that have surrounded school psychology's rise to prominence are examined, including values conflicts within various dimensions of the field and the historical and current differences between the two primary organizations representing the field. The chapter ends with some discussion of what lessons and trends have been apparent in the history of the field and what these issues may portend for the future.

## PHILOSOPHICAL, INTELLECTUAL, AND SOCIAL–CULTURAL FOUNDATIONS

The most influential historian of the field of school psychology, Thomas Fagan, has stated that "no significant aspect of contemporary school psychology, including its practitioners, was present before the 1890s" (Fagan & Wise, 2000, p. 23). Thus at first glance it appears that there may not be any point to tracing the historical context of the field prior to the late 19th century. However, it is important to recognize that school psychology did not develop in a social or cultural vacuum. Rather, its emergence was the product of a confluence of forces and timing. Therefore, it is useful to look at some of the more notable historical forces that contributed not only to the birth of school psychology but also to the larger fields of psychology and education in general.

## Classical Greek Influences

Psychology is considered to be a "Western" discipline, given that its philosophical, intellectual, and cultural foundations stem from ancient and modern forces flowing from the classical world of ancient Greece to modern Europe. It has been said that there is no distinctive aspect of psychology that cannot be traced to the philosophical world of the Greeks (Leahey, 1987). Specifically, most modern psychological thought can be traced to the various philosophies espoused and shaped in succession by three prominent Greek philosophers: Socrates (470–399 B.C.), his student Plato (428–348 B.C.), and particularly Plato's student Aristotle (384–322 B.C.), a founder of the philosophy of science who was known as the "first professor."

Socrates was an itinerant teacher whose work focused on inquiring about the meaning of general ideas or constructs, especially *Truth*, *Justice*, and *Beauty*. Socrates was antagonistic toward the Sophists, a group of Athenian teachers who espoused a view of the world that we might today term humanistic relativism or postmodernism. The Sophists proposed that "man is the measure of all things," meaning that all experience is subjective and that it is not possible to derive an ultimate reality because of individual differences in the way that reality is perceived. Socrates believed that the ideas of the Sophists were dangerous and could lead to moral anarchy. By posing provocative questions that contrasted sharply with the views of the Sophists, he promoted the notion that ultimate general truths existed and that there were enduring laws or principles that could lead to such truth. However, Socrates did not provide answers to most of his own questions. Rather, it was his famous student Plato who provided answers through written dialogues based on Socrates' questions.

Plato extended Socrates' quest for general universal truths to encompass a quest for all forms of knowledge. Thus *epistemology*, or the study of theories of knowledge or various ways of knowing, was born. Although Plato was concerned with ways of deriving knowledge, his focus and methods did not lend themselves very well to the scientific study of human behavior. It was Aristotle who first promoted the philosophy of empiricism that ultimately became a foundation of modern psychology. Aristotle's views were in many ways antithetical to those of his teacher, Plato. Aristotle moved away from the somewhat mystical ideas of Plato and firmly established a foundation for scientific thought that was based on observation. It is worth noting that Aristotle was the first to conduct a systematic "literature review" of earlier thinkers (Leahey, 1987), a technique for laying the groundwork for particular problems that later became a bedrock practice of psychological science and a practice that is certainly familiar to any graduate student in school psychology.

The cultural, artistic, and philosophical activity of the Greek and Roman worlds began to decline noticeably around A.D. 300. By the fall of Rome in the late fifth century, the intellectual energy characterized by the work of the Greek philosophers had largely dissipated, and it was centuries before there was a revival of significant cultural and intellectual life in the Western world. The "dark ages" marked a long period of retrenchment in these areas, and it affected every level of society. However, despite the ending of the incredible accomplishments of the classical era, an important legacy was left to influence future generations. In particular, one of the hallmark intellectual tensions that emerged in the Greek period—the conflict between rationalism and empiricism—carried into greater European culture and became one of the primary foundational influences that led to the emergence of psychology.

## Modern European Influences

By the time that the new discipline of psychology emerged in the late 19th century, and by the time that public education was becoming an increasingly important aspect of American society, the Western world had emerged from centuries of intellectual and artistic retrenchment. During the church–state-controlled medieval period, virtually the only persons who could read and write in most of Europe were clerics, and rigid rules were imposed regarding the development and dissemination of written literature. In addition, questions regarding the structure, function, and meaning of human behavior, which had flowed with great energy during the classical period, became the nearly exclusive province of the religious orthodoxy, and individuals who dared challenge the status quo often put their liberty and even their lives at risk. However, the new energy and ideas that began to flow during the Renaissance period did stem from some roots that were established during the middle ages. It is interesting to consider that the comingling of Christianity, Islam, and Judaism in the Near East produced and preserved some important written works and that the unauthorized translation of the Bible into vernacular language was an important intellectual development.

By the 17th century, the modern scientific revolution had begun. Prominent figures such as René Descartes (1596–1650) and John Locke (1632–1704) emerged and revitalized the philosophy of science and its empirical and epistemological roots. Descartes wrote and taught regarding the process of seeking truth in a skeptical manner, of the native physical or material structure of the world, and, importantly, of the *dualism* of the body and mind of humans, which he saw as distinct elements. Locke, on the other hand, dismissed the notion of innate moral and metaphysical truths and advocated discovering truth through personal experience. An important aspect of Locke's work for the formation of psychology and the advancement of education was his focus on the mind and on the process of using reflection or introspection to gain knowledge. In many ways, Locke's work was a precursor to the science of the mind, paving the way for theories of intelligence, learning, and cognitive processing. Other 17th-century thinkers also provided important foundations for the emergence of psychology and the refinement of educational pedagogy. For example, Thomas Hobbes (1588–1679) was the first intellectual who explored the connection between the development of speech and the development of reasoning. He also introduced the concept of *Natural Law*, the notion that there were regulations inherent in nature, whether or not humans recognized them. This concept was a precursor to the psychological principle that behavior is lawful and is governed by basic principles, a concept that became especially important in behavioral psychology.

The 18th century is considered a period of enlightenment, with major developments (and revolutions) in science, philosophy, art, and politics. Many of the developments of this period provided a further foundation for the emergence of psychology during the next century. David Hume (1711–1776) was a moderate skeptic who wrote extensively on the notion of *habit* or *custom*, the propensity to behave, think, and feel in customary and predictable ways. Hume desired to apply Newtonian-like laws to predict human behavior, using the technique of introspection to generate his ideas. One of the particularly psychological contributions of Hume was his development of a classification of the contents of the human mind, which focused on perceptions and distinguished between impressions and ideas.

In opposition to the notions espoused by Hume and various other skeptics, a school of thought emerged out of Scotland by the mid-18th century that espoused "common sense" in analyzing and understanding human behavior. This assertion of common sense, typified by the writing of Thomas Reid (1710–1796) and his student, Dugald Stewart (1753–1828), ridiculed the claims of philosophy and posited that everyday experience provides a better foundation for understanding human thought and behavior than the theories of skeptics, which they considered to be absurd. The writings of both these men dissected the mind into component faculties and advocated the practical value of the study of human behavior and thought. One of the foremost thinkers of the century was Immanuel Kant (1724–1804). Kant developed a science of understanding humanity, which he called anthropology but which actually bears more similarity to psychology. He studied human intelligence, moral character, the notion of self, and other constructs that would become important within psychology. Kant's work greatly influenced fellow German Wilhelm Wundt, who later developed the first psychology laboratory. Another Enlightenment-era figure whose writings proved to be highly influential in psychology (and in education and politics) was Jean-Jacques Rousseau (1712–1778). Rousseau became known for many things, including his influence on political revolutionaries Marx and Engel, who were intrigued with his notions of free will and of the innate freedom of humans and with his criticism of Enlightenment-era scientific and technological advances, which Rousseau viewed as chaining or enslaving people. He advocated for education as the means of overcoming the corrupt state of civilization. Rousseau was one of the first intellectuals to discuss in detail the *nature vs. nurture* dichotomy of the influence on human behavior, and he weighed in on the side of nurture, believing that external conditions and influences shaped the individual rather than innate drives. Interestingly and somewhat paradoxically, his belief in human malleability foreshadowed B. F. Skinner's advocacy of using a carefully controlled society to enhance human potential (as espoused in his book *Walden II*) and also served as inspiration for "whole child" education advocates, who rejected highly structured and sequenced teaching of basic skills as advocated by Skinner.

In sum, 17th- and 18th-century intellectual developments, which are often referred to as the *Age of Reason* and the *Age of Enlightenment*, helped move Western thinking out of the Dark Ages and the medieval period and provided the intellectual foundation for the birth of psychology, as well as developments in education, that would provide an impetus for school psychology. And unlike the classic Greek philosophers, whose work was foundational for psychology, many of the prominent intellectuals of the 17th and 18th centuries overtly concerned themselves with issues and constructs that were distinctly psychological, regardless of the fact that the field had not yet emerged.

## THE EMERGENCE OF PSYCHOLOGY

Although the foundation of psychology had been laid in the preceding centuries, the discipline formally emerged in the mid- to late 19th century, first in Europe, and then in

America. Certain 19th-century influences made a strong impression on the emerging field. One of the foremost influences was the work of Charles Darwin (1809–1882), whose elucidation of a scientific theory of natural selection in evolution revolutionized science. His 1859 seminal work *On the Origin of Species* broadly influenced Western intellectual circles, and his later works on the descent of humans and the expression of emotions in humans and animals became cornerstone literature in the fledgling field of psychology. Franz Joseph Gall (1758–1828) developed the science of phrenology, or the description and prediction of human traits from bumps on the head and the shape of the cranium. Although phrenology is now relegated to a status only slightly higher than an amusing footnote, it must be understood that it was an enormously popular enterprise. More important, phrenology focused the seat of human behavior clearly on the brain, correlating specific regions of the brain with specific behavioral functions. In a sense, Gall's phrenology was the first formal expression of physiological psychology, especially the study of brain–behavior relationships.

By late in the 19th century, the discipline of psychology became formally established and legitimized, and three forms of psychology had emerged: the *psychology of consciousness*, the *psychology of the unconscious*, and the *psychology of adaptation*. The German scientist and philosopher Wilhelm Wundt (1832–1920) is credited with establishing the first psychology laboratory in 1879 and establishing psychology as an independent experimental science. Wundt's work focused on the experimental study of individual consciousness. On the other hand, Viennese physician Sigmund Freud (1856–1939), who is credited as being the father of psychiatry, introduced ideas as radical as Darwin's by suggesting that unconscious desires and motives shape much of human behavior. Freud's deterministic view of human behavior and the unconscious was truly revolutionary. Although many of his theories have now been rejected even by proponents of the psychodynamic approach he pioneered, one must not overlook the enormity of his contributions and influence. Even today, his metaphor of the conscious mind as being the "tip of the iceberg" of human experience is widely used, and the influence of his work in Western cultures cannot be minimized. In addition, the psychology of adaptation, with roots in Darwin's theory of natural selection, focused on how the individual adjusts to the environment and, ultimately, how the environment shapes behavior. This psychology later developed into behaviorism, which became perhaps the most influential force of the 20th century in academic psychology.

By the end of the 19th century, there was no question that psychology had moved from an emerging to an established field. American and European universities established psychology curricula and began awarding academic degrees in psychology. The American Psychological Association was established in 1891. Seminal texts were published, and scientific journals were established. Although the clinical or practical application of psychology was not yet established, all the pieces were in place for that to happen. Through these events and forces, the conditions that allowed for the development and establishment of school psychology were established.

# DEVELOPMENTS IN AMERICAN EDUCATION

We have tried to make it clear that the field of school psychology was hatched from a confluence of intellectual and social developments in both psychology and education. This section provides some additional discussion regarding some of the important historical developments in American education that were important in this confluence.

## Colonial Foundations

Although most educational historians have identified the period of about 1825 to 1875 as the era during which the building blocks of American public education were put into place (i.e., Butts, 1978; Calhoun, 1969), there were important historical antecedents during the prior two centuries that led to this series of developments. During the American colonial period in the 17th century, although public schools as we now know them did not exist, the idea of public education began to sprout, particularly in the New England colonies. Although there was generally no public taxation for schools or compulsory education during this period, the notion of education for the public good became more prominent, and the idea that formal education of youths would serve a greater civic purpose began to take hold. Most of the formal efforts to educate young people involved a primary component of religious instruction, and the preparation of future clerics was a major emphasis in this regard. By the early to mid-1700s, colonial society was becoming increasingly pluralistic with respect to religious views (albeit within the general Christian worldview, particularly the Protestant version of it, see Smith, 1967). Tensions were increasing regarding the appropriate place of religious instruction and influence within civic or public life and the legitimacy of public efforts to promote the superiority of one religion over another (Butts, 1978). These tensions ultimately helped lead to the "establishment" clause in the U.S. Constitution and to the weakening of legal bonds between established churches and new states following the Revolutionary period. With the establishment of the first state constitutions in the late 1700s, some states (such as North Carolina, Georgia, and Pennsylvania) adopted specific provisions for public schooling, although it would be many years before these efforts resulted in a strong system of public education. During this same time period, there was considerable national tension between those leaders who favored a strong centralized role for national government and those who advocated for a weaker federal system and the sovereignty of individual states. Interestingly, during this late-18th-century debate regarding the proper role of the federal government, several prominent voices argued in favor of the establishment of a strong national system of public education, something that never occurred. Ultimately, the framers of the U.S. Constitution left somewhat vague the appropriate role of the federal government in public education, with education considered a "creature of the states," and as the 19th century emerged, conditions varied greatly from state to state regarding public education efforts, which had not yet emerged as a visible, identifiable entity (Butts, 1978; Calhoun, 1969).

## 19th-Century Steps

During the 1800s, significant steps were taken toward the development of systems of public education. Underlying these developments was the growing belief that voluntary and private efforts to formally educate America's young citizens were insufficient and that the new democracy could not flourish under such conditions. As many of the cities in the northeastern United States grew rapidly with industrialization, so did the numbers of poor and uneducated youths, along with deteriorating social conditions and a public outcry to improve the situation. As a result, "common schools," the precursor to today's public schools, began to be established (Butts, 1978; Ravitch, 1974), primarily in the mid-Atlantic and New England states but also in Virginia and the Carolinas. The growth of the abolition movement and the relative lack of common schools in the southern states further set the stage for future development of public systems of education. Following the horrors of the Civil War and the end of the institution of slavery, the nation was in massive debt, many of the southern cities were in shambles from the war, and the industrialization that had swept the northern cities slowly began to move to the urban areas southward. Thus the reconstruction period saw further expansion of the common schools, increasing efforts to assure that African American youths received a public education, and an expansion of compulsory schooling laws, particularly in urban centers (Best & Sidwell, 1967; Tyack, 1967). This period of expansion was aided by the increasingly centralized power of governments at both the state and national levels. As governmental authority became more centralized, typically a concurrent increase occurred in efforts to promote common schools and to provide a financial base from which to support them (Berlin, 1974).

## 20th-Century Developments, Persistent Issues

By the early 1900s the combination of (1) systems of public and compulsory education in the United States, (2) the social conditions following industrialization and reconstruction, and (3) the emergence of new educational tools and scientific technologies was becoming extremely complex. The field of public education began to grow rapidly at the same time that the budding discipline of psychology was emerging in the United States. Thus the conditions were in place that allowed, or perhaps required, the incipient field of school psychology to begin to make a toehold during what has come to be known as the *progressive era* in American social history (Tyack, 1967). One of the biggest impacts the progressive era had on education was the combination of more far-reaching child labor laws and compulsory education laws. By the end of the first decade of the 20th century, all states had compulsory education laws of some type in place, and by 1920, almost all American children attended schools, at least through the grammar school level (History of American Education Web Project, 2004; Tyack, 1967).

Before we move directly into the beginnings of the field of school psychology, it is worth considering that by the first quarter of the 20th century two persistent and significant issues in American education had developed that would have long-lasting implications (even to the present day) for school psychology: the development of the IQ or mental ability testing movement and the common state of racial segregation and inequality in schools. We consider these two issues in more detail, as they both have had a major impact on school psychology.

The movers in the mental ability testing arena had, by the end of World War I, developed a great confidence in the potential of IQ tests to measure the human mind, and this confidence spread throughout much of public education. Most of the individuals who were influential in this movement, such as Lewis Terman and Henry Goddard, held a *nativist* view of intelligence, viewing it as inherited, essentially fixed, and difficult if not impossible to modify in any meaningful way through education. The power of the IQ testing movement became enormous and led to what Ravitch (2000) has termed "a brutal pessimism" regarding educational programming, tracking, and opportunities. In essence, the results of IQ tests were used—initially with little criticism—to determine in great measure individuals' opportunities and future. "The intelligence testers promoted fatalism, a rueful acceptance that achievement in school is the result of innate ability, not sustained effort by teachers and students. The cult of the IQ became an all purpose rationale for students' lack of effort and for poor teaching: Why study hard in school if IQ predicts outcomes? Why work hard to teach slow learners if their IQ's predict they cannot do well in school?" (Ravitch, 2000, p. 161). As anyone familiar with school psychology knows, the development of the field ultimately became inextricably linked to the IQ testing movement, a connection that, we would argue, plagues the field to this day and that is commonly cited as the greatest barrier to moving the role of school psychologists to a greater focus on prevention, intervention, and consultation. This issue is discussed in greater detail in several other chapters of this volume. It is also worth considering that the IQ movement influenced American education well beyond the practice of school psychology. The practices and notions that came from this movement were often used as a basis for excluding children with disabilities from public schools (an issue discussed in more detail in Chapter 6), for routing students into vocational versus academic tracks, and for reducing the focus on alterable variables (such as student and teacher effort, curriculum delivery, school structure) within schools (Ravitch, 2000).

With respect to racial segregation, tension, and inequalities in American public education, the struggle has been long and divisive, and it has taken legal precedents from the nation's highest courts to steer improvements and precedents that are still evolving and trying to fulfill their promise. During the colonial period and early years of the nation, public education efforts were aimed almost exclusively at white children: Native Americans were essentially left out, Asians and individuals of Hispanic descent did not yet exist in large enough numbers to develop a critical mass for advocacy, and laws throughout the southern states prohibited educating African American slaves, who existed in large numbers. There were relatively few exceptions to this state of affairs. By the advent of the reconstruction era in the late 1800s, African American children began to be offered formal opportunities for public schooling in increasingly greater numbers, but for the most part and for many years these opportunities existed in separate systems that were operated at a severe disadvantage, with far fewer resources than other public schools. As educational opportunities for African Americans increased, serious debates took place within the community of black leaders regarding what direction was best, as typified by the debates between Booker T. Washington (who advocated for a practical, industrial education for blacks) and W. E. B. Du Bois (who advocated for an intellectually rigorous education for blacks and derided practical education efforts as second class). As the 20th century evolved, two forces began to merge that gradually began to chip away at these historical antecedents. First, American society was becoming increasingly diverse and pluralistic due to patterns of immigration dating to the late 1800s. Second, legal advocacy and public discourse regarding the education of children from minority group backgrounds increased. The 1954 landmark ruling of the U.S. Supreme Court in *Brown v. Board of Education* was the culmination of many years of advocacy to change inequity. This ruling held that segregated educational environments were bad for children and that the notion of "separate but equal" treatment in America (which became the law of the land in the Court's 1892 *Plessy v. Ferguson* decision) was a cruel myth. Now, as the 50th anniversary of *Brown* has been recently celebrated, it is apparent that, notwithstanding the substantial gains made following this and other court decisions, the full promise of equality has yet to be fulfilled. School psychologists are currently dealing with two major issues related to race, ethnicity, and social class: (1) The "achievement gap" (between white/Asian and black/Hispanic/ Native American students) in educational attainment is becoming an increasingly serious issue for educators and policymakers, and (2) minority overrepresentation in special education programs (particularly among African American youths) continues to present significant challenges. In addition, the past two decades have witnessed increased emphasis on developing and using culturally and linguistically appropriate assessment and intervention techniques. Issues related to ethnic and cultural issues in public schools are addressed in more detail in other chapters of this volume, particularly Chapters 3 and 5.

# BEGINNINGS OF SCHOOL PSYCHOLOGY

Fagan's assertion that no significant aspect of school psychology existed before the 1890s (Fagan & Wise, 2000) is accurate, but the seeds from which the field would spring were already planted by that time. In addition to the establishment of psychology as a unique discipline by the late 1800s, other forces paved the way for the emergence of school psychology. As we have noted, the industrialization and urbanization of America, increased support for public education, the beginnings of the compulsory schooling movement, and post-Civil War social changes all contributed to a need for professionals to focus on education, child development, mental health, and other aspects of providing supports, training, and supervision for children in an increasingly complex society.

One of the seminal events in the beginnings of school psychology was the 1896 establishment of a psychological clinic by Lightner Witmer at the University of Pennsylvania in Philadelphia. This clinic has been referred to as the first child guidance clinic. Witmer's goal was to prepare psychologists to help educators solve children's learning problems (Bardon & Bennett, 1974). Based on this contribution, Witmer has been credited with being the founder of both school psychology and clinical psychology. This clinic was clearly the first effort of its kind in North America. However, a somewhat similar laboratory clinic had been established by Sir Francis Galton at University College in London in 1884, predating Witmer's American clinic by 12 years. Although the primary purpose of Galton's laboratory was the measurement of individual human differences rather than direct service, one of its first endeavors was to assist local schools in selecting and classifying pupils. Thus some writers have argued that the birth of school psychology may be more appropriately credited to Galton's laboratory in England (White & Harris, 1961).

One of the events almost always mentioned in the same breath as the beginning of school psychology is the publication of the Binet–Simon scales in 1905. We have previously addressed the impact of the IQ testing movement on American education and school psychology, but it is worthwhile to consider the beginnings of this movement in more detail. Psychologist Alfred Binet and psychiatrist Theophile Simon were commissioned by the Minister of Public Education in Paris to develop a methodology for classifying and sorting children who were not successful in the general education settings and who could not profit from the regular curriculum for the purpose of providing them specially designed training in other settings. Together, they developed the Binet–Simon scales, the first modern intelligence test, which was not only used in France but also later adapted by Lewis Terman of Stanford University into an English-language version for use in the United States. Thus the early history of school psychology became inextricably linked to intelligence testing and individual assessment and classification. These efforts proved to be instrumental in expanding the field of school psychology in later years and also served to entrench many school psychologists in a psychometric-driven role of sorter or gatekeeper. Of course, part of the early entrenchment of school psychologists in the psychometric-gatekeeper role could also be attributed to the fact that the field of psychology had not yet developed a technology for effective intervention selection and implementation.

In the United States, the 1890s and early 1900s marked an increasing emphasis on providing educational and mental health services for youths whom we would today consider as being "at risk." Most urban public school districts in the larger cities of the eastern United States had established special educational programs and classes by this time, aimed at assisting students with significant learning problems. In 1899, William Healey established a clinic in Chicago for a juvenile court in the public school system, perhaps the precursor to today's special programs for students with emotional and behavioral disorders. The mental health field became formally established by 1910, with the founding of the "mental hygiene" movement that year. A primary focus of the incipient mental health field was the founding of child guidance clinics to help prevent and treat juvenile delinquency. Although these efforts were not necessarily specific to the field of school psychology nor conducted by individuals who were known as school psychologists, they nevertheless were early manifestations of activity in the field.

By the 1920s, the terms "school psychology" or "school psychologist" had emerged, indicating that the field was becoming increasingly established, with the signs of a distinct profession. Arnold Gesell became the first person to be appointed to position of "school psychologist," and he served in that role in Connecticut between 1915 and 1919. The term "school psychologist" also had appeared in the literature by this time. Thus the field of school psychology, though barely in its infancy and without any formal structure or specific professional organization, had arrived.

## DEVELOPMENT AND PROFESSIONALIZATION OF THE FIELD

By the late 1920s, the first efforts to establish training programs and credentialing for school psychologists had occurred, and during the 1930s, these efforts were expanded. During this decade, the young field was beginning to grapple with increasing regulation and recognition, a sign that it had arrived. However, the practice of psychology in the schools was still largely unregulated, and individuals who fulfilled psychological service roles in schools had a wide range of professional training and went by a plethora of titles, such as psychological examiner, psychoclinician, and clinical or consulting psychologist. The first book on school psychology, *Psychological Service for School Problems*, authored by pioneering school psychologist Gertrude Hildreth, was published in 1930. Interestingly, one of the features of this book was the illustration of a typical day for a school psychologist and of the division of different activities within a work day. Hildreth's view on school psychology service delivery was fairly broad. Although individual testing and diagnosis played a prominent role in her breakdown of a professional day, consulting with teachers, administrators, parents, and other individuals through conferences appeared to be the single activity that consumed the most time.

During the 1940s and 1950s, the field of school psychology continued to expand. During this era, two important professional conferences with strong implications for the future of school psychology were held. The Boulder Conference on Clinical Psychology was held in 1949, shortly after the end of World War II, and during the time when the practice of psychology was expanding greatly due to the development of the Veterans Administration hospitals and clinics to provide medical services to personnel who had served in the military during the war effort. The Boulder Conference resulted in the articulation of the scientist-practitioner model of psychology training and in models for credentialing of psychologists. The impact of the Boulder Conference was to further legitimize the applied professional practice of psychology, which had previously taken a back seat in status to the academic or scientific aspect of the field. The Thayer Conference of 1954 was held for the purpose of advancing and shaping training, credentialing, and practice in school psychology. The proceedings of the Thayer Conference provided the first comprehensive picture of the field of school psychology and its circumstances. During this era, a division of the APA emerged (Division 16) that was specifically focused on school psychology, and the first few state school psychology associations were started. However, there was no strong link between national and state organizations and efforts such as was increasingly enjoyed by the field of clinical psychology during this time. Part of the reason for lack of a cohesive school psychology organizing body stemmed from the huge disparity in procedures for credentialing of school psychologists across the various states. Many states still did not have any formal recognition or training standards for psychologists to practice in schools. In addition, the doctoral versus nondoctoral conflict in psychology had begun to emerge, and it clearly affected the status and organization of school psychologists. Unlike clinical psychologists, who were increasingly trained at the doctoral level and followed similar routes to credentialing and practice across states, school psychologists were almost entirely nondoctoral practitioners, and there was little consistency from state to state with regard to credentialing.

During the 1950s and 1960s, a social or demographic development occurred that had a major impact on American education and culture and ultimately on the development of school psychology. The "baby boom" began in 1947 at the conclusion of World War II. Because such a large percentage of young American men were involved in military service, and because of the war effort in general (due to which a large percentage of young American women were working in civilian-military roles and war-related industries), marriages and birth rates declined substantially during this time. As the war ended, an enormous number of young men and women, whose lives had been "on hold" during the war, resumed normal life. Most married, many pursued higher education with the assistance of the new G.I. Bill, and almost all members of this generation began to raise their own families. Thus a period of extensive growth in the numbers of children and youths in the United States began. By the mid-1950s, this growth spilled into the public schools, which began to expand at an unprecedented rate that continued into the 1970s. At the same time, federally funded efforts were made to improve mathematics and science education, which in part led to the expansion of school guidance services.

As the numbers of schoolchildren expanded greatly, so did the numbers of students who had disabilities or who otherwise struggled with respect to their academic and behavioral adjustment in the school setting. These rapidly expanding numbers of "exceptional" students spurred the growth of school psychology, as parents, teachers, and administrators looked for solutions to learning and behavioral problems. Although no federal law for the education of students with disabilities was passed until 1975, most states and larger school districts expanded and refined their programs for meeting the needs of exceptional children, and school psychologists were usually a part of these efforts. The passage of new laws for the education of students with disabilities ultimately proved to be a watershed set of events for the field of school psychology.

The era of increasing emphasis on awareness and laws for education of students with disabilities corresponds to a great extent with the emergence of a new era of growth in school psychology. According to school psychology historian Thomas

Fagan, the field's historical development can be divided into two distinct eras: the *hybrid years* of 1890 to 1969, when school psychology was emerging and beginning to develop an identity, and the *thoroughbred years* of 1970 to 2000 and beyond, when school psychology had clearly emerged as a unique field with a stable professional identity. Without question, the culminating symbol of the bridge between the two eras was the establishment of the National Association of School Psychologists (NASP), which held its first convention in St. Louis in 1969. The founding of NASP was significant not only because it signaled that the field had achieved a strong professional identity and professional structure but also because it represented the beginnings of a shift in the voice of the field (Fagan & Wise, 2000). Division 16 of APA had previously served as the only national-level voice of the field of school psychology and was the first national organization within the field (Fagan, 2002). However, after NASP was established, its membership numbers quickly surpassed those of Division 16, giving it increased credibility and visibility. Division 16, through its connection with APA and its advocacy of the doctoral degree as a necessity for independent practice, positioned itself as the voice of psychology within the greater body of American psychology. NASP, on the other hand, was a freestanding organization representing what was viewed as a unique field and as a mission to advocate for the interests of master's- and specialist-level school psychologists. These differences between APA and NASP had enormous implications for some of the later tensions and dynamics that would shape the field and that continue today.

# RECENT HISTORY OF SCHOOL PSYCHOLOGY

It is important to consider that history is constantly being written and rewritten. The history of school psychology consists not only of the foundations and early period but also of recent events and issues. The beginning of Fagan's thoroughbred years in 1970 can be considered a starting point for a brief overview of some of the recent history of the field. This section provides a brief overview of two aspects of recent history within the field: the impact of the public law for education of students with disabilities and the impact of the development of training and credentialing standards for school psychology training programs and practitioners.

## Public Law 94-142/Individuals with Disabilities Education Act

Some of the most important recent historical developments in the field of school psychology have been attributable to the impact of new laws and court decisions. These legal issues and related ethical issues are covered in more detail in Chapter 6, but they are briefly introduced in this section with an emphasis on how they have been critical in shaping the field. Specifically, the passage by the United States Congress of Public Law 94-142 in 1975, originally referred to as the Education for All Handicapped Children Act, proved to be hugely important in the development of school psychology. For the first time, there was a unified federal law rather than a patchwork of state laws and policies mandating a free and appropriate public education for students with disabilities. Three areas show the immediate and continuing impact of this law on the recent history of the field of school psychology.

First, because of the mandates for appropriate special education eligibility assessment of students, significantly greater numbers of school psychologists were needed. This need resulted in a significant expansion of school psychology training programs and of the numbers of practicing school psychologists from the 1970s through the 1990s. For example, it has been estimated that the number of training programs doubled from about 100 to more than 200 during this period and that the number of members of NASP likewise more than doubled. In short, the significant expansion of school psychology can be attributed in large measure to the impact of the federal law.

Second, the legal mandate for eligibility assessment not only expanded the field but also served to further entrench school psychologists in the gatekeeper or sorter role, a legacy that is proving to be highly resistant to being changed to the broad expanded role that we advocate. Many of the generation of school psychologists who entered the field within the few years immediately after the enactment of Public Law 94-142 were trained with the expectation of functioning primarily as psychometricians, and their expectations were in many cases further shaped in this direction by school administrators. The entrenchment in the gatekeeper/sorter role has proven to be a continued source of great frustration to many in the field who desire to engage in a broader range of services and to play an intervention-focused role.

Third, some of the specific mandates of Public Law 94-142 and its successors (the Individuals with Disabilities Education Act [IDEA] 1990, 1997, and 2004) have shaped professional practice. Perhaps the most singular example is the original definition of learning disabilities (LDs) in the Public Law, which defined LDs primarily on the basis of a significant discrepancy between a student's intellectual ability and academic achievement. This definition not only further entrenched the field in the psychometric gatekeeper model but also actually resulted in day-to-day practice constraints. A generation of school psychologists has learned to live with a standardized intelligence test kit in one hand and a standardized academic achievement test in the other, much to the chagrin of many who believe that this type of assessment activity is not only questionable in terms of the premises on which it is based and the results it produces but also does little or nothing to help children other than give them access to services (Reschly & Ysseldyke, 2002). Although the most recent (2004) reauthorization of IDEA reduces dependency on the ability–achievement assessment paradigm, it is too early to tell whether this change will result in a significant broadening of roles for school psychologists. Another example of specific mandates of the public law shaping practice is the requirement of conducting a functional behavioral assessment (FBA) for students with severe behavioral problems, which was added to the law in its 1997 reauthorization. Although we view this mandate as positive and needed, it is interesting to see how it so quickly influenced professional practice. Prior to 1997, the only school psychologists who knew anything about FBA were those who were trained and practiced in behavioral school psychology models and who were reasonably competent in the principles of applied behavior analysis. However, within a short time following the 1997 reauthorization, FBA became an issue of interest to the entire field. Journal articles, books, book chapters, and professional conference presentations on this topic that were previously barely visible at the national level suddenly became "hot topics." Some school psychologists learned to implement the FBA mandate with integrity and positive results and used it to help establish effective intervention plans for students. Sadly, others viewed the mandate as one more hoop that must be gone through in the gatekeeper role. Without question, the public law will continue to evolve, and as it does so, it will certainly affect the role of school psychologists in one way or another.

## Training Standards and Credentialing

Chapter 4 discusses training and credentialing of school psychologists in detail. As a precursor to that chapter, it is worth noting that the recent history of the field has seen some important developments in this arena. This section details some of the important historical developments related to training standards and credentialing of individual school psychologists and training programs.

### APA Accreditation of Doctoral Programs

Although Division 16 of APA began to pursue efforts for the accreditation of doctoral programs in school psychology in the 1960s, it was not until 1971 that the first program was accredited (Fagan & Wells, 2000). Before then, no nationally accredited training programs in school psychology existed at any level. In the decade following the first accreditation of a school psychology program, interest and activity in this area moved slowly, and most doctoral programs in the field either did not meet the minimum criteria for accreditation or were not interested in pursuing accreditation. By 1980 there were 20 accredited doctoral programs. However, the perceived importance of APA accreditation gradually built steam. By 1990 38 programs had received accreditation, and by 2000, the number was 52. By 2004, there were 58 APA-accredited doctoral programs in school psychology and an additional 13 APA-accredited doctoral programs in the combined professional–scientific psychology category, which lists school psychology as one of its focus areas.

### NASP Approval of Specialist Programs

With respect to master's and specialist programs (i.e., 60-semester-credit graduate programs in school psychology), Fagan and Wells (2000) have noted that the use of standards specifically for school psychology training did not occur within the relationship of NASP and the National Council for Accreditation of Teacher Education (NCATE) until the 1980s and that the NASP folio review for program accreditation was implemented in 1988. By the end of that decade, NASP program approval could be gained by adherence to the training standards developed by NASP, either through an institution's NCATE review process for all education credentialing programs or separately through the NASP training program review board. Like APA accreditation for doctoral programs, NASP approval for specialist programs increasingly became perceived as important. By 2005, 121 specialist-level programs and 54 doctoral-level programs were approved by NASP. Currently, an agreement exists between NASP and APA that allows for doctoral programs to receive joint APA accreditation and NASP approval within the same accreditation process. Thus, when a doctoral program receives APA accreditation in school psychology, it may also be awarded doctoral-level program approval by NASP.

### The NCSP Credential

Credentialing of individual practitioners is another area in which recent history has witnessed significant developments that have affected both training and practice. Because individual states dictate their own standards and procedures for both psychological board licensing for independent practice and department of education certification to practice in the schools, there has been much variation among the states, which has sometimes created difficulties for practitioners who train in one state and then want to work in another state. One important recent development in this area was the establishment by NASP in 1988 of the National School Psychology Certification System. This system leads to the granting of the Nationally Certified School Psychologist (NCSP) credential to those individuals who are ascertained to have completed minimum standards of training and competence. Obtaining this credential requires practitioners to have completed a NASP-approved training program or its equivalent (consisting of at least 60 semester credits of graduate-level coursework in an identified school psychology program, plus a 1,200 clock hour internship under the supervision of a credentialed school psychologist) and passing a standardized national examination. The purpose in enacting this system was to promote the NASP training standard for quality assurance and to make it easier for holders of the NCSP credential to receive state department of education certification to practice as school psychologists as they move from one state to another.

Initially, the national certification program took off slowly, and few states signed agreements allowing certification or license reciprocity for holders of the NCSP credential. However, after nearly two decades of existence, it has gradually increased in visibility and influence. By 2005, 21 states recognized the NCSP credential as a complete or partial basis for awarding their own state practice licenses or certificates. It is also worth noting that the number of practitioners holding the NCSP credential has continued to rise steadily, with more than 8,600 individuals listed by 2005. This figure represents approximately one third of the membership of NASP and a reasonably large percentage of all school psychologists.

## GROWTH THROUGH TENSION AND OPPOSITION

It has been said that stress, tension, and opposition are natural prerequisites to growth and development. If this notion is true, then the field of school psychology has had ample opportunities for growth! Perhaps more so than the other areas of professional psychology (clinical and counseling), school psychology has experienced not only the general tensions inherent in all of psychology but unique turmoil as well. This section explores some of these tensions or "culture wars."

### Two Cultures of Psychology

In a 1984 study published in *American Psychologist*, Gregory Kimble identified a "scientist–humanist" dimension in belief systems and values among psychologists that has created an underlying tension in the field for many years. The scientist–humanist dimension was his label for the dichotomy that he found through a survey of psychologists that utilized sophisticated sampling and survey techniques. The implication is that psychologists can be roughly divided into two distinct cultures: one representing the scientist end of the dimension, and the other representing the humanist end. Because school psychology is part of the larger field of psychology and is certainly included in this dichotomy, it is worth reviewing the six major areas in which this cultural division is said to be manifest.

## Scientific versus Human Values

This conflict involves the tension between the principles of objective science and the values of some practitioners who might be consumers of the science. A good illustration in the field of school psychology involves the use of behavioral theory to increase positive reinforcement within a classroom to increase appropriate behavior and decrease inappropriate behavior. Although there is a virtual mountain of evidence that increasing reinforcement for positive behaviors of students will lead to positive results, doing so goes against the value systems of many teachers and some school psychology practitioners, who might be opposed to the notion of "bribing" or otherwise hold the belief that external reinforcement systems are mechanistic and inappropriate, an idea that was popularized by journalist Alfie Kohn's (1993) book *Punished by Rewards*.

## Determinism versus Indeterminism

This second area of conflict has been in existence for centuries or longer. It is reflected in the tension between the notion that behavioral or personal outcomes are the result of fixed laws or determinants and the notion that outcomes are malleable and that individuals can alter their personal destinies. A good example of the unfolding of this conflict in our field is the hoopla that surrounded the publication of *The Bell Curve* by Herrnstein and Murray (1994). The conclusion of these authors was that intelligence was for the most part hereditary or native and that educational achievement and related outcomes of individuals low in ability cannot be meaningfully affected through well-meaning intervention programs. Strong advocates of this view argue that early intervention programs such as Head Start are a poor use of resources. However, there is an impressive array of evidence to the contrary, as detailed in Hart and Risley's (1995) book *Meaningful Differences*, which documents in painstaking detail that intellectual skills of young children are significantly affected by their early environments and that early life experiences set the stage for later accomplishments.

## Objectivism versus Intuitionism

This area of conflict is self-explanatory. Those who value objectivism use the axiom "in evidence we trust," whereas those who value intuitionism may reject data-driven approaches and instead make evaluations based on subjective feelings. A good example of this conflict within school psychology involves the selection and use of projective-expression assessment techniques for evaluating children's social–emotional status. Although objective data in this area overwhelmingly raise caution regarding the questionable technical properties of many tools, such as drawing and sentence completion tests, many practitioners continue to have a strong allegiance to such methods and view their intuitive value as compensating for their technical flaws (Merrell, 2003).

## Laboratory versus Field

This dimension of conflict is between results and methods refined in laboratory settings and those applied in naturalistic field settings. Because school psychology, as opposed to some branches of psychology, is an extraordinarily applied field, this conflict does not rear its head to a significant extent in our world. However, instances exist.

When FBA became a mandated assessment practice through the 1997 reauthorization of the IDEA, many practitioners were frustrated with and perhaps resented the necessity of implementing in school settings a technology that had been developed primarily in laboratory or clinic settings with individuals who had low-incidence disabilities.

### Nomothetic versus Idiographic

This interesting conflict will require some background for most readers to fully understand it. These two terms were first proposed in 1894 by Wilhelm Windelband, a German philosopher of science, as the two primary and somewhat opposing methods of scientific inquiry. Nomothetic inquiry involves procedures and methods designed to cover general laws and is concerned with similarities among phenomena such as population averages, aggregate statistical methods, and psychometrics. Idiographic inquiry involves attempts to understand a particular event or individual or the uniqueness of a phenomenon. Idiographic inquiry would support the use of qualitative analysis and single-case designs. The reality in school psychology is that both methods of inquiry are used by most practitioners and researchers, and for most it does not pose a significant conflict. For example, a school psychologist might assess a student's reading ability using curriculum-based assessment methods (an idiographic approach) but place the results in context for intervention planning by comparing the results with averages from the classroom or group (a nomothetic approach).

### Elementism versus Holism

Elementism is reflected in the notion of looking at very small parts or elements of human behavior and in isolation, whereas holism involves looking at the "whole" person and not considering any particular aspect of their characteristics or behavior in isolation. Like the conflict between laboratory and field, this particular conflict has not been as much of a controversy in school psychology as it has been in some other branches of psychology. However, there are clear precedents for this conflict in our field. A good example is the use of individual subtest or item-level analysis of assessment data versus relying on total scores. Some practitioners may find a great deal of intuitive value in the former, whereas psychometric fundamentalists will likely decry such practices as being fraught with unreliability.

   In sum, school psychology is not immune to the tensions that have existed within the field of psychology in general. The two cultures of psychology identified by Kimble (1984) still appear to be distinctive enough to warrant this discussion, and they appear to have some very specific manifestations within school psychology. Again, it is important to recognize that the stress produced by this tension is not a bad thing for school psychology. Not only can it help the field to grow but also can work like a system of checks and balances—advocates at each end of the dimension help to curb possible excesses of the opposite end.

## NASP and APA

No discussion of tensions within the field of school psychology could be complete without an examination of the historic and ongoing tension between NASP and APA that has waxed and waned over the years but has never gone away. This discussion is not provided to inflame any wounds or to promote a particular point of view. Rather, it is considered to be an essential part of the recent history and ongoing development of this dynamic field.

Although there are several historical issues that characterize the conflict, in many ways the tension that has existed between NASP and APA comes down to one overriding issue: disagreement and debate regarding the doctoral versus the specialist level of training. NASP was founded in 1969 for the purpose of providing an organized voice to practicing school psychologists, the vast majority of whom did not have doctoral degrees in psychology. Although the percentage of school psychologists who have earned the doctoral degree has increased slightly over the years, it is still true that the vast majority of school psychologists (currently about 75%) do not have doctoral degrees. APA is the oldest and largest organization of psychologists, and it has attempted to be the advocate and voice of the broad field of psychology in America. NASP, on the other hand, was specifically founded to represent the interests of practicing school psychologists. Because the founding of NASP was brought about in great part by perceptions among many school psychologists that APA was either an ineffective voice for them or was actively ignoring or excluding them, it did not take long for tensions to arise.

The position of APA in the mid- to late 20th century was always implicit in contending that the doctoral degree should be the minimum level for the use of the term "psychologist" or "professional psychologist." Within only 6 years following the founding of NASP, this position was formally codified by APA's 1977 stance that the doctoral degree in psychology is the minimum level of training needed for engagement in independent practice, state board licensing, and use of the term "psychologist." However, the APA position statement and the language of most state psychology licensing boards included a provision for individuals who were trained at the master's or specialist level and were appropriately credentialed by their state department of education to use the term "school psychologist" within the scope of their school-based practice. In other words, the stance of APA and general professional psychology was that one must be a doctoral-level psychologist to receive a board license and to practice independently and call oneself a psychologist, but one could use the term "school psychologist" with less than doctoral-level training providing the work was specifically limited to school settings and conducted under the authority of a state department of education certificate. This statement represents the current APA position.

APA's position has never been accepted by NASP, and it has always been a point of some tension between the two organizations. In fact, NASP has supported the efforts of its state affiliates to promote legislation allowing specialist-level school psychologists to become licensed for independent practice, whereas APA and its state affiliates have continued to oppose such efforts. Although it has waxed and waned over the years, this conflict has always been present and is enormously complicated, especially given that many school psychologists are members of both APA and NASP and support both organizations.

This conflict has been complicated by several developments and issues over the years. Fagan and Wells (2000) noted that the U.S. Department of Education resurrected the jurisdictional conflict between APA and NASP by questioning the designation of two separate accrediting bodies for the same profession. In response, APA and NASP established a joint task force in 1978 (the Inter-Organization Committee, or IOC) to work cooperatively to resolve the conflict. This body established a collaborative pilot effort in 1983 for joint APA and NASP/NCATE accreditation of doctoral programs. However, whereas APA supported this effort, NCATE did not, and joint site visits were discontinued. Even with these tensions, doctoral programs accredited by APA have still been able to automatically qualify for NASP program approval, although the future of this historical cooperative process is still uncertain. One of the interesting questions of the doctoral versus nondoctoral conflict is whether there is any evidence that supports one position over the other. In general, there has not been any such evidence, although a review by Reschly and Wilson (1997) opined that the specialist level of training was not sufficient for the independent practice of school psychology in nonschool settings. In 1988, at the NASP convention in Chicago, one of us (KWM) attended a "town hall meeting" on the doctoral versus nondoctoral issue, moderated by then-NASP president Thomas Fagan. What was striking about this meeting were the large numbers of participants who attended, whose impassioned arguments at the open microphones appeared to surprise even the moderator. Clearly, this issue will not simply go away anytime soon, and some leaders in the field have even acknowledged that it appears to be intractable (Short, 2002).

It is probably simplistic to view the historical and continuing rift between APA and NASP as being exclusively the result of the entry-level-training disagreement. Rather, the tension seems to include differences in the broader culture and worldviews of the two organizations. According to Short (2002), there are distinct cultural differences in how the two organizations perceive school psychology within the broader context of professional psychology, with APA representing a culture of school psychology as part of professional psychology and NASP representing a culture of school psychology as a separate profession. Thus "APA views school psychology as a specialty within American psychology, sharing significant commonalities with other specialties in terms of skills, knowledge, and competencies," whereas NASP asserts "that school psychology is a separate profession from professional psychology" (Short, 2002, p. 111). To an outsider or someone newly initiated to the field, these differences may seem to be trite, even pointless, yet they persist and continue to have ramifications for the development of the field, siphoning off tremendous energy that might otherwise be used to move the practice and science of school psychology forward. In 2002, APA's board of directors voted to withdraw their participation from the APA–NASP Inter-Organizational Committee, based on the conclusion "that the IOC had failed in its mission to gain consensus on important issues" (Clark, 2002, p. 40). It is evident that history is continuing to be written in this arena and that the APA–NASP tension has not yet subsided.

# LEAVING ADOLESCENCE: TOWARD THE MATURATION OF THE FIELD

Some of the most important dates and landmark events in the history of school psychology that have been described in this chapter are detailed in Table 2.1. It is clear that school psychology is a very young field. It has a relatively brief history that is inseparable from the fields of both psychology and American education. If we accept that school psychology is a young field, just how young is it in developmental terms? School psychology is clearly out of the infancy state, having emerged as a distinctive profession with strong voices, major influences, and extensive numbers of professionals. One can also easily make the case that the field has left its childhood, given that we have moved from Fagan's hybrid years to the thoroughbred years. If identity confusion and turmoil are essential components of adolescence, as some influential developmental psychologists have proposed, then it would be hard to argue that school psychology has left ado-

**TABLE 2.1. Some Important Dates and Landmark Events in the History of School Psychology**

| | |
|---|---|
| 1892 | American Psychological Association is founded. |
| 1896 | Lightner Witmer establishes first psychological/child guidance clinic at University of Pennsylvania. |
| 1899 | First school-based psychological clinic is established in Chicago public schools. |
| 1905 | Binet–Simon intelligence scales are published in Paris, France. |
| 1915 | Arnold Gesell of Connecticut becomes first person hired as "school psychologist." |
| 1916 | American/English-language revision of Binet–Simon scales is published by Lewis Terman at Stanford University ("Stanford–Binet"). |
| 1928 | First school psychology training program is established at New York University. |
| 1930 | First book on school psychology, *Psychological Service for School Problems*, is published by Gertrude Hildreth of Columbia University. |
| 1943 | Ohio School Psychologists Association is founded, becomes first state school psychology organization. |
| 1945 | APA is reorganized into divisions, and first national organization for school psychology (APA Division 16) is established. |
| 1954 | Thayer conference, first national school psychology conference, is held in West Point, New York. |
| 1962 | *Journal of School Psychology* is founded, becomes first school psychology journal. |
| 1969 | National Association of School Psychologists is founded at organizational meeting in St. Louis, Missouri. |
| 1971 | PhD program in school psychology at University of Texas at Austin becomes first APA-accredited doctoral program in school psychology. |
| 1975 | Public Law 94-142, Education of All Handicapped Children Act, is enacted by U.S. Congress and takes effect in 1977. |
| 1977 | APA council resolution declares that doctoral degree is required for use of "professional psychologist" title and increases tension with NASP. |
| 1978 | Joint APA–NASP Inter-Organizational Committee is established to work out differences between two organizations. |
| 1988 | NASP begins training program approval process with folio review system and approves first training programs. |
| 1988 | NASP institutes Nationally School Psychology Certification Board and administers first national certification exam; first NCSP certificates are granted in 1989. |
| 1997 | APA grants specialty recognition to school psychology. |
| 2002 | Future of School Psychology Invitational Conference is held in Indianapolis, Indiana. |
| 2002 | APA board of directors votes to withdraw from joint APA–NASP Inter-Organizational Committee. |

lescence. Rather, like the 20- or 30-something young adult "twixter" who continues to live in his or her parents' basement and is not quite ready to take on the full responsibilities of adult life, our field appears to be in a delayed or extended period of adolescence. Adulthood and full maturity appear to be just around the corner and even in sight, but the field still seems hesitant or unsure regarding making the next steps to get there.

The Spanish philosopher and poet George Santayana is credited with making the statement "those who forget the past are doomed to repeat it." Our foray into school psychology's brief history in this chapter might well be concluded by considering the accomplishments and disappointments of the field to date and pondering when it will take leave of the basement of postadolescence and move into maturity. We believe that a "paradigm shift" is taking place in the field (Reschly & Ysseldyke, 2002) and that the past is not necessarily the future. However, the past is important, even critical, to our current understanding of the field. We have provided a background in this chapter that we hope the reader will not forget within the context of the road map that subsequent chapters present regarding moving the field forward.

## DISCUSSION QUESTIONS AND ACTIVITIES

1. Go to the "Today in the History of Psychology" website at www.cwu.edu/~warren/today.html and use the search engine to locate important historical events in the chronology of psychology that occurred on your birthday (day and month). Are any of the events you identified specifically relevant to the history of school psychology?

2. Select an individual who played a prominent role in the history of school psychology and write or present a brief overview of his or her life and accomplishments.

3. For those who have recently entered a graduate program in school psychology, what were the features of this field that attracted your interest? Why did you choose to train for a career in school psychology rather than other professional fields of psychology (clinical or counseling psychology) or related educational or mental health fields (such as school counseling, social work, or teaching)?

4. The history of school psychology has clearly been tied to the role of gatekeeper or sorter and to the work of psychoeducational assessment. What are your views regarding the opportunities, risks, and barriers to moving school psychologists into broader roles that reduce substantially the amount of time spent conducting individual psychoeducational assessments?

5. The ongoing conflict between the sometimes opposing views and values represented by APA and NASP has clearly taken up a tremendous amount of time, talent, and energy that might otherwise be used to move the field forward in other ways. How do you view this cultural tension, and what do you think it will take for the field to settle these concerns and rise above them?

# 3

# The Changing Face of School Psychology

RESPONDING EFFECTIVELY TO CULTURAL
AND LINGUISTIC DIVERSITY

with ELSA ARROYOS-JURADO

The title of this chapter recognizes the importance of including a discussion of issues related to cultural and linguistic diversity. As the field of school psychology continues to establish a professional identity, it does so in the face of an ever-changing population of children, adolescents, and their families and of the consequent responsibility to meet their educational and mental health needs. The United States is currently experiencing rapid and unprecedented changes in the demographic makeup of its population. Ethnic groups that have historically been in the minority of the population are quickly becoming a majority. In addition, although the United States has historically been a linguistically diverse society, it is also experiencing a new and powerful influx of persons whose native languages are not English (U.S. Bureau of the Census, 1998). These demographic shifts are being reflected in our school systems, and this diversification of the student body clearly affects the delivery of school psychological services.

In this chapter, we provide an introductory discussion of the relevant issues and concepts related to cultural and linguistic diversity and related implications for school psychology practice. The chapter begins with a brief overview of the demographic shifts and changes that are occurring in the United States, highlighting the implications of these changes for the field of school psychology. With this change in the population it is inevitable that "differences" will become more pronounced. However, in order to

**Elsa Arroyos-Jurado, PhD,** is an assistant professor in the Department of Counseling and Educational Psychology at New Mexico State University, Las Cruces, New Mexico.

avoid the pitfall of equating differences with stereotypes, a discussion of within-group and between-group differences is included. The need to recruit and retain school psychologists from diverse backgrounds is highlighted as a significant challenge facing the field, given the ever-changing student population and the need to provide culturally responsive school psychological services. In addition, some key concepts and issues related to cultural and linguistic diversity in general are provided to highlight the important variables that school psychologists need to consider in their work with diverse groups and/or individuals. This chapter includes a brief overview of the components of culturally competent or culturally effective school psychology practice, as well as a discussion of the issue of minority overrepresentation in special education programs. Finally, the chapter concludes with an introduction to the data-driven problem-solving model that we promote throughout this volume and a discussion of why this approach may be particularly beneficial in helping school psychologists to reduce bias in their practice and to better aid children and their families without regard to their cultural and linguistic background.

## DEMOGRAPHIC TRENDS: THE CHANGING LINGUISTIC, ETHNIC, AND CULTURAL LANDSCAPE

Although the United States has been a multicultural and multilingual nation since its inception, recent trends indicate substantial diversification of its demographic makeup. In 1992, it was estimated that by the year 2050 the Latino population would become the largest minority group in the United States (Pratt & Rittenhouse, 1998; U.S. Bureau of the Census, 1992) and that individuals from an Anglo/European heritage would constitute no more than 50% of the U.S. population (U.S. Bureau of the Census, 1998). This recent substantial increase in diversity of the U.S. population has been driven by the influx of individuals of color (non-Caucasian) whose native languages are not English at rates that have not previously been experienced in this nation (U.S. Bureau of the Census, 1998). Data from the 2000 census confirm these trends and show that Latinos currently make up the largest non-European ethnic group in the United States, exceeding those individuals who identify as African American or black (U.S. Bureau of the Census, 2002). Currently, Latinos make up approximately 12.5% of the population, whereas African American/blacks, Asian American/Pacific Islanders, and American Indian/Alaskan Natives make up about 12.3%, 3.6%, and 0.9% of the population, respectively. Furthermore, 17.9% of the U.S. population speaks a language other than English, and 11% of individuals in the United States are foreign born (U.S. Bureau of the Census, 2002).

These demographic trends are also being paralleled in our school systems. Thus there is a tremendous and unprecedented need for school psychologists to develop more culturally competent and responsive practices. In general, our schools are even more diverse than the U.S. population as a whole, largely because of demographic characteristics previously discussed and due to birthrates across ethnic groups. For example, recent immigrants to the United States are more likely to be younger than the U.S. population in general, and some of the ethnic minority groups in the United States have higher birthrates than the U.S. population in general. Thus we are more likely to see an even more diverse population in our public schools than in other avenues of life. According to the U.S. Department of Education (2000), 53 million students are entering public and private elementary and secondary schools in the United States (as cited in

Meece & Kurtz-Costes, 2001). Approximately 27% of the U.S. population is under 18 years of age, and racial and intragroup diversity in this segment of the population is even more pronounced than in the general population.

The field of school psychology has not been blind to these expansive demographic shifts. Many writers in our field have clearly recognized the need to employ more culturally responsive practices in an increasingly diverse society (e.g., Gopaul-McNicol, 1997; Halsell, 2002; Ortiz & Flanagan, 2002; Ysseldyke et al., 1997). With these changes in demographics comes a diversity of experiences from the increasingly diverse groups and the individuals within the population. These individuals bring with them a multitude of cultural and linguistic experiences that add richness to our population and that need to be recognized and valued in our schools and by society as a whole.

# BEYOND STEREOTYPES: WITHIN-GROUP AND BETWEEN-GROUP DIFFERENCES

The rapid changes occurring in the linguistic, cultural, and ethnic makeup of the U.S. population accentuate the differences that make these groups diverse in the first place. Although we need to recognize these differences in our work as school psychologists, we also must be careful not to equate these differences with stereotypical descriptions and/or expectations for individuals from diverse groups. That is, there is a fine line between acknowledging differences and interpreting these differences in stereotypical fashion. It is critical to understand the role that within-group and between-group differences play in working with culturally and linguistically diverse individuals.

## Stereotypes

Humans have a natural inclination to socially categorize individuals based on some salient feature such as age, gender, race, ethnicity, socioeconomic status, and so forth. There is a purpose to socially categorizing, or stereotyping, individuals, as the case may be, in that it serves as a means of simplifying a complex social world. However, in doing so, we run the risk of minimizing or even erasing the individuality of people, including what makes them different, if we stereotype their identity and behavior based solely on their group membership.

By way of definition, the action of stereotyping is to categorize people based on an artificial construction (i.e., a fixed or conventional notion or conception) of a certain group that is designed to impart the "essence" of that group and that blends the group, erasing individuality and difference (Neufeldt, 1989). By engaging in stereotyping we are in essence engaging in a form of prejudicial behavior. Although stereotyping may sometimes be benign, it may also lead to discrimination against groups to which one does not belong in favor of one's own group. Furthermore, one runs the risk of overstating differences between groups or highlighting the similarities between self and other members of one's own group. Finally, stereotypes can serve as a means to "justify" the behavior of individuals from a particular group, which can further eradicate the individuality of the individual by reinforcing a "they're all alike" attitude or perception. Stereotypes may also lead to the development of certain expectations about an individual's abilities, behaviors, and so forth that can lead to interpreting subsequent behavior(s) in a manner that "fits" expectation for a person from "that" group. As practitioners working with the general public (i.e., schools and their associated members) it becomes our responsibility to acknowledge differences but in a manner that does not alienate or harm individuals. This is a challenging responsibility. It requires a conscious effort to overcome one's own stereotypic expectations and not to rely on general stereotypes as professional judgments are formed.

## Within- and between-Group Differences

To move beyond stereotypic representations of individuals from various cultural and linguistic groups, we must understand the implications or relevance of within- and between-group differences. Individual differences obviously refer to how individuals differ from one another in some aspect, whereas group differences refer to how individuals from one group typically differ from those of another group. In understanding individual and group differences, there are two important considerations: (1) there is significant variability *within* any one group and (2) there is always significant overlap *between* groups (Merrell, 2003). Given these facts, it becomes essential for professionals to be careful not to draw undue inferences about students' characteristics, abilities, behaviors, and so forth simply on the basis of their group membership (e.g., gender, ethnic background, and/or cultural background). Furthermore, in understanding the overlap between groups it is crucial to consider that the typical differences between groups do not necessarily apply to individual members of those groups. In other words, although there may be characteristics that describe a group as a whole (e.g., whether a group is individualistic or collectivistic), the characteristic does not automatically get ascribed to *all* individuals within the group (e.g., not all Latinos or Latinas are collectivistic).

By understanding that individuals from the same group are not necessarily alike in every respect and that there may be similarities across different groups, we become less prone to making stereotypical interpretation of individuals. It comes down to understanding our clientele on an individual, case-by-case basis. We are not suggesting that you need not take into account individuals' group memberships; on the contrary, it is still crucial to understand their group memberships and the role these played in their personal development. However, at the same time you still need to acknowledge your clients' individuality by taking into account factors other than their group memberships. For example, many school psychologists may be prone to automatically using nonverbal assessment methods for students whose native language is not English and/or who are considered bilingual. However, one must also consider other variables, such as the student's generational status, level of acculturation, and so forth. It may be appropriate to use traditional tests such as standardized ability and achievement tests that have been normed primarily on individuals from the dominant (Anglo) culture with a Latino student, for example, who was born and raised in the United States, is highly acculturated, and is fluent in English and Spanish (and prefers English). What is especially important is to understand the individual as both a part of his or her own ethnic/cultural group and family group, as well as part of society at large, and to understand what the intermingling has been or continues to be between them. There are many factors that may distinguish individuals from their cultural groups and from mainstream culture, as well as other factors that make them similar to those from their cultural group and mainstream society. It is the responsibility of multiculturally competent and effective school psychologists to evaluate these factors in the most culturally sensitive manner possible

## ETHNIC MINORITY UNDERREPRESENTATION AMONG THE RANKS OF SCHOOL PSYCHOLOGISTS: A MAJOR CHALLENGE FOR THE FIELD

Professionals in our field have long recognized the disparity in numbers of culturally and linguistically diverse (CLD) school psychologists to serve the needs of students in ever-changing school settings. Reschly (2000) noted that CLD school psychologists have historically been vastly underrepresented in the field. In a recent survey of practicing school psychologists (Curtis, Hunley, & Grier, 2004; Curtis, Hunley, Walker, & Baker, 1999), it was found that school psychologists of color represented only 5.5% of the field (1.1% African American, 1.7% Hispanic, 0.9% Asian/Pacific Islander, and 0.7% Native American/Alaskan), and only 9.7% (1 out of 10) reported fluency in a language other than English. Furthermore, if we consider other characteristics that "match" the clientele we serve, only 2.6% reported having a disability. Clearly, these figures indicate that the demographic makeup of professionals in school psychology is much different from that of the population that is served by school psychologists (Fagan, 2002). In addition, when considering that more than 70% of school psychologists are women, yet boys are disproportionately more likely to be recipients of special education and other remedial educational services, the demographic disparity between school psychologists and the children we serve is even more striking.

Based on a recent survey of members of NASP (2003a), there is additional support for the notion that practicing school psychologists do not reflect the diversity of the U.S. population in general. The ethnic breakdown from this survey was as follows: 91% white, 1.7% Hispanic/Latino, 2.4% black/African American, 1.1% Asian American/Pacific Islander, and 0.6% American Indian/Alaskan Native. With regards to linguistic diversity, this survey indicated that 612 school psychologists who are members of NASP speak at least one foreign language, with 97 school psychologists speaking more than two languages (NASP, 2003a). The face of school psychology is predominately white, middle class, and female and is expected to become more so in the next few decades (Curtis et al., 1999; Hosp & Reschly, 2002).

According to Reschly (2000), some studies indicate that minority representation in graduate programs and faculty has increased during the past decade (1990–2000); however, because this increase in minority representation has not kept pace with the demographic changes of the U.S. population in general, the makeup of the field will still remain overwhelmingly European American for the next decade. There is no denying that many of these white, middle-class females are committed to working with issues of diversity and becoming more informed about best practices with a diverse student population, but there is still the possibility of a cultural mismatch between them and individuals from CLD backgrounds (Reschly, 2000).

Reschly (2000) sums up the current (and future) status of the field with the following statement:

> There is reason to believe that school psychology is becoming more ethnically diverse; however, the pace of change is not sufficient to improve markedly the current imbalance in the characteristics of school psychologists and the populations they serve. . . . School psychologists can expect to be challenged in the next decade and beyond by issues relating to disproportionate minority representation, valid and culturally sensitive assessment and interventions, and improved outcomes for all children. (p. 519)

Other professionals in the field also refer to the importance of a paradigm shift in order to meet the new demands of a changing population. For example, Sheridan and

Gutkin (2000) reiterated the importance of making necessary changes to the field, via a paradigm shift, to meet the needs of the populations we serve:

> School psychology must be reflective of, responsive to, and proactive toward the multiple and changing systems within which we operate (e.g., school, family, societal, legislative systems) including the increasingly diverse populations whom we serve (e.g., children, families, educators, administrators, community leaders) and the settings in which they function (e.g., homes, schools, agencies, hospital). (p. 489)

One way in which the field of school psychology can be "reflective of, responsive to, and proactive toward" the changing systems in which we work is through the recruitment and retention of culturally and linguistically diverse school psychologists at all levels—from practitioners to administrators to trainers. These individuals would not only become valuable new assets to the field, but they would also facilitate and reinforce work already being done regarding culturally responsive service delivery (Curtis et al., 1999). NASP, along with many leaders in the field, has already taken on this challenge to recruit and retain more CLD school psychologists. Although the ultimate outcome of such efforts is yet to be seen, these steps are crucial if the field of school psychology is to make progress in the arena of cultural and linguistic diversity.

To better serve our youths and meet their mental health and educational needs, NASP has recognized the need to "actively increase" the number of culturally and linguistically diverse school psychologists to work with these students. Furthermore, the organization also sees the need to recruit and retain culturally and linguistically diverse trainers in school psychology programs. In its current position statement regarding this issue, NASP delineates its recruitment and retention efforts that are being put into place to meet to meet their goal of remedying the "disproportionately few culturally and linguistically diverse school psychologists available to serve regular education and special education students" (NASP, 2003b). Other efforts include the NASP-minority scholarship program, as well as instituting the Multicultural Affairs Committee and the presidential initiative of the Minority Recruitment and Retention Task Force, both of which have the goal of increasing the number of CLD school psychologists at all levels in the field.

These efforts are similar to those put forth by other governing bodies, such as the APA and its Division 16. As a major organization in the field of psychology, APA has committed itself through many efforts to increase the number of culturally and linguistically diverse trainers and practitioners in the field of psychology, as well as to enhance services to diverse populations. For example, APA has put out *Guidelines on Multicultural Education, Training, Research, Practice, and Organizational Change for Psychologists* (APA, 2002c) and *Guidelines for Providers of Psychological Services to Ethnic, Linguistic, and Culturally Diverse Populations* (APA, 1990). APA also established the Office of Ethnic Minority Affairs (OEMA) in 1979, which, among its many efforts, also seeks to promote recruitment, retention, and training opportunities for ethnically diverse individuals in psychology. Other APA organizational initiatives in this area include the Committee on Ethnic Minority Affairs, the Commission on Ethnic Minority Recruitment, Retention, and Training in Psychology Task Force, and the Council of National Psychological Associations for the Advancement of Ethnic Minority Interests. Finally, Division 16 also supports recruitment and retention efforts, as is indicated in the objective of the division to "encourage opportunities for the ethnic minority participation in the specialty [of school psychology]" (www.indiana.edu/~div16/G&O.htm). More recently, NASP and Division 16 of APA have joined forces to develop a joint position article that addresses the overall shortage of school psychologists in the field by drafting guidelines for professional psychologists trained with a clinical or counseling psychology focus to "respecialize" in school psychology (Tharinger & Palomares, 2004). It is unclear whether this effort will result in more diversity within school psychology, but it may help somewhat in alleviating overall personnel shortages. It is important to appreciate that these efforts to diversify the ranks of professionals in the field require a shift in thinking about diversity and approaches to working in diverse school and learning environments.

## KEY CONCEPTS AND ISSUES IN CULTURAL AND LINGUISTIC DIVERSITY

Although there is currently a call to increase the number of culturally and linguistically diverse school psychologists in the field to help serve an even more diverse student population, it may take many, many years for the field to meet this goal. However, it must also be acknowledged that increasing the number of CLD school psychologists in the field is only one means of increasing cultural responsiveness of practitioners in the field. We must recognize that *all* school psychologists need to be aware of key issues in working with culturally and linguistically diverse clientele. Stated simply, we cannot assume that the challenge of responding effectively to increasing cultural and linguistic diversity of students and families in our schools will be met by enhanced recruitment and retention of diverse professionals within the field. Rather, it is incumbent on all school psychologists to enhance their own multicultural competence or effectiveness.

One starting point is in how we define *culture*. We would agree with other professionals in the field who call for consideration of diversity from a broad perspective as part of the need for school psychologists to change their role to meet the demands of the new millennium (Bradley-Johnson & Dean, 2000). For example, Bradley-Johnson and Dean (2000) concur with other professionals in the field (e.g., Nastasi, Varjas, Sarkar, & Jayasena, 1998) that "culture" should be more broadly defined to include place of residence (urban vs. rural), geographic location (native vs. international), age, gender, socioeconomic status, sexual orientation, and specific family traditions, along with the more limited definition of culture as race and ethnicity. A "broader" definition of culture would compel practitioners to take account of many more factors that could be potential contributors to current functioning that would not have otherwise been considered if the focus had simply been on race or ethnicity. The drawback on focusing exclusively on the latter could be an overinterpretation of characteristics based on race or ethnicity alone to the exclusion of other important factors.

Second, there is also a need to consider other moderating variables in working with culturally and linguistically diverse individuals. Moderator variables such as *acculturation*, *worldview*, and *identity* (Dana, 1993) differentiate and help to deepen understanding of within-group and between-group differences and similarities in theory and research (Vázquez, 1997). By taking moderator variables into account in your work with culturally and linguistically diverse individuals, you are better able to obtain a more reliable estimate of the potential contribution of cultural variance in your evaluation procedures (Dana, 1993). Acculturation, worldview, and identity are discussed briefly in this section.

## Acculturation

Acculturation is the process of psychological change in values, beliefs, and behaviors when adapting to a new culture (Takushi & Uomoto, 2001). With school populations increasing in diversity, this process is an important issue that warrants consideration. School psychologists need to be aware of this process and to interpret students' behavior in light of it so as not to assume that a particular response is necessarily associated with a learning disability, emotional disability, or other form of within-person pathology. It may be the case that the students' behavioral responses may be associated with the process of acculturation or adaptation to a new cultural environment such as the school. It may also be true that individuals who are less acculturated into the dominant culture—those who have more of a traditional cultural orientation—are more likely to function in ways that are more consistent with some of the known generalizations regarding their particular ethnic or cultural minority group. Competent evaluation of culturally and linguistically diverse individuals needs to account for the contribution of culture; therefore, it is necessary to know to what level the person has acculturated to an environment. Many acculturation instruments have been developed to assist school psychologists in evaluating this construct with their clientele.

However, as with many constructs in psychology, there is no single measurement model of acculturation. These acculturation measurement models consist of conceptualizing acculturation along a single unilinear continuum (e.g., Berry & Annis, 1974) or using a bilinear model (e.g., Szapocznik & Kurtines, 1980; Szapocznik, Kurtines, & Fernandez, 1980) and can further be classified as based on a single or on multiple cultures (i.e., monocultural or dual-cultural; Kim & Abreu, 2001). Kim and Abreu (2001) recently conducted a search of acculturation instruments and found 33 instruments for use with either African Americans, Asian Americans, Hispanic Americans, Native Americans, or Native Hawaiians and 1 instrument for all ethnic minority groups (p. 399). Acculturation scales for Hispanic populations by far are the most developed, which is not surprising given the rapid growth of this segment of the population. In addition, many acculturation scales had initially been developed on the adult population, but more recently a focus on children and, in particular, adolescents has been noted.

Rhodes, Ochoa, and Ortiz (2005) suggest using interviews and observations in addition to the questionnaire/survey method of assessment, to assess level of acculturation. Using an interview helps you to determine or judge the level of acculturation (i.e., distance between individual's own acculturation and that of the mainstream culture). In addition, observation as a tool for assessing acculturation allows you to observe patterns of preference, identification, participation, and affiliation with mainstream culture, as well as language preference, manner/style of dress, celebration of holidays, and explicit expressions of cultural knowledge. Although some methods may be better (i.e., interviews and surveys) than others (observations) for assessing acculturation, what is most important is that acculturation level is assessed in the first place. Another variable to consider besides level of acculturation is the stress that can be directly associated with it.

The process of acculturation itself can be a stressful encounter for individuals. The effect of experiencing what has been termed "acculturative stress" may lead to certain problems, such as anxiety, depression, marginality and alienation, or identity confusion (e.g., Williams & Berry, 1991). Therefore, it is critical as part of our work with culturally diverse individuals that we take the process of acculturation and possible stressors associated with it into account in order to best meet the needs of these individuals.

## Worldview

Another important moderator variable is *worldview*. The concept of worldview has been defined as *people's insight regarding their culture and individuality* (Sue & Sue, 1999), or how they perceive the world given their own experiences, culture, and so forth. People's beliefs and assumptions are rooted in their worldview (Takushi & Uomoto, 2001). Furthermore, worldview encompasses group identity, individual identity, beliefs, values, and language. It influences all perceptions, including what and how we learn. Thus culture and worldview can have an impact on how individuals perform on evaluative procedures and on their communication style (e.g., verbal and nonverbal behaviors). It is also critical for school psychologists to be aware of their own worldviews and subsequent beliefs and assumptions, as they may differ significantly from those of their clientele. Many times school psychologists acknowledge the importance of taking cultural diversity into account in their work but do little to put aside or even examine their own cultural assumptions, values, and beliefs to consider how their clients might view the world differently than they do (e.g., Savage, Prout, & Chard, 2004).

Many of the practices in school psychology, as well as the systems in which school psychologists work, adhere to a "Western" worldview. The Western worldview can be described as being influenced by Judeo-Christianity and "concerned with individualism, autonomy, and the need to control and survive" (Ibraham, Roysircar-Sodowsky, & Ohnishi, 2001, p. 441). Because of the pervasive influence of this worldview in American society, there is often a general expectation that all students need to adhere to it in order to function and/or succeed in a society that also adheres to a Western worldview. But are we doing more harm than good by expecting certain groups of students to put aside their beliefs and assumptions in order to stay within the status quo? This is a difficult question.

Because worldview encompasses an individual's group and individual identities, beliefs, values, and even language(s) used, it directly influences his or her perceptions, including what and how he or she learns. Thus it follows that it is important to take an individual's worldview into account because it can have a significant impact on a student's performance in a classroom. Expecting students to adopt a Western worldview is in some ways an unfortunate practice given that students' worldviews are directly related to their cultural and ethnic identities (i.e., a shared cultural heritage, social relatedness, and cultural ties; Sodowsky, Kwan, & Pannu, 1995); ethnic identity has also been identified as an important moderator variable. What message are we sending to these students about the value of their own culture or ethnicity? Unfortunately, perhaps the message that is being received by many students is that they are not valued. If this is indeed how this message is being received, then perhaps the implication of that is a self-fulfilling prophecy related to poor academic and social performance at school.

To become culturally responsive, competent, and effective, all practitioners need to start with an exploration of their own cultural beliefs and assumptions, as well as to understand how their worldviews may differ from those of their clients, to assure that this "difference" will not interfere with meeting the needs of the student. It is also critical that practitioners be aware of their own ethnic identity development to best serve their diverse clientele.

## Identity

Being aware of where a student is regarding his or her identity development will give a school psychologist a better indication of that student's cultural background and characteristics, as well as his or her perspective on how he or she will approach the world. It is through acknowledgement of a student's identity that a school psychologist can avoid stereotyping students or approaching students in a stereotypical manner. It is through understanding identity development that school psychologists can learn about and appreciate the experience of their culturally and ethnically diverse clientele. As a result of much research, several models of racial and ethnic identity development have been developed. This section highlights some of the prominent models and/or experts in this area.

Cross (1971, as cited in Atkinson, Morten, & Sue, 1998) was one of the first individuals to develop the idea of the racial identity model (Negro-to-Black Convergence Experience) that dealt with the issues of racial oppression and African Americans' identity development in relation to it. Cross's models addressed the notion that individuals have varying racial and cultural levels of identity, which allowed service providers to clearly identify the client's level of racial identity and encouraged them to be culturally competent in order to provide effective services. Because of this positive influence (i.e., service providers' consideration of racial/cultural variables), Cross's models had a profound impact on the profession of psychology. Many identity development models designed for various ethnic groups were patterned after Cross's original models (e.g., Atkinson et al., 1998; Sue & Sue, 1999).

Cross's model (1971, 1972; Hall, Cross, & Freedle, 1972, 1995, as cited in Sue & Sue, 1999) outlined four stages of black identity development: *preencounter, encounter, immersion–emersion*, and *internalization*. Individuals move from a white frame of reference to a positive black frame of reference as illustrated by the *preencounter* stage, in which a person consciously or unconsciously diminishes his or her "blackness," to a sense of inner security as conflicts between "old" and "new" identities are resolved during *internalization* (Sue & Sue, 1999). In sum, "global anti-White feelings subside as the person becomes more flexible, more tolerant, and more bicultural/multicultural" (Sue & Sue, 1999, p. 124).

Atkinson, Morten, and Sue (1998) developed a five-stage minority identity development model. Unlike Cross's model, this model is based on the assumption that all minority groups experience the common force of oppression and that, as a result, all will generate attitudes and behaviors consistent with a natural internal struggle to develop a strong sense of self- and group identity. These authors conceptualized their model as a continuous process in which the stages blend into one another without clear or abrupt separation: *conformity, dissonance, resistance and immersion, introspection*, and *synergetic articulation and awareness*. A person's development follows from a preference for dominant cultural values (*conformity*) to a sense of self-fulfillment regarding his or her ethnic identity (*synergetic articulation and awareness*). This model again has implications for the school psychologist in understanding the impact of cultural experiences on a person's behavior.

D. W. Sue and D. Sue (1990, as cited in Sue & Sue. 1999) elaborated on this model and developed the racial/cultural identity development model (R/CID). Like the previous model, it includes five stages of development that "oppressed people experience as they struggle to understand themselves in terms of their own culture, the dominant culture, and the oppressive relationship between the two cultures: conformity, dissonance, resistance and immersion, introspection, and integrative awareness" (Sue & Sue, 1999). The authors further delineate attitudes and beliefs at each stage of development that help service providers understand their clients more thoroughly. These attitudes and beliefs relate to how the client views himself or herself, others of the same ethnicity, others of differing minority ethnicity, and those from the majority culture.

In summary, the commonality across these ethnic identity development models is the importance of outlining the cultural experience of individuals from minority backgrounds. That is, in order to provide proper services to individuals from culturally diverse backgrounds, school psychologists need to understand their clients' and their own ethnic identities.

# MODELS FOR BEST PRACTICE IN SCHOOL PSYCHOLOGY SERVICE DELIVERY

## Assessment

One of the first things that comes to mind when someone mentions what a school psychologist does is that they are assessment experts. We do advocate that school psychologists should be prepared and expected to provide a broad range of important services, including assessment; however, despite continuing professional efforts to promote role expansion, the primary function of the practitioner in school psychology has traditionally been that of psychoeducational evaluator or "sorter" (Fagan & Wise, 2000). There is no denying that assessment plays a large role in defining what school psychologists do, but it is important to understand that we are not limited to being solely diagnosticians. As assessment experts, we are required to make informed decisions regarding our choice of evaluation procedures with any student or group we are assessing. In particular, we need to attend to the various cultural, ethnic, and linguistic variables that influence the evaluations that we complete. Not only is it best practice to consider cultural, ethnic, and linguistic variables in assessment, but it is also mandated by the IDEA, as well as by NASP and APA, all of which make reference to the need to assess these factors. Yet many school psychologists do not receive adequate training in this area (Ochoa, Rivera, & Ford, 1997; Padilla, 2001).

### Nondiscriminatory Assessment

A long line of research in the field of psychology and assessment has shown many tests to be biased against individuals from minority (racial and ethnic) backgrounds. As such, there has been a significant push to develop assessment procedures and tests, in particular, that are "culturally sensitive," "culture reduced," and/or "culture free." However, it has been argued that it is impossible to eliminate the influence of culture (Ortiz, 2003), as it is a multifaceted, multidimensional construct that is too complex to be able to completely account for in our evaluations. Thus many researchers in the field argue not only for the development of assessment instruments that take into account issues of culture and diversity but also that evaluation is a process that we strive to make as "nondiscriminatory" as possible (Ortiz, 2003). Ortiz (2003) suggests that nondiscriminatory assessment is a process that guarantees that every individual is evaluated in the least discriminatory manner possible, rather than just the search for "the" best unbiased test. He further contends that this process is applicable to all individuals, not just those who are "different" in some way or are from a minority cultural background.

Another prominent researcher in the field, Padilla (2001), argued that assessment of psychological variables is made culturally sensitive through a "continuing and open-ended series of substantive and methodological insertions and adaptations [e.g., development of instruments, administration, to interpretation] designed to mesh the process of assessment and evaluation with the cultural characteristics of the group being studied" (p. 6). So it is not sufficient solely to incorporate instruments that have been designed by considering cultural variables; we must also engage in a "process" that leads to evaluations being culturally responsive to our clients. Padilla (2001) advocates for a paradigm shift in which evaluation takes into account the unique value of specific ethnic groups, which in turn does not necessitate comparison with other groups, especially if the comparison is likely to be biased.

When it comes to nondiscriminatory assessment of culturally and linguistically diverse students, there are no clear-cut formulas for what to do (i.e., a "use this test with this student" type approach). Rather, one has to consider each case individually, while keeping cultural, ethnic, and linguistic factors in mind, to develop a hypothesis regarding that individual's functioning. Therefore, the goal is to develop and follow strategies that can be implemented with any student; as such, general guidelines have been developed to help accomplish just this. For example, Ortiz (2003) offered a comprehensive framework for nondiscriminatory assessment that includes the following components: assessing and evaluating the learning ecology (i.e., extrinsic cause of learning difficulties); opportunity for learning; educationally relevant cultural and linguistic factors (e.g., exposure to different cultures and languages); evaluating, revising, and retesting hypotheses (i.e., to reduce making incorrect inferences about assessment data based on preconceived notions); determining the need for and language(s) of assessment; reducing bias in traditional testing practices (i.e., either administering tests in a standardized way and attempting to evaluate results in a nondiscriminatory manner or modifying testing in way that is less discriminatory initially); utilizing authentic and alternative assessment procedures; evaluating and interpreting all data within the context of the learning ecology; and linking assessment to intervention. Although this model provides a very thorough assessment of cultural factors, one must still consider the application of this model on a case-by-case basis.

## Assessing Language

Aside from the assessment of cultural variables such as acculturation, worldview, and ethnic identity, a school psychologist also must be competent in assessing language and language proficiency. However, before the actual assessment process begins, a school psychologist needs to have fundamental knowledge regarding language proficiency and development. Oftentimes, what is deemed abnormal or a language deficit is actually a natural consequence of developing two languages simultaneously or acquiring a second language. During second-language acquisition, children may go through some learning processes such as *code switching* (i.e., mixing languages), *interference* (i.e., having one language interfere with the other, such as when a child has to translate from one language to the other cognitively), and *silent periods* that could be perceived as deficits (Rhodes et al., 2005). These are normal processes and should not be taken as signs of language delays or disorders. Frequently, some behaviors of bilingual students or second-language learners are interpreted as being similar to those of children with learning disabilities: being withdrawn, distractible, moving more during English class, hesitating to speak, making mistakes in verbal or written English due to use of L1 (first language) phonetic system, difficulty in math because of limited vocabulary in English, and making similar mistakes in reading, such as losing his or her place, making substitutions, repeating words, and so forth. However, it is critical to assess where a student is with regard to language development and proficiency to better inform your practice as a school psychologist.

Cummins's (1984) work is central to understanding development of language proficiency. He has suggested that it takes 2–3 years to develop basic interpersonal communication skills (BICS), or what is equated with "social" language, whereas it may take 5–7 years for acquirement of cognitive academic language proficiency (CALP), or the language of "school" (i.e., that which facilitates academic success). BICS and CALP help us understand why a student learning a second language is able to converse in the second language much sooner than he or she succeeds with written and oral language related to schoolwork and learning in academic areas. Thus oral language proficiency can be deceiving, because a student may appear to be very fluent in a social context (Yansen & Shulman, 1996) but may be challenged in other facets.

Language proficiency has typically been measured on a continuum from nonspeaker of a language to a fluent speaker (Yansen & Shulman, 1996). According to Yansen and Shulman (1996), language proficiency can be classified under five levels of proficiency: level 1, nonspeaker; level 2, very limited speaker; level 3, limited speaker; level 4, functional speaker, and level 5, fluent speaker. In addition to assessing language development and proficiency, it is equally important to assess language dominance. A school psychologist can use a home language survey (Ortiz, 1992, as cited in Yansen & Shulman, 1996) to assess information regarding language use patterns, language first learned, and language preference. Yansen and Shulman (1996) recommend an additional method of using story narration stemming from picture or book prompts that helps give an indication of a student's capacity for self-expression in both languages. More formal methods of assessments that have been used include the Language Assessment Scales (De Avila & Duncan, 2005), the Bilingual Syntax Measure (Burt, Dulay, & Hernandez-Chavez, 1976), the Bilingual Verbal Abilities Test (Cummins, Muñoz-Sandoval, Alvarado, & Ruef, 1998), and La Batería Woodcock–Muñoz–Revised (Woodcock & Muñoz-Sandoval, 1995; New Mexico Department of Education, 2001). Again, method of choice will be dependent on several factors, including the referral question and other sources of information related to language development and proficiency

### Use of an Interpreter

Another consideration for school psychologists is whether to use an interpreter during evaluation procedures or for other facets of school psychological services. However, using an interpreter takes serious consideration, given the complexity inherent in bringing in an additional person to serve as an intermediary. Not only must the interpreter be competent in interpretation, but also the school psychologist must be competent in working with interpreters. Castle (1984; as cited in Lopez, 2003) outlined several competencies for interpreters: They must have high levels of language proficiency in the source and target languages, knowledge of cultural backgrounds of those they are translating for, and knowledge and skills in the different types of translation styles; they must conduct themselves professionally and ethically (including adherence to confidentiality); and they must be excellent listeners with great memories. Additionally, effective interpreters must understand the context in which translation takes place (e.g., school) and the developmental and psychological principles and issues, especially when working with children and families (Lopez, 2003). Figueroa, Sandoval, and Merino (1984; as cited in Lopez, 2003) further delineated competencies for school psychologists: cross-cultural awareness, skills in nondiscriminatory assessment, knowledge of language development and second-language acquisition, and knowledge of interventions appropriate for second-language learners. In addition, school psychologists must be able to establish rapport with students and families, to interview, to conduct meetings, and so forth, *through* an interpreter (Lopez, 2003). If you do not have a bilingual school psychologist at your disposal—which would be the first step—then you need to be able to train an individual to interpret. In using an interpreter, various potential problems can arise, and one must be able to anticipate issues such as the interpreter's lack of "psychological" knowledge or his or her attitudes and beliefs that may interfere with the process (Vázquez, 2003). In sum, the use of interpreters in school psychology practice—particularly in assessment—is an extremely complex matter that has only recently begun to receive the detailed attention it requires.

## Consultation

Another area of focus for service provision by school psychologists is consultation. Consultation is an indirect service delivery model emphasizing prevention and problem solving of student issues. School consultation is a critical component of our work as school psychologists. It is highly likely that we will engage in consultative work, whether in schools or other educational and mental health settings. In schools, consultation involves interaction between school personnel (including school psychologists) and families in conferring and collaborating as a team to identify the needs of students (Dettmer, Dyck, & Thurston, 2002). Furthermore, school consultants aid in the implementation, evaluation, and revision of educational programs that have been designed to serve the learning and behavioral needs of the students they serve. As such, the role of the consultant is important in providing not only an indirect service to the students we serve but also a direct service to those we consult with (e.g., teachers, administrators, counselors).

Recently attention has been given to further understanding and explicitly outlining the need to incorporate multicultural variables into the consultation framework (e.g., Ingraham, 2000; Rogers, 2000; Sheridan, 2000). Ingraham (2000, p. 323) stated that there is a need for a conceptual framework for multicultural school consultation that "considers diversity issues in the structures, processes, context, and their interactions for practice." Ingraham suggested that a multicultural framework for consultation is needed that incorporates diversity in its broadest form, that focuses on all individuals involved in consultation (and their interrelationships), that takes into account the cultural context of consultation, that considers issues and constructs resulting from consultation across and within cultures, that clearly articulates competencies of consultants and consultees alike, and that increases attention to areas of much-needed research. A multicultural school consultant regards culture as influencing the "thoughts, expectations, and behaviors for each party in the consultation and makes adjustments to develop and maintain rapport and understanding with the consultee(s) and client(s)" (Ingraham, 2000, p. 326). Ingraham offered five components of a multicultural school consultation (MSC) framework that underlie the theory and practice of MSC. These domains are related to consultant learning and development, consultee learning and development, cultural variations in the consultation constellation, contextual and power influences, and hypothesized methods for supporting consultee and client success. In addition, Sheridan (2000) considered the impact of multiculturalism and diversity in behavioral consultation with parents and teachers and noted that much empirical support exists for the use of behavioral or conjoint behavioral consultation in the schools but that much less research exists on the use of this model when the individuals involved in the consultation process represent different areas of diversity.

Rogers (2000) summarized the themes related to cross-cultural competencies in consultation that have been identified as "important and necessary for effective consultation" (p. 415). These competencies refer to understanding one's own and other's cultures. It is necessary to be aware of your own beliefs, assumptions, and prejudices, as well as to understand the cultural and sociopolitical backgrounds of your client(s), to understand and respect their perspectives, values, and histories. Another competency identified is that of developing cross-cultural communication and interpersonal skills. A school consultant must be effective in bridging diverse perspectives and building relationships with those involved (i.e., stakeholders). Additionally, it is necessary to examine the cultural embeddedness of consultation. Just as in the assessment role, school psychologists must consider the context (i.e., using your cultural lenses throughout the process of consultation). School consultants also need to be skilled in using qualitative and quantitative methodologies for the purpose of data gathering, which is a central component of the consultation process. School consultants are also competent in acquiring culture-specific knowledge (e.g., acculturation, second-language acquisition or bilingualism, bilingual education, emigration, culture-specific issues in assessment, education, and mental health). Finally, school consultants understand and are skilled in working with interpreters (i.e., from finding an interpreter to training and working with him or her).

It has been recognized that consultation frameworks themselves need to incorporate multicultural and diversity issues, and this recognition also needs to be translated into systematic training in graduate training programs. Martines (2003) outlined specific suggestions related to training cross-cultural consultant school psychologists. Martines reiterated the importance of integrating Sue's (1981) cross-cultural competencies (i.e., attitude, knowledge, and skill competencies related to culture and ethnicity) into the course objectives, as well as incorporating instructional strategies and assignments related to further understanding and applying these issues. According to Martines (2003), it is not sufficient just to provide "on-the-job training"; students must also be provided with a framework to be able to continue to develop their multicultural competency in their profession (p. 13).

## SCHOOL PSYCHOLOGY AND THE OVERREPRESENTATION OF MINORITY STUDENTS IN SPECIAL EDUCATION PROGRAMS

In direct contrast to what is occurring in the field of school psychology related to the underrepresentation of minority individuals practicing in the field, we are continuing to see overrepresentation of minority students in special education. Thus responding effectively to cultural and linguistic diversity as school psychologists becomes even more salient.

For over three decades the overrepresentation of ethnic minority students in special education programs has been a prominent and controversial issue. Zhang and Katsiyannis

(2002) evaluated data from the 22nd Annual Report to Congress on the Implementation of IDEA (U.S. Department of Education, 2000) from the National Center for Education Statistics, as well as poverty rates in the United States (U.S. Census Bureau, 1999), to examine minority representation across states and regions for all disabilities and to address such variability in light of minority representation in the total student population and state poverty rates. These authors' findings support previous concerns (e.g., Patton, 1998, as cited in Zhang & Katsiyannis, 2002) regarding African American students' historic disproportional classification as having disabilities, especially mental retardation. Even today, African American students continue to have the highest representation of all groups in the mental retardation category. Concurrently, educators must ensure that minority students who qualify have access to appropriate services despite calls to achieve proportionate representation. Zhang and Katsiyannis's (2002) study also supported previous reports for Hispanic American students regarding representation across all disabilities, including mental retardation (MR). Of importance is the finding that American Indian/Alaskan Native students were the second most overrepresented group in special education, after African American students. Zhang and Katsiyannis (2002) further described concerns regarding the large regional variations in minority representation for emotional–behavioral disturbance (EBD). For example, higher percentages of Hispanic American students from the Northeast region were represented in EBD than from the West and South regions. The authors concluded that, despite an increased emphasis on curbing minority overrepresentation in special education, national data indicate limited success in reducing this overrepresentation. They emphasized the importance of agencies being vigilant in ensuring a nonbiased identification and placement process through the expanded use of prereferral teams (also supported by the New Mexico Department of Education, 2001). In addition, Zhang and Katsiyannis (2002) recommend improvement of prereferral, multidisciplinary, and placement team training and the use of technically sound, norm-referenced instruments, along with the expanded use of curriculum-based measures.

Rhodes and colleagues (2005) recommend solutions to minority overrepresentation in five areas. These five areas include teacher training at both the preservice and in-service levels in instructing diverse students; improvement in early intervention/prereferral activities; research to test the "differential susceptibility" versus the systematic-bias hypothesis and related to the interaction between a child's ecology and culture; activities that need to be undertaken by the U.S. Office of Civil Rights (e.g., collecting data and writing reports); and factors that should be considered by the profession (e.g., identification procedures).

In sum, the issue of overrepresentation in special education programs is complex. It may take years of systemic changes at the federal, state, and local levels to address adequately this concern. However, in the absence of such far-reaching efforts, school psychologists can ensure that they engage in best practices in service provision to culturally, ethnically, and linguistically diverse groups so as not to become a part of the problem. As a means to aid both practicing and future school psychologists in the effort to become leaders in the field, ensuring that disparities such as those described earlier dissipate, we offer several suggestions for increasing one's own multicultural competency and effectiveness. These suggestions are listed in Table 3.1. To those who have already begun this journey, we commend your efforts in understanding that "diversity is a gift to be cherished and not a fear to be destroyed because of lack of knowledge" (Vázquez, 1997).

# DATA-DRIVEN PROBLEM SOLVING: AN APPROACH
# FOR SUPPORTING ALL STUDENTS

In Chapter 7 we introduce the data-driven problem-solving model for school psychology practice. The problem-solving approach is a keystone of this volume, and it permeates the view we seek to promote for advancing the science and practice of school psychology. In this model, school psychologists move from simply being diagnosticians and sorters to using their professional and scientific training to become integral players in determining student needs, selecting appropriate interventions, and evaluating the efficacy of these interventions in an ongoing manner.

So what does data-driven problem-solving have to do with cultural and linguistic diversity? We chose to initially introduce the problem-solving model—albeit briefly—at the conclusion of this chapter on diversity because we believe it has great potential to enhance the ability of school psychologists to respond effectively to the needs of students, families, and school systems, regardless of the cultural and linguistic characteristics of those involved. We recognize that human cultural and language differences will always provide a unique challenge to effective delivery of educational and psychological services and that professionals in our field are under special obligation to enhance their awareness of their clients' unique backgrounds, of their own values and biases, and of

---

**TABLE 3.1. Suggestions for Strengthening the Multicultural Competency of School Psychologists**

1. Be aware of your own values, beliefs, and worldview so as to understand how your perceptions may help or hinder your work with others (families, students, colleagues, administration, etc.).

2. Be aware of where you are in your own ethnic identity development so as to understand your comfort level within your own and others' cultures/backgrounds.

3. Be aware of any potential bias(es) (you may have) related to cultural variables (e.g., race, ethnicity, gender, socioeconomic status, disability, etc.) to best meet the needs of your clientele.

4. Understand your limitations and be willing to seek out consultation from others who may have more multicultural knowledge and/or experience.

5. Be willing to learn about others' cultural backgrounds and experiences to avoid stereotyping and to consider within- and between-group differences and similarities.

6. Seek out information regarding your clients' worldviews, values, and beliefs in order to establish and sustain a productive working relationship.

7. Always consider students' and families' cultural contexts when collecting and interpreting evaluation data.

8. Understand how to use and seek out interpreters and/or translators to assist you in your work with linguistically diverse clientele.

9. Understand individual's preferred method of communication (e.g., preferred language) and understand cultural variations in communication (e.g., showing respect for others).

10. Understand the strengths and limitations of traditional assessment techniques such as the use of tests with individuals from culturally and linguistically diverse populations.

---

models for culturally sensitive service delivery. That said, we propose that many of the current issues we face in this regard (such as bias in our assessment tools, barriers to effective communication, and minority overrepresentation in special education programs) may be reduced when we begin to move away from a focus on within-child pathology and move toward a focus on environments, contexts, desired outcomes, and assets.

The basis for the data-driven problem-solving approach is that problems are not necessarily viewed as forms of pathology or disorder but are considered to be discrepancies between *what is occurring* and *what is expected within a given context* (e.g., a classroom or a family). This model is *outcome-focused*, meaning that the emphasis is on a solution or outcome to the problem rather than simply offering an elegant description of the problem. It is *context specific*, meaning that what constitutes a problem or a viable solution to it may differ across settings or contexts, just as expectations and social ecologies differ across settings. Moreover, the problem-solving approach is driven by *ongoing data collection*, which is essential not only to defining the problem and developing potential solutions but also to determining whether the solutions are resulting in the desired effect. In addition, the problem-solving model we advocate is integrally linked to intervention. It includes assessment and description, but only to the extent that it helps clarify what is needed and what is effective. The four basic steps of this model, as outlined in Chapter 7, include identifying and validating the problem (what is the problem?), analyzing the problem (why is it occurring?), determining what should be done about the problem (developing and implementing an intervention), and evaluating the efficacy of the intervention through follow-up and ongoing data collection.

Some recent examples of innovative problem-solving-based service delivery systems in education have been shown to reduce bias and enhance outcomes for students of various backgrounds. Some of these examples include the problem-solving model developed by the Heartland Area Education Agency in Iowa (see Tilly, 2002), and the Screening to Enhance Educational Performance (STEEP), a multiple-gating system for defining problems and developing targets for intervention (see www.lsu.edu/steep/themes/services.htm for more details) developed by Joseph C. Witt and colleagues. These innovations show that it is possible to increase the success of students in general education environments while reducing the need for placing so many students in already overburdened special services programs. As data-based problem-solving models—including the recently developed response to intervention (RTI) approach—have become more widespread, there is increasing evidence that they hold great promise for promoting academic and behavioral success of all students (e.g., VanDerHeyden, Witt, & Barnett, in press). Some of the promises of problem-solving RTI models include enhancing academic performance of students from minority backgrounds and from low-performing schools and reducing errors stemming from teacher misidentification of learning problems (e.g., Shinn, Collins, & Gallagher, 1998; VanDerHeyden & Witt, in 2005). Although our field is still in the formative stages of learning to use innovative data-based problem-solving models to enhance school and student outcomes, the potential is tremendous. As our society becomes increasingly diverse and pluralistic, the field of school psychology must not only honor and embrace diversity but must also adopt practices and service delivery models that reduce bias, meet individual needs, and result in better outcomes for all children and their families.

## DISCUSSION QUESTIONS AND ACTIVITIES

1. Based on the discussion presented in this chapter, list what you consider to be three important things that you can do to ensure that culturally or linguistically diverse students and/or families are comfortable in your office. Provide your rationale for your choices.

2. Observe different school settings and decide whether the school includes a diverse population of students and, if so, what forms of diversity are present. What indicators, if any, are present that show respect for and value of the diversity?

3. Reflect on your own behavior (e.g., language and dialect) and determine which of your own behaviors are consistent with mainstream American culture. Reflect on your own biases and/or assumptions.

4. Seek out an experience that will enable you to get to know an individual or group that is different from you in some way, such as culture, ethnicity, religion, sexual orientation, race, nationality, or social/economic class. The experience needs to be a new one and one that you would not normally encounter if not for this specific assignment. Write a reaction paper describing the experience and relating to one or more concepts or issues discussed in this chapter.

5. What do you consider to be the most important personal or professional characteristic for a culturally competent school psychologist? Provide a rationale for your answer.

6. As a way to begin to understand your own cultural experiences, keep a weekly journal documenting what you read, hear, or experience regarding diversity during the week. Some questions to consider may include: What impact did it have on you? How did the information fit with your existing knowledge and/or experiences? What, if anything, did you learn about someone else who is different from you?

7. Refer to NASP's website on culturally competent practice and complete the "self-assessment" questionnaire (http://www.nasponline.org/culturalcompetence.html).

# Becoming
# a School Psychologist
TRAINING AND CREDENTIALING ISSUES

The previous chapters in this volume have addressed general characteristics and background regarding the field of school psychology: an introduction to the field, the historical context of the fields of psychology and education as they have influenced school psychology, and an overview of issues pertaining the cultural and linguistic diversity–the changing face of school psychology. With that background as a foundation, we now move into the process of becoming a school psychologist. This chapter comprehensively addresses a variety of issues related to the process of professional entry into the field. At the onset of the chapter, we explore how individuals make the decision to become school psychologists. An extensive discussion of school psychology training programs and of the characteristics of students and faculty in these programs makes up a substantial portion of this chapter. We also explore a myriad of issues related to the training of future psychologists and the regulation of the programs that provide the training. An important and unique aspect of preparation to enter the field–practicum and internship training–is detailed, along with an exploration of the considerations involved in selecting and finding an appropriate internship. The various processes for credentialing school psychologists (certification and licensure) are also discussed, and the chapter concludes with a brief discussion of continuing professional development expectations and opportunities within the field.

## BECOMING A SCHOOL PSYCHOLOGIST

Collectively, we interview or field inquiries from hundreds of individuals who are interested in learning more about the field of school psychology, are seeking admission to graduate programs in the field, or are trying to find answers to questions about the roles and functions of school psychologists. Most of these interactions are with prospective graduate students who are considering careers as school psychologists. In some cases, these individuals are well informed about the field and have a fairly good understanding of what a school psychologist is and how one becomes a member of the profession. We also find many misconceptions about both issues. These experiences, as well as our own experiences that led us personally to the field of school psychology, have caused us to reflect on the paths that lead to our field. Although it is true that everyone's path is somewhat unique, we have found many similarities on the road to becoming a school psychologist.

One typical commonality among individuals who seek entry into the field of school psychology is a strong interest in both psychology and education, because the field is a unique hybrid of both disciplines. Our experience has been that, increasingly, individuals who apply for admission to graduate programs in school psychology have earned undergraduate degrees in psychology. We estimate that at least 80% of applicants to our respective training programs in recent years have their undergraduate degrees in psychology, with the remaining 20% in the fields of education, sociology, or a variety of other disciplines. A minority of applicants to our graduate programs in recent years—maybe 15–25%—have previously earned graduate degrees (usually master's degrees) in psychology, education, social work, or counseling, and some who enter the field have had previous professional experience in one of these fields or in another area. However, prior graduate degrees and professional experience are not necessarily the norm for entering the field, and it is our experience that the percentage of applicants to graduate programs in school psychology who have extensive professional experience and a prior graduate degree has declined in recent years. Although we have no hard data to prove this point, our perception is that the "typical" newcomer to the field of school psychology in recent years is one who enters graduate school in his or her early to mid-20s, having earned an undergraduate degree in psychology within the past year or two.

The motivations of individuals who enter the field of school psychology are varied and diverse, but there are some common threads tying them together. Primarily, most budding school psychologists have a strong desire to help provide support to children and their families and to assist them as they struggle with the challenges of the educational experience. With this general motivation almost always comes a particular interest and desire to support and assist children and families who are struggling academically or behaviorally or who are otherwise at risk for negative educational and life outcomes. In other words, those attracted to the field of school psychology tend to have a strong humanitarian or service orientation, coupled with a strong sense of social responsibility. Beyond these general motivations, there are certainly some differences among those who desire to enter the profession. Some aspiring school psychologists move into the field with a burning desire to make a major impact in improving educational and social systems, whereas others are content to work within systems as they are. Some are attracted to the field because of the continuing strong job market, stable employment situations, and their perceptions of reasonable compensation and benefit packages, whereas others appreciate the good employment opportunities and general stability of the profession but settle for what they consider disappointing compensation packages. Almost all school psychologists enjoy the generally regular work hours, which typically are similar to a school day or business day. Those who work in public school settings often have 9- or 10-month employment contracts, with additional vacation and holiday time off during the school year.

Regardless of the varied backgrounds, aspirations, and motivations of individuals who enter the field, the highway to the profession invariably begins with acceptance to a graduate training program in school psychology. The 3- to 5-year graduate school experience (depending on whether one pursues specialist or doctoral-level training) provides the foundation for working as a school psychologist and is an important socializing factor in developing an initial model of practice and a worldview of the field. Thus graduate training programs in the field, as well as the faculty who staff them, are of particular interest in the process of becoming a school psychologist, and these are the focus of the next section.

# SCHOOL PSYCHOLOGY TRAINING PROGRAMS, STUDENTS, FACULTY

Without successfully completing a graduate training program in school psychology, it is not possible in most states to become a school psychologist. The training programs not only function as the initial point of entry into the profession but also serve the essential role of professional socialization into the field, as well as transmission of values and practices for new professionals. It is the training programs that have responsibility for implementing the training standards of the national organizations (NASP and APA) and for endorsing graduates of the programs for licensure and certification from state departments of education and from state psychology licensing boards. Given the critical role that school psychology training programs play in the development and well-being of the field, we cover in detail various aspects of graduate training programs and the faculty and graduate students who are connected to these programs. In addition, some of the emerging issues and trends that affect training programs are addressed.

## School Psychology Training Programs

### Characteristics

It is quite difficult to obtain a highly accurate picture of school psychology training programs across the United States and Canada because two separate national organizations (NASP and APA) accredit or approve programs across North America and because many programs are not accredited and thus do not appear on lists of approved programs, nor do they have reporting responsibilities to the national organizations. Furthermore, it is complicated to generalize what we do know about training programs and to make inferences about the students and faculty within them. That said, with the information currently available, as well as previous detailed efforts to describe the characteristics of school psychology training programs, it is possible at least to make some generalizations about training programs, their host institutions, and the faculty and students who are involved in these programs.

   The most comprehensive recent lists of school psychology training programs have been compiled by Alex Thomas, author of a NASP-published guide to training programs in the late 1990s (Thomas, 1998), and compiler of a comprehensive appendix of training programs in his coedited two-volume *Best Practices in School Psychology: IV* (Thomas & Grimes, 2002). According to this information, there are more than 200 institutions of higher education in the United States and Canada that provide graduate-level training in school psychology at some level and more than 300 different training programs at these institutions. Why are there so many more training programs than institutions? The reason is that many institutions have both doctoral and specialist-level training programs and that these programs are counted separately in attempts to define and accredit training programs. For example, Thomas and Grimes's (2002) appendix lists 7 training institutions but 10 training programs for the state of Florida, because three of the institutions listed provide both specialist and doctoral training programs. The majority of the current training programs are at the specialist-degree level or other nondoctoral levels, such as master's degree or certification/licensure-only programs. Based on our review of the most recent accredited-programs lists from both NASP and APA and of previous attempts to consolidate the information on training programs (e.g., Thomas, 1988; Thomas & Grimes, 2002), we can infer that there are slightly more than two specialist-level training programs for every doctoral-level training program in existence. Given that numerous unaccredited training programs exist and that these programs are more likely to be specialist than doctoral programs, the ratio of specialist to doctoral level programs most likely ranges from about 2.2:1 to about 2.5:1. The number of graduates produced by these programs each year is likely to be even more skewed in the direction of nondoctoral programs because specialist programs tend to be larger than doctoral programs in terms of the number of new students accepted each year.

A review of the lists of accredited training programs from NASP and APA indicates that the large majority of school psychology training programs—roughly 60–70%—are found at public rather than private institutions of higher education. Within these institutions, about 75% of the training programs are located within colleges of education (often within departments of educational psychology), whereas about 25% are located within colleges of arts and sciences in departments of psychology. With a few exceptions, doctoral programs are more likely to be found at national research universities than at regional universities or liberal arts colleges, where specialist-level programs are the norm. Regionally, school psychology programs at all levels exist across the United States and Canada, but they are not necessarily distributed evenly by region. For example, the midwest and northeast regions of the United States have a large number of training programs, whereas there are fewer training programs in the western United States and only a small number of programs in Canada. Table 4.1 provides a comprehensive listing of the master's- and specialist-level school psychology training programs in the United States and Canada, and Table 4.2 provides a comprehensive listing of doctoral training programs. We developed these tables based on information provided to us by Alex Thomas (personal communication, January 19, 2004), as well as on our own 2004 review of NASP and APA program listings and Internet searches for additional training programs. We recognize that there may be some inaccuracies in these listings, because there is a constant flux in program status over time. However, these data were the most recent and complete currently available as we prepared this chapter.

## Models of Training

Although there are many commonalities among the various school psychology training programs, each program has unique characteristics and a unique identity and tradition. Even two training programs that claim to use the same broad training model and have similar training philosophies may differ substantially. As prospective students research various training programs and make decisions regarding where to apply, the array of choices can be overwhelming, particularly if one is not exclusively focused on a specific location or region. One of the ways to distinguish training programs is to identify the model of training they utilize, as well as the specific focus or philosophy to which they adhere. In this regard, there are existing models of training that provide a framework for looking at the similarities and differences among programs.

**TABLE 4.1. Listing of Master's- and Specialist-Level School Psychology Training Programs in the United States and Canada**

| University | Master's/Specialist degree | NASP/ NCATE |
|---|---|---|
| Alabama | | |
| Auburn University | EdS | |
| University of Alabama | EdS | Full |
| Arizona | | |
| Northern Arizona University | EdS | Full |
| University of Arizona | EdS | |
| Arkansas | | |
| University of Central Arkansas | EdS | Full |
| California | | |
| California State University–Chico | MA | Full |
| California State University–Fresno | MS | Full |
| California State University–Hayward | MS | Full |
| California State University–Long Beach | MA | |
| California State University–Los Angeles | MA | Full |
| California State University–Northridge | | |
| (educational psychology) | MS | |
| California State University–Sacramento | MS | |
| Full California State University–San Bernardino | PPS | |
| Chapman University | EdS | |
| Fresno Pacific University | MA | |
| Humboldt State University | MS | Full |
| La Sierra University | EdS | |
| Loyola Marymount University | MA | |
| San Diego State University | MS | Full |
| San Francisco State University | MS | Full |
| University of California–Riverside | MA | |
| University of California–Santa Barbara | MEd | Full |
| University of the Pacific | EdS | |
| Colorado | | |
| University of Colorado–Denver | EdS | Full |
| University of Denver | EdS | |
| University of Northern Colorado | EdS | Full |
| Connecticut | | |
| Fairfield University | MA | |
| Southern Connecticut State University | MS | Full |
| University of Connecticut | MA/6th-year equivalent | Full |
| University of Hartford | MS | Full |
| Delaware | | |
| University of Delaware | MA | Full |
| District of Columbia | | |
| Gallaudet University | PsyS | Full |
| Howard University | MA/MEd | |
| Florida | | |
| Barry University | SSP | Full |
| Florida International University | EdS | |

*(continued)*

**TABLE 4.1.** (continued)

| | | |
|---|---|---|
| Florida (continued) | | |
| Florida State University | EdS | |
| University of Central Florida | EdS | Full |
| University of Florida | EdS | Full |
| University of South Florida | EdS | Full |
| Georgia | | |
| Georgia Southern University | EdS | |
| Georgia State University | EdS | |
| Valdosta State University | EdS | Full |
| Idaho | | |
| Idaho State University | EdS | Full |
| University of Idaho | EdS | Full |
| Illinois | | |
| Eastern Illinois University | SSP | Full |
| Governors State University | MA | Full |
| Illinois State University | SSP | Full |
| Loyola University of Chicago | EdS | Full |
| National-Louis University | EdS | Full |
| Northern Illinois University | MA | Full |
| Southern Illinois University–Edwardsville | SSP | Full |
| Western Illinois University | SSP | Full |
| Indiana | | |
| Ball State University | EdS | Full |
| Indiana State University | EdS | Full |
| Indiana University | EdS | Full |
| Valparaiso University | EdS | |
| Iowa | | |
| University of Northern Iowa | EdS | Full |
| Kansas | | |
| Emporia State University | Ed | Conditional |
| Fort Hayes University | EdS | |
| Pittsburg State | EdS | |
| University of Kansas | EdS | Full |
| Wichita State University | EdS | Full |
| Kentucky | | |
| Eastern Kentucky University | PsyS | Full |
| University of Kentucky | EdS | Full |
| Western Kentucky University | EdS | Full |
| Louisiana | | |
| Louisiana State University–Shreveport | SSP | Full |
| McNeese State University | MA | |
| Nicholls State University | SSP | Full |
| Northeast Louisiana University | SSP | Full |
| Maine | | |
| University of Southern Maine | MS | Full |
| Maryland | | |
| Towson University | MA | Full |
| University of Maryland | MA | Full |
| Massachusetts | | |
| American International College | C.A.G.S. | |

| | | |
|---|---|---|
| Northeastern University | MS | Full |
| Tufts University | MA | Full |
| University of Massachusetts–Amherst | MEd | Full |
| University of Massachusetts–Boston | MEd | Full |
| Michigan | | |
| Andrews University | EdS | Conditional |
| Central Michigan University | SSP | Full |
| Michigan State University | EdS | |
| University of Detroit–Mercy | EdS | |
| Wayne State University | MA | |
| Western Michigan University | EdS | Full |
| Minnesota | | |
| Moorhead State University | EdS | Full |
| University of Minnesota | EdS | Full |
| Mississippi | | |
| Mississippi State University | EdS | Full |
| Missouri | | |
| University of Missouri–Columbia | EdS | |
| Montana | | |
| University of Montana | EdS | Full |
| Nebraska | | |
| University of Nebraska–Kearney | EdS | Full |
| University of Nebraska–Lincoln | EdS | Full |
| University of Nebraska–Omaha | EdS | Full |
| Nevada | | |
| University of Nevada–Las Vegas | EdS | Full |
| University of Nevada–Reno | EdS | |
| New Jersey | | |
| Fairleigh Dickinson University | MA | |
| Kean University | MA | Full |
| Montclair State University | Certification | |
| Rider University | EdS | |
| Rowan University | EdS | Full |
| Seton Hall University | EdS | |
| New Mexico | | |
| New Mexico State University | EdS | |
| New York | | |
| Alfred University | MA | Full |
| City University of New York, Brooklyn College | MSE | Full |
| City University of New York, Queens College | MSE | Full |
| College of New Rochelle | MS | |
| Columbia University | EdM | |
| Fordham University | Professional Diploma | Full |
| Marist College | MA | |
| New York University | Certification | |
| Rochester Institute of Technology | MS | Full |
| St. John's University | MS | Full |
| State University of New York–Albany | Certification | |
| State University of New York–Buffalo | MA | Full |

*(continued)*

**TABLE 4.1.** (*continued*)

| | | |
|---|---|---|
| New York (*continued*) | | |
| State University of New York–Oswego | MS | Full |
| State University of New York–Plattsburgh | Certification | |
| Touro College | MS | |
| North Carolina | | |
| Appalachian State University | MA | Full |
| East Carolina University | MA | Full |
| North Carolina State University | MS | |
| University of North Carolina–Chapel Hill | MEd | Full |
| Western Carolina University | MA | Full |
| North Dakota | | |
| Minot State University | EdS | Full |
| Ohio | | |
| Bowling Green State University | EdS | Full |
| Cleveland State University | PsyS | Full |
| John Carroll University | MEd | Full |
| Kent State University | EdS | Full |
| Miami University | EdS | Full |
| Ohio State University | MA | Full |
| University of Cincinnati | MEd | Full |
| University of Dayton | EdS | Full |
| University of Toledo | EdS | |
| Oklahoma | | |
| Oklahoma State University | EdS | Full |
| University of Central Oklahoma | MA | |
| Oregon | | |
| Lewis and Clark College | MS | Full |
| University of Oregon | MS | |
| Pennsylvania | | |
| Bucknell University | MSEd | |
| California University of Pennsylvania | MS | |
| Duquesne University | MSEd | Full |
| Edinboro University of Pennsylvania | MEd | |
| Immaculata College | Certification | |
| Indiana University of Pennsylvania | MS | Full |
| Lehigh University | EdS | Full |
| Marywood University | MA | |
| Millersville University of Pennsylvania | MS | Full |
| Temple University | EdM | Full |
| Rhode Island | | |
| Rhode Island College | MA | |
| Conditional University of Rhode Island | MS | Full |
| South Carolina | | |
| Francis Marion University | MS | Full |
| The Citadel | EdS | Full |
| Winthrop University | SSP | Full |
| South Dakota | | |
| University of South Dakota | EdS | Full |
| Tennessee | | |
| Austin Peay State University | EdS | |

| | | |
|---|---|---|
| Middle Tennessee State University | EdS | Full |
| Tennessee State University | EdS | |
| Tennessee Technological University | EdS | |
| University of Memphis | EdS | Full |
| University of Tennessee–Chattanooga | EdS | |
| University of Tennessee–Knoxville | EdS | Full |

**Texas**

| | | |
|---|---|---|
| Abilene Christian University | MS | |
| Baylor University | EdS | |
| Our Lady of the Lake University | LSSP | |
| Sam Houston State University | MA | Full |
| Southwest Texas State University | MA | Full |
| Texas A & M University | MS | Conditional |
| Texas Women's University | MA | Full |
| Trinity University | MA | Full |
| University of Houston–Clear Lake | MA | Full |
| University of North Texas | MA/MS | |
| University of Texas–Pan American | MA | |

**Utah**

| | | |
|---|---|---|
| Brigham Young University | MS | |
| University of Utah | MS | |
| Utah State University | MS | Full |

**Virginia**

| | | |
|---|---|---|
| College of William and Mary | EdS | Full |
| George Mason University | MA | Full |
| James Madison University | EdS | Full |
| Radford University | EdS | Full |

**Washington**

| | | |
|---|---|---|
| Central Washington University | MEd | Full |
| Eastern Washington University | MS | Full |
| Seattle Pacific University | MS reactivating 2005 | |
| Seattle University | EdS | Full |
| University of Washington | MEd | Full |

**Wisconsin**

| | | |
|---|---|---|
| University of Wisconsin–Eau Claire | EdS | Full |
| University of Wisconsin–La Crosse | EdS | Full |
| University of Wisconsin–Milwaukee | EdS | |
| University of Wisconsin–River Falls | EdS | Full |
| University of Wisconsin–Stout | MSE | Full |
| University of Wisconsin–Whitewater | EdS | Full |

**Canada**

| | | |
|---|---|---|
| Mount St. Vincent University | MA | |
| Ontario Institute of Studies, University of Toronto | MA | |
| University of British Columbia | MA/MEd | |
| University of Calgary | MEd/ MSE | |
| University of Saskatchewan | MEd | |

**TABLE 4.2. Listing of Doctoral-Level School Psychology Training Programs in the United States and Canada**

| University | Doctoral degree | APA accreditation | NASP/ NCATE |
|---|---|---|---|
| Alabama | | | |
| Auburn University | PhD | | |
| University of Alabama | PhD | | Full |
| Arizona | | | |
| Argosy University/Phoenix | PsyD | | |
| Arizona State University | PhD | Full | Full |
| Northern Arizona University | EdD | | Full |
| University of Arizona | PhD | Full | Full |
| Arkansas | | | |
| University of Central Arkansas | PhD | | |
| California | | | |
| University of California–Berkeley | PhD | Full | |
| University of California–Riverside | PhD | | |
| University of California–Santa Barbara | PhD[a] | Full | |
| University of the Pacific | EdD | | |
| Colorado | | | |
| University of Denver | PhD | | |
| University of Northern Colorado | PhD | Full | Full |
| Connecticut | | | |
| University of Connecticut | PhD | Full | Full |
| District of Columbia | | | |
| Howard University | EdD/PhD | | |
| Florida | | | |
| Florida State University | PhD[a] | Full | |
| University of Florida | PhD | Full | Full |
| University of South Florida | PhD | Full | Full |
| Georgia | | | |
| Georgia State University | PhD | Full | Full |
| University of Georgia | PhD | Full | Full |
| Illinois | | | |
| Illinois State University | PhD | Full | Full |
| Loyola University of Chicago | PhD | Conditional | |
| National-Louis University | EdD | | |
| Northern Illinois University | PhD | | |
| Indiana | | | |
| Ball State University | PhD | Full | Full |
| Indiana State University | PhD | Full | Full |
| Indiana University | PhD | Full | Full |
| Iowa | | | |
| University of Iowa | PhD | Full | Full |
| Kansas | | | |
| University of Kansas | PhD | Full | Full |
| Kentucky | | | |
| University of Kentucky | PhD | Full | Full |

| Louisiana | | | |
|---|---|---|---|
| Louisiana State University–Baton Rouge | PhD | Full | Full |
| Tulane University | PhD | Full | |
| **Maryland** | | | |
| University of Maryland | PhD | Full | Full |
| **Massachusetts** | | | |
| Northeastern University | PhD[a] | Full | |
| University of Massachusetts–Amherst | PhD | Full | Full |
| **Michigan** | | | |
| Andrews University | PhD/EdD | | |
| Central Michigan University | PhD | Full | Full |
| Michigan State University | PhD | Full | Full |
| Wayne State University | PhD | | |
| Western Michigan University | PhD | | |
| **Minnesota** | | | |
| University of Minnesota | PhD | Full | Full |
| **Mississippi** | | | |
| Mississippi State University | PhD | Full | Full |
| University of Southern Mississippi | PhD | Full | Full |
| **Missouri** | | | |
| University of Missouri–Columbia | PhD | Full | |
| **Nebraska** | | | |
| University of Nebraska–Lincoln | PhD | Full | Full |
| **Nevada** | | | |
| University of Nevada–Reno | EdD | | |
| **New Jersey** | | | |
| Fairleigh Dickinson University | PsyD | | |
| Rutgers University | PsyD | Full | |
| **New York** | | | |
| Alfred University | PsyD | Full | |
| City University of New York, Graduate School and University Center | PhD | Full | |
| Columbia University | PhD/EdD | Full | Full |
| Fordham University | PhD | Full | Full |
| Hofstra University | PsyD[a]/PhD[a] | Full | Full |
| New York University | PsyD/PhD | Full | Full |
| Pace University | PsyD[a] | Full | Full |
| St. John's University | PsyD | | |
| State University of New York–Albany | PsyD | Full | |
| State University of New York–Buffalo | PhD[a] | Full | |
| Syracuse University | PhD | Full | |
| Yeshiva University | PsyD[a] | Full | Full |
| **North Carolina** | | | |
| North Carolina State University | PhD | Full | Full |
| University of North Carolina–Chapel Hill | PhD | Full | Full |
| **Ohio** | | | |
| Kent State University | PhD | Full | Full |
| Ohio State University | PhD | | Full |
| University of Cincinnati | PhD | | Full |

*(continued)*

| | | | |
|---|---|---|---|
| **Oklahoma** | | | |
| Oklahoma State University | PhD | Full | Full |
| **Oregon** | | | |
| University of Oregon | PhD | Full | Full |
| **Pennsylvania** | | | |
| Bryn Mawr College | PhD | | |
| Duquesne University | PhD | | |
| Immaculata College | PsyD | | |
| Indiana University of Pennsylvania | EdD | | Full |
| Lehigh University | PhD | Full | Full |
| Pennsylvania State University | PhD | Full | Full |
| Temple University | PhD | Full | Full |
| University of Pennsylvania | PhD | | |
| **Rhode Island** | | | |
| University of Rhode Island | PhD | Full | Full |
| **South Carolina** | | | |
| University of South Carolina | PhD | Full | Full |
| **South Dakota** | | | |
| University of South Dakota | PhD | | |
| **Tennessee** | | | |
| Tennessee State University | PhD | | |
| University of Memphis | PhD | | |
| University of Tennessee–Knoxville | PhD | Full | Full |
| **Texas** | | | |
| Texas A & M University | PhD | Full | Full |
| Texas Women's University | PhD | | Full |
| University of Texas | PhD | Full | Full |
| **Utah** | | | |
| University of Utah | PhD | Full | Full |
| Utah State University | PhD[a] | Full | |
| **Virginia** | | | |
| James Madison University | PsyD[a] | Full | |
| University of Virginia | EdD/PhD | | Full |
| **Washington** | | | |
| Seattle Pacific University | EdD | | |
| University of Washington | PhD | Full | Full |
| **Wisconsin** | | | |
| University of Wisconsin–Madison | PhD | Full | Full |
| University of Wisconsin–Milwaukee | PhD | Full | Full |
| **Canada** | | | |
| McGill University | PhD | Full | |
| Ontario Institute of Studies, University of Toronto | PhD | | |
| University of Alberta | PhD | | |
| University of British Columbia | PhD | | |
| University of Calgary | PhD | | |

[a]School psychology training provided within a combined program in professional–scientific psychology that also includes a clinical and/or counseling psychology focus.

The APA has supported numerous efforts since the 1940s to articulate and define models of training for doctoral programs in professional areas of psychology. The best known of these models is the *scientist-practitioner* model, a training model that is presumed to apply to programs that train their students in a solid foundation in research and scientific aspects of psychology and to apply these foundations to the professional practice or application of the discipline. This model was initially articulated in a clinical psychology training conference held in Boulder, Colorado, in 1949 (Frank, 1984). Hence the scientist-practitioner model of training is sometimes referred to as the "Boulder model." In addition to this model, other models of training emerged beginning in the 1970s. The *practitioner* model of professional psychology emerged from the Vail conference on graduate training in psychology in 1973, partially through dissatisfaction with the scientist-practitioner model, which some trainers and practitioners contended did not provide sufficient attention to the preparation of practitioners in psychology and did little to alleviate personnel shortages during that era. The practitioner model of training places the primary focus of graduate education on professional or clinical practice and does not emphasize conducting independent research (e.g., an original dissertation or thesis) as an integral aspect of preparing psychologists. In this respect, the practitioner model is more similar to the training that physicians receive during their time in medical school, which is typically built on a foundation of basic science and clinical practice but does not require the completion of a research dissertation or extensive research methodology courses for receipt of the MD degree.

Besides the two best-known training models, newer models have emerged within American psychology since the 1980s. The *clinical science* model of training reflects a focus on training scientists who have interests in clinical problems, such as childhood psychopathology or prevention science. The *practitioner-scholar* model is a recent model that seeks to bridge the difference between the scientist-practitioner and practitioner models of training. Within this model, the primary emphasis is placed on training graduate students to become practitioners, but more emphasis is placed on the production of scholarly work than would be expected in a practitioner model program.

The four training models that have just been described are not specific to school psychology. Rather, they have evolved out of the broad area of professional psychology doctoral training, which includes many more training programs in clinical and counseling psychology than in school psychology. Within school psychology doctoral programs, there is probably a smaller variety of training models currently used. We are not aware of any PhD programs in school psychology that claim to follow the clinical science model, and the practitioner-scholar model, although promising, has not yet been formally adopted by many programs at this point in time (although we suspect that many doctoral programs that list "scientist-practitioner" as their model are actually more closely aligned to the practitioner-scholar model). Most doctoral programs in our field tend to list either the scientist-practitioner or practitioner models as the training model they adhere to.

Because a majority of school psychology programs are at the specialist rather than doctoral level of training, it is doubtful that the four training models that have emerged in American psychology apply as much to them as they do to doctoral programs. Within a specialist-level program (which typically consists of at least 60 semester or 90 quarter hours of coursework), it is simply not as feasible to be as highly specialized as within a doctoral program (which typically consists of about 100 or more semester hours or 150 or more quarter hours). We doubt that the clinical science model of training fits outside of doctoral-level training. Rather, the specialist-level programs in school psychology tend to fit within the practitioner, practitioner-scholar, and, in some cases, scientist-practitioner models. In addition, Fagan and Wise (2000) have articulated another model of training, the *pragmatic* model, which they view as a relevant choice for nondoctoral programs. Their view of the pragmatic model is that it reflects an orientation toward meeting accreditation standards (of NASP and state departments of education) and is highly prescriptive in terms of specific courses and competencies that must be covered for someone to become a practicing school psychologist. "This prescriptiveness can result in a high degree of similarity among programs" (Fagan & Wise, 2000, p. 203), which the authors consider to be an unavoidable tradeoff with the specificity inherent in accreditation standards. Certainly, there is something to be said for this pragmatic model of training, although we think that it is still quite possible for specialist-level programs to focus on one of the general training models, particularly the practitioner-scholar and practitioner models. The five training models that have been described in these paragraphs are summarized in Table 4.3.

## Curricula

Although individual training programs may establish whatever curricula and course work requirements they deem to be appropriate, the reality is that there is a great deal of similarity among programs in this regard, because of the need to adhere to prescribed standards from national accrediting bodies and from state departments of education (which often use national accrediting standards as a basis for their internal requirements for school psychology licensure or certification). As a result, training programs may vary substantially in terms of their models of training and the philosophical underpinnings of the program faculty, but there tends not to be much difference in terms of credit hour requirements, general curriculum domains, and, in many cases, even the content and title of specific courses.

The specialist-level training standard advocated by NASP (and adopted by numerous state departments of education for program approval) requires a minimum of 60

TABLE 4.3. Overview of Five General Training Models in School Psychology

| Training model | Brief description |
|---|---|
| Scientist-practitioner | Emphasizes research and scientific aspects of psychology and application of these foundations to the professional practice or application of the discipline |
| Practitioner (professional practice) | Emphasizes professional or clinical practice of discipline; does not include substantial requirements for research |
| Practitioner-scholar | Primary emphasis on professional or clinical practice of discipline, but also has extensive expectations for production of scholarly work, such as dissertation research |
| Clinical scientist | Emphasizes scientific research in areas of psychology that have direct application to clinical practice, such as developmental science, prevention science, and child psychopathology |
| Pragmatic | Main emphasis is on alignment with state department of education and/or NASP training standards to ensure that program meets all relevant criteria and receives program approval |

semester credits or 90 quarter credits and includes a full-time (1,200 clock hour) internship. The complete criteria for this standard are found in the NASP publication, *Standards for Training and Field Placement Programs in School Psychology* (NASP, 2000b). Full-time enrollment in a specialist-level program typically requires 2 years of full-time study on campus, in which students complete 12–16 credit hours of course work each semester or term and also complete practicum or field training requirements. In terms of specific course work required, NASP has adopted a general approach wherein several content domains are specified and programs are required to demonstrate that their curricula sufficiently cover these domains. In some instances, state departments of education are more prescriptive of specific course work requirements and may require the completion of specific courses rather than general domains. The following 11 domains of training practice are included in the NASP (2000b) *Standards*:

- Data-based decision making and accountability
- Consultation and collaboration
- Effective instruction and development of cognitive/affective skills
- Socialization and development of life skills
- Student diversity in development and learning
- School and systems organization, policy development, and climate
- Prevention, crisis intervention, and mental health
- Home/school/community collaboration
- Research and program evaluation
- School psychology practice and development
- Information technology

At the conclusion of the 2 years of course work and practicum training, students in specialist-level programs complete a full-time internship for 1 academic year (1,200 clock hour minimum) under the supervision of a licensed or certified school psychologist. NASP training standards also allow a student to complete the internship on a half-time basis over a 2-year time frame and provide some flexibility in the settings in which the internship may be completed. At least 600 of the 1,200 clock hours must be completed in a school setting, a requirement that allows students to complete their remaining hours in a non-school setting (such as a clinic or research center) under the supervision of an appropriately credentialed professional. Although several states have school psychology certification standards that are well below the NASP standards, few training programs adopt curriculum requirements below the NASP standard, because doing so would preclude them from pursuing NASP program approval and because graduates of programs with lower standards may have difficulty obtaining jobs outside of the state in which the training program is located.

Separate standards for doctoral-level training in school psychology have been developed by both NASP and APA. The doctoral standards advocated by NASP include the basic standards for all training programs and coverage of the 11 domains listed in the previous paragraph but also specify that "Doctoral programs provide greater depth in multiple domains of school psychology training and practice as specified in these standards" (NASP, 2000b, p. 14). In addition, the NASP standards stipulate that doctoral programs must include a minimum of 4 full-time years of training beyond the bachelor's degree, consisting of a minimum of 90 semester credits (or 135 quarter credits) and a minimum of 1,500 clock hours for the internship. If a doctoral student has previously completed a specialist-level internship in school psychology in accordance with

NASP standards, then he or she may complete the doctoral internship in a non-school setting, such as a clinic, residential treatment facility, or child guidance center. Otherwise, the same rule for a minimum of 600 school-based clock hours during the internship holds true for doctoral internships.

The doctoral program training standards espoused by APA and required for accreditation from this organization differ from NASP's in terms of specificity and design but are otherwise similar in terms of general expectations and credit hour requirements. APA does not have separate accreditation requirements for doctoral programs in clinical, counseling, school, and combined professional-scientific psychology. Rather, the accreditation standards, which are detailed in *Guidelines and Principles for Accreditation of Programs in Professional Psychology* (APA, 2002b), are generic, but they specify that "A program or institution has the right to be evaluated in terms of its own education and training philosophy, models, goals, objectives, and methods, insofar as they are consistent with those generally accepted as appropriate to the profession" (p. 5). Thus it is assumed that doctoral programs in school psychology that seek APA accreditation will adhere to the general psychology training guidelines and will also be consistent with what is generally deemed to be appropriate specialty training in school psychology. Like NASP's doctoral training standards, the APA guidelines specify that doctoral programs must include at least 3 years of full-time academic study beyond the bachelor's degree, plus an additional year of full-time internship training. APA's specification of domains that are expected to be covered through course work and other experiences within the doctoral training program differ considerably from NASP's 11 domains. The APA domains that are expected to be covered through course work and other training experiences include the following areas (APA, 2002b):

- Biological aspects of behavior
- Cognitive and affective aspects of behavior
- Social aspects of behavior
- History and systems of psychology
- Psychological measurement
- Research methodology
- Techniques of data analysis
- Individual differences in behavior
- Human development
- Dysfunctional behavior of psychopathology
- Professional standards and ethics
- Theories and methods of assessment and diagnosis
- Effective intervention
- Consultation and supervision
- Efficacy of interventions
- Issues of cultural and individual diversity relevant to all of the above areas

In comparing the NASP and APA standards and domains for doctoral training programs, we certainly find some identifiable differences but also many similarities. Regardless of whether doctoral programs in school psychology are accredited by APA, approved by NASP, or have joint program approval, students who enter these programs can expect that their training will take at least 4 years beyond the bachelor's degree (5 years is more typical); that their course work will include broad coverage of scientific, theoretical, and professional practice issues; that they will engage in extensive practicum or fieldwork experiences during the years in which they complete their course work; and that their experience will culminate in a full-time internship for 1 year in a school setting or a related youth-serving setting. Doctoral students can also typically expect to complete a dissertation research project toward the end of their program. Some programs (particularly PsyD, EdD degree programs and programs that adhere to a professional training model) may require a comprehensive or terminal project in lieu of the doctoral research dissertation, but the dissertation requirement seems to be much more typical than the alternatives.

### Specialist or Doctoral Training? Where?

As well-qualified prospective school psychology students consider applying to graduate programs, they have a bewildering array of choices to make concerning which programs to target. One of the first decisions that must be considered is whether to pursue training at the doctoral level or at the specialist level. There is no question that the specialist level of training will continue to serve as the entry level into the field in most, but not all, respects. The large majority of practitioner positions within public school systems do not require more training than the master's/specialist degree, and in many systems there is no financial incentive for investing the additional time and money required to obtain a doctoral degree. However, there are some very good reasons to consider doctoral-level training. One cannot become a core faculty member in a school psychology training program without a doctoral degree, and this level of training is also usually required for school psychologists who desire to work in clinic or medical practice settings. Although some states allow school psychologists with specialist degrees and appropriate credentials to engage in independent or private practice, most states do not have such a provision and require the doctoral degree and a Board of Psychological Examiners license as well for this role. In addition, some supervisory positions in larger school systems, such as school psychology coordinator, director of pupil personnel services, or director of student services, may require a doctoral degree.

Aside from these practical considerations, there are other reasons for prospective students to consider doctoral-level training. Although the 2 years of university-based training and the additional year of internship training required for the specialist degree may provide an excellent foundation for a career as a school psychologist, the additional 2 years of training that are typically required for doctoral degree programs may greatly enhance a student's background and competence in research methods, specialized assessment and intervention techniques, and clinical expertise with specialized populations. These benefits may be important to consider in selecting the level of training one aspires to. In addition, we have observed that many of our students in master's- or specialist-level programs have the desire to obtain a doctoral degree but decide that it would be best to first work for 3–5 years or so and then return to graduate school. Although having such professional experience can be a great asset to a student in a doctoral program, the reality is that there are many potential barriers than can get in the way of returning to graduate school once a school psychologist is employed full time. Not the least of these barriers to returning to the role of a full-time student (with its accompanying lifestyle changes) are the practical issues of becoming accustomed to a full-time professional income, starting a family, taking on greater financial obligations, and so forth. For these reasons, graduate students interested in pursuing doctoral-level training may want to think twice before deciding to work for a few years after the specialist degree and then returning to school. Although some doctoral programs in school psychology are tailored to the needs of working professionals who decide to pursue the doctoral program while still maintaining their employment and a handful of doctoral programs cater to the needs of returning professionals, such programs are still the exception and are not available in most regions of the United States, particularly outside of large urban areas.

The other choice that prospective students must make is which specific institutions or programs to consider. Certainly, there are practical issues to consider in this regard, such as relocating to a distant state or region, the cost of tuition, availability of financial assistance, and so forth. There are also important professional and conceptual issues to consider in the selection of a program. Although a great deal of similarity exists among various training programs in terms of training and curricula offered, there are also many important differences. Typically each program has its own unique philosophical orientation and training model. Thus programs may vary greatly in their approach to teaching assessment and intervention techniques, in their view of the role of school psychologists, in the types of training settings available, and so forth. Prospective students would be wise to carefully research potential graduate programs and apply to programs that have the type of training model, course offerings, and practice or research specialties that they are seeking. Another important element in program selection is to learn about the faculty who staff particular programs. What are their research, teaching, and clinical interests? How many are there, and what is the faculty-to-student ratio and availability of faculty for advising students? For students who enter doctoral programs considering the possibility of becoming a school psychology faculty member, the selection of a program with faculty who can provide them with the appropriate mentoring and experiences in research and publication is especially critical. Finally, there is an important climate or environmental element to consider when selecting admission offers to training programs. Given that one is investing 3–5 years of his or her life in the program, it is wise to consider such issues as level of collegiality among faculty and students, how satisfied and positive current students seem to be, and what it would be like to live in the community where the program is located. These are important issues, and we consider them so essential that we advise potential graduate students to do whatever they can to visit the program and community in person if at all possible before making their decision.

## Characteristics of Faculty and Students

For the same reasons that it is difficult to obtain a highly accurate picture of school psychology training programs, it is quite complicated to accurately portray the characteristics of graduate students in school psychology training programs, as well as the faculty (or "trainers" as they are commonly called) that staff these programs. In many respects it is even more difficult to gather highly accurate data on students and faculty, because the numbers are so much greater than the numbers of programs and because there is not a common metric or reporting system for programs to provide this information. Given these caveats, attempting to portray an accurate representation of the graduate students and faculty in school psychology training programs is an activity that is of great worth to the field, because the faculty serve a role as the gatekeepers and socializing agents into the profession, whereas the current student population represents an important part of the future of the profession.

## Students

The most recent membership data available from NASP during the time this volume was being prepared (from a 2000 membership survey and a 2004 listing of NASP membership) indicates that there were just over 5,000 members of NASP in the "student" and "student in transition" categories. The most recent complete membership data available from APA's Division 16 (the 2004 membership list) indicate more than 600 student affiliates of the division. Although there is some overlap between the student membership of the two organizations, we can assume that these data underestimate the total number of students preparing to enter the field of school psychology because not all students become student members or affiliates of the professional organizations. A very conservative estimate, then, would be approximately 6,000 students currently in graduate training programs in school psychology in the United States and Canada. If we look at this estimate as a percentage of the estimated number of 30,000 school psychologists in the United States and Canada that we presented in Chapter 1, the implications are revealing: if these figures are reasonably close, then about 20% of the individuals who are currently aligned with the profession of school psychology are students who are at some point of preparation. A small percentage of these students are undoubtedly going back to school for doctoral degrees after having previously worked full time as school psychologists, but even taking this possibility into account, the percentage of students affiliated with the field is both sizeable and healthy. These data give us reason to believe that there is a continual infusion of new talent into the field, with new generations of school psychologists continually emerging.

Previous efforts to analyze the demographic characteristics of graduate students in school psychology (such as Thomas's 1998 training directory) have indicated that a large majority of school psychology students at all levels—80% or more—are female. A strong shift in gender balance in the field has been noticeable since about the 1970s, and the percentage of school psychologists who are women surpassed the percentage of school psychologists who are men in about 1980 (Curtis, 2002). Since then, the percentage of female students and practitioners in the field has been rising and may continue to do so. The other two fields of professional psychology—clinical psychology and counseling psychology—have also experienced a similar gender shift among graduate students in recent decades, although not to the same level as is evident in school psychology. When considering only doctoral training programs, some interesting comparative data are available. The most current federal report on doctoral recipients from U.S. universities indicates that in 2002 (the most recent reporting year) about 67% of all PhD recipients in psychology were women, and women made up 66% of counseling psychology PhD recipients, 70% of clinical psychology PhD recipients, and 76% of school psychology PhD recipients, respectively (Bailey, 2004). Over time, as graduate students enter the field and older members retire, the gender composition of the field will look increasingly more like the current composition of graduate students.

In terms of race or ethnicity, the field of school psychology is also quite dissimilar to the population of children that are served by professionals within the field and to that of American society in general. Although members of racial or ethnic minority groups currently make up 35% or more of the general population within the United States (U.S. Bureau of the Census, 2001), they make up only about 17% of the population of graduate students in school psychology (Thomas, 1998) and only 19% of the population of graduate students in all fields of psychology (Bailey, 2004). NASP, APA, various state-level organizations, and many university training programs have enacted initiatives during the past two decades to increase the racial/ethnic diversity of school psychologists, and it is important to recognize that the current student data represent an increased percentage of members of ethnic minority groups from early periods of time in the field and that the racial/ethnic proportionality of the current graduate student population is substantially more diverse than that of the field in general, in which only about 6% are from a racial or ethnic minority group (Curtis et al., 1999; Fagan & Wise, 2000). However, even though the percentage of school psychologists who are members of racial or ethnic minority groups may continue to increase as the more diverse graduate student population enters the field, the diversity of the field is not growing nearly as fast as the diversity of the U.S. population in general. These demographics illustrate a significant challenge for the field: Even with the increasing diversity of individuals entering the field, the profession of school psychology is not currently on track to achieve anything like ethnic or racial similarity to the larger population in the foreseeable future.

What characteristics make for a successful graduate student and ultimately a successful school psychologist? Although a few attempts have been made over the past decades to describe the desirable personal attributes of school psychology students and practitioners, no consensus, overarching survey, nor scientific findings exist. However, based on some of the common elements of lists compiled by previous authors (e.g., Bardon, 1986; Bardon & Bennett, 1974; Fagan & Wise, 1994; Fireoved & Cancelleri, 1985), as well as our own take on what is required for a successful educational and professional experience in school psychology, we view the following characteristics as being highly desirable (and essential in many respects) for school psychology graduate students and practitioners to possess:

- Strong academic aptitude
- Intellectual curiosity and the ability and desire to apply scientific methods in conceptualizing and solving problems
- Excellent interpersonal and social skills
- The ability to communicate clearly and effectively, both verbally and in writing
- A sense of personal, social, and ethical responsibility
- Intrapersonal strength, including insight into ones' own behavior and motivations, emotional stability, and the ability to persist and persevere when circumstances are difficult
- A strong desire to assist and support children, their families, and other professionals through educational and psychological processes
- Understanding of and respect for persons from diverse backgrounds and with varying experiences and worldviews
- The ability to provide leadership and facilitate effective problem solving within small groups
- The ability to adapt successfully to changing conditions and expectations and to be resilient in stressful situations
- The ability to be well organized and to complete a high volume of tasks in a timely manner

To some extent, these skills and personal characteristics may be taught, learned, or refined within a graduate training program in school psychology. There is also the reality that many of these attributes are developed and refined over one's lifetime and that it may be difficult to simply "teach" the characteristics during the graduate training years. For example, if a new graduate student begins his or her training with noticeable deficits in social and interpersonal skills, there may be limits to how much these characteristics can be improved during a 3- to 5-year period of graduate education. Thus school psychology training program faculty are likely to carefully consider an applicant's possession of these desired personal attributes during the admission process for graduate school.

## Faculty

Each school psychology training program must have faculty to teach courses, admit and advise students, administer the program, supervise student research and field training, and assist students in their transition from internship to regular employment, including endorsing them for licensure or certification after they have completed all program requirements. This list is only partial. School psychology trainers do not operate independently or within a vacuum (although they may sometimes feel that this is the case!). Rather, they are typically part of a broader faculty within a college of education or department of psychology and as such have faculty responsibilities within the larger context outside of the program. School psychology faculty may teach undergraduate courses or other graduate courses outside of the school psychology program. They may have departmental, college, or university committee responsibilities, such as serving on the faculty senate or being on a personnel or facilities committee. They may have administrative responsibilities outside of the program, such as budget planning, program development, and review of personnel decisions, such as tenure and promotion or hiring. In addition, school psychology faculty members are typically expected to contribute to their field outside of the college or university context. They may provide leadership or other service in state or national school psychology organizations and collaborate with state departments of education in developing the standards for the profession within that state. School psychology faculty may be asked to serve as editorial board members or editors of professional journals or newsletters within the field. Faculty who work at institutions in which research and the production of scholarly work are considered primary activities are expected to conduct research, publish articles in peer-reviewed journals, and present their research at professional meetings. They may also be expected to write books, develop products (e.g., assessment tools and intervention programs) for use in the field, and secure funding for their research or training efforts through submitting grant proposals to government agencies or private foundations. In some cases, school psychology faculty may provide professional services in schools or clinics on a part-time basis or work as consultants to school districts or other organizations. Indeed, the roles and expectations of school psychology faculty are many and varied, and this role requires creativity and the ability to juggle multiple responsibilities.

Faculty in school psychology programs typically work full time for the institutions in which the programs are housed, although many programs hire part-time "adjunct" faculty to teach courses and assist in supervising the training of students in other ways. In many cases, these adjunct faculty members are full-time practitioners or administrators in school districts and clinics. Given that there are more than 200 institutions of higher education in the United States and Canada that support school psychology training programs, a very conservative estimate is that at least 600 full-time school psychology faculty and many adjunct faculty are employed at these institutions. We reach this conclusion by examining the training and accrediting standards of the national organizations and through our own experience examining what is typical practice in training programs. NASP's *Standards for Training and Field Placement Programs in School Psychology* (NASP, 2000d) state that each approved program must have "at least three full-time equivalent faculty members" (p. 12). APA's *Guidelines and Principles for Accreditation of Programs in Professional Psychology* (APA, 2002b) do not have a specific requirement in terms of number of faculty in accredited programs, but instead state that programs must have "an identifiable core faculty responsible for its leadership who . . . are sufficient in number for their academic and professional responsibilities" (p. 10). In practice, programs differ in the number of faculty they have, a figure that is usually correlated with the number of students in a program. Usually, the more students a program admits, the more faculty members the program has. Data from a 2003 policy clarification document from APA indicate that APA-accredited PhD programs in school psychology have an average of 4.5 core faculty per program and a mean ratio of 8.8 students for each faculty member in the program (APA, 2003).

As training standards and professional expectations have evolved over the years, the doctoral degree has become the entry-level educational attainment to work as a school psychology faculty member, at least on a full-time basis (some programs may employ specialist-level adjunct faculty to assist in supervising students or teaching courses). The few surveys of characteristics of school psychology trainers that have been published in recent years (e.g., Reschly & Wilson, 1995; Thomas, 1998) indicate that the demographic characteristics of school psychology faculty differ to some extent from those of graduate students and the field in general. For example, although women make up about 80% of graduate students in school psychology and about 70% of practitioners, they account for just slightly more than half of school psychology trainers (Curtis, 2002). For whatever reason, the percentage of women in school psychology faculty positions has lagged behind that of the field in general. However, the percentage of women who enter faculty positions has increased substantially from the 18% reported in 1969–1970 (Curtis, 2002), and we anticipate that this trend will continue to the point at which the percentage of female trainers will be considerably larger than the percentage of male trainers within the next decade or two as the number of new graduates continues to reflect at least 80% women. However, it has also been our observation that the gender representation of trainers is related to more than just the demographics of doctoral graduates entering the field. In our collective experience as trainers, we have observed that a smaller percentage of female than male doctoral graduates aspire to obtain full-time faculty appointments, or even view this role as desirable. This trend mirrors the percentage of female faculty members in psychology fields in general—that is, the percentage of female students does not match the percentage of female faculty members. Perhaps this trend will change in future years as more women enter faculty positions and become role models and mentors for graduate students.

In terms of ethnicity, the most recent estimates indicate that about 15% of program faculty are members of racial or ethnic minority groups, a figure that is close to the percentage of minority graduate students in school psychology training programs and more than twice as high as the percentage of minority school psychologists in general but that still is considerably lower than the 35% figure for racial or ethnic minority group members in U.S. society in general. It is our observation that diversity of school psychology faculty helps greatly to enhance diversity within student recruitment and retention. Programs that specifically emphasize multicultural diversity within their curricula and mission statements and that have faculty members of color are often more successful in recruiting minority students to their training programs. In terms of other demographic characteristics of school psychology faculty, such as age and prior experience as school psychology practitioners, no national or comparative data exist of which we are aware. There appear to be a substantial number of school psychology program faculty approaching retirement age within the next several years, and the employment market for well-qualified doctoral graduates who desire to become trainers is currently considered to be very strong. It was common for faculty who joined training programs two decades ago or longer to have had several years' experience as school psychologists in practice settings prior to becoming trainers. Certainly, there is much to be said for the mentoring and role modeling qualities of school psychology trainers who have extensive experience as practicing school psychologists. It is our observation that it is becoming increasingly typical for new program faculty to enter their first academic jobs directly out of graduate programs, with only practicum and internship experiences as practitioners, and less common for new faculty members to have had several years' prior experience as practitioners. Perhaps the increased demands on academicians in recent years to establish prominent research and publication records—regardless of the type of institution at which they work—has been responsible in part for this perceived trend. The "publish or perish" nature of faculty positions at many institutions certainly may drive this phenomenon.

What are the personal characteristics or attributes necessary to help one become a successful faculty member in a school psychology training program? To start with, the characteristics we have previously noted as desirable for graduate students and practicing school psychologists would be of great value in making an excellent trainer. To these qualities, we add a few more that we believe are especially relevant to the unique demands and expectations of being a faculty member:

- A desire to mentor graduate students into the profession and to serve as a professional guide and role model for them
- The ability to juggle multiple—and often conflicting—role demands and expectations (for example, staying current in practice within the field while also establishing a strong program of scholarly work)
- The ability to think creatively and establish innovative programs of teaching, scholarly work, and clinical training
- The ability and desire to stay current on trends and findings within the field of school psychology and to continually incorporate new ideas into teaching and scholarly work
- The ability to work effectively and positively within systems that often have what we call a "lean schedule of reinforcement," understanding that some important efforts and roles required to be a good trainer and faculty member will not necessarily be rewarded or highly valued by the institution
- For faculty who work at research universities or other institutions at which research and scholarly work is an essential expectation, it is absolutely necessary for one to have the desire to engage in these activities on a continual basis and to produce the expected results (publications, products) at regular intervals and sometimes in large volume

After reading this list of desired characteristics (and some of the implications), some graduate students may wonder why one would want to become a faculty member in the first place! Although there some aggravations and frustrations built into the role of a trainer—just as there are the role of a practitioner—we do not intend to discourage graduate students from considering careers as faculty members. On the contrary, we view this role as exciting, tremendously rewarding, and usually quite enjoyable. Having the opportunity to shape the future of the field and to mentor graduate students into the profession is a great privilege, and we think that being a school psychology trainer is a great career path for those graduate students who are so inclined and have the necessary characteristics.

# PRACTICUM AND INTERNSHIP TRAINING

In the applied or professional areas of psychology and education, students develop expertise in the practice of their particular field through supervised field experience. The field of school psychology has particularly strong traditions and practices in this area. Both NASP and APA have been active in shaping field experience standards for the field and have addressed expectations for practicum and internship training at length in their respective guidelines for training and credentialing (APA, 2002b; NASP, 2000b). Although there are some differences in the standards of the two organizations with respect to field training (especially with regard to differences between specialist- and doctoral-level training standards), there is also a great deal of similarity.

## Practicum Training in School Psychology

Practicum training generally begins early during the graduate training experience. It is not unusual for school psychology training programs to have students begin a limited practicum placement during their first year in the program. Practicum training provides an opportunity for students to receive an orientation to the culture and expectations of schools and related systems, to become familiar with professional practice in the field through observing and shadowing a practicing school psychologist, and to take on gradually increasing responsibilities for providing professional services. Professional services provided during the practicum experience may include assessment, consultation, and direct interventions conducted under the supervision of an experienced credentialed professional.

Training programs vary in terms of their specific expectations and opportunities for practicum training. Some programs maintain university-based clinics or service centers in which students practice their clinical skills by providing direct services to the public under the supervision of program faculty. Other programs do not maintain such clinics but place their students in practicum settings in the community. These settings are primarily in public schools, but they are not limited to such settings, particularly in doctoral programs. For example, training programs that are located in universities with medical centers may also provide practicum opportunities for their students in specialty medical clinics under the supervision of licensed psychologists. In addition, training programs that have relationships with child guidance, mental health, or residential treatment facilities may create practicum opportunities for their students in these agencies.

By definition, practicum training occurs on a time-limited basis while students also complete academic course work, research, and other program requirements. A practicum experience may be tied to a specific academic course (such as a consultation or assessment course), or it may be broader in scope. In a typical arrangement, practicum placements require anywhere from 6 to 10 hours per week, and they might be done in one or more time blocks per week. Practicum experiences typically include time for on-site supervision with the field supervisor, but by definition they are conducted under the direction of the training program and may include weekly supervision and training seminars with program faculty . The best available survey on the practicum requirements of school psychology training programs is found in Thomas's (1998) NASP-published directory of training programs. This resource indicates a median of 225 clock hours of practicum training for master's-level training programs, 360 clock hours for specialist-level programs, and 600 clock hours for doctoral-level programs, with a wide variation in clock-hour requirements within each level.

## Internship Training in School Psychology

Internship training differs from practicum training in four major ways. First, rather than being integrated within the academic course work, internships are conducted at the end of a student's program of study, after all course work, practica, and other program requirements have been completed. Second, rather than being a part-time experience with limited involvement, internships require a full-time commitment over the course of an academic or calendar year (although both NASP and APA allow for internships to be conducted on a half-time basis over 2 years by special arrangement). Third, whereas supervision of practicum experiences is usually the direct responsibility of faculty within the training program (with assistance from field supervisors on site), internship training is conducted under the direct supervision of a field supervisor, with the training program playing a more limited role, such as progress monitoring, communicating with the student and supervisor, and student evaluation. And fourth, although practicum training experiences may focus on limited types of professional skills, interns are expected to provide a comprehensive range of professional services, using and integrating a broad range of skills. In essence, the internship is a capstone experience of student's graduate training in school psychology, one of the final steps toward independence as a professional.

Definitions of what constitutes a full-time internship in school psychology vary somewhat based on training programs, organizational training standards, and level of training. As long as they meet the training standards of relevant professional association(s), and assuming that they satisfy the credentialing requirements of the states or provinces in which they are located, training programs may establish their own unique guidelines for internship training in order to make this experience appropriate to the specific objectives of the program. Some of the primary general principles and guidelines for internship training in school psychology are as follows:

- For specialist-level internships, NASP requires that the internship must be at least 1,200 clock hours, which is equivalent to full-time work for an academic year or half-time work over a 2-year period.
- For doctoral-level internships, both APA and NASP require a minimum of 1,500 clock hours. Some predoctoral internships (particularly those in non-school settings or consortiums) may require as many as 2,000 clock hours.
- NASP training standards stipulate that approximately half of the internship time (600 hours minimum) must be conducted in school settings. APA has no such setting-specific requirement, a difference that has been a point of contention between the two organizations with respect to doctoral training programs.

- Internships must be conducted under the supervision of an appropriately credentialed school psychologist or, in the case of non-school settings, a board-licensed psychologist. Supervision duties may be split among two supervisors if needed. Supervisors of specialist-level interns are expected to hold at least a specialist degree, whereas supervisors of predoctoral interns are expected to hold a doctoral degree.
- A minimum of 2 hours per week of individual, face-to-face supervision between interns and their supervisors is the general expectation.
- The internship experience is considered to be a training experience, not just full-time employment. Thus the internship should be based on a written internship plan and include a broad range of activities, including activities such as group supervision seminars, professional development workshops, opportunities for observation of supervisors, and so forth.
- The training program monitors the student's internship experience to ensure that the objectives of the program are realized. The internship supervisors and training program faculty communicate as needed for problem solving and evaluation of the student's progress.

The process of securing an internship placement is as variable as the training and internship programs. NASP has yet to adopt any accreditation or approval program for specialist-level internships, so there is no central clearinghouse for posting internship positions. School psychology training programs typically develop their own network of internship settings on an informal basis, and it is not unusual for students from particular training programs to intern at these sites. Information on internship opportunities is often sent to training program directors and then posted for potential interns to consider. Attending state school psychology association conferences and networking with psychologists and administrators from potential internship sites is a time-honored way to get one's foot in the door for an internship. If a student is willing to look nationally rather than regionally for internship opportunities, attendance at a national convention (NASP or APA) often provides similar networking opportunities on a broader scale, and such national opportunities are sometimes advertised in professional newsletters such as the NASP *Communiqué* or APA *Monitor on Psychology*. In addition, students who desire to stay or to locate in a particular geographical area are often successful in securing internships by contacting school psychologists and administrators early in the year prior to their internships, letting them know of their interest and availability and initiating a dialogue.

Potential interns in doctoral programs in school psychology often secure their internships through the same methods as were discussed for specialist-level internships. However, for many doctoral-level internships, an established network is available for accreditation and posting of internships. APA accredits predoctoral internships and posts a listing of accredited sites on its website (www.apa.org) and in each December issue of the *American Psychologist*. APA-accredited internships operate their posting, applications, and notification process through the Association of Psychological Postdoctoral and Internship Centers (APPIC; www.appic.org. APPIC listings include APA-accredited internships, as well as many other doctoral-level internships that are not APA-accredited but that agree to operate under the conditions established by APPIC, which are similar to those of APA. Although many of the internship opportunities in this network are not appropriate or relevant for school psychology students (i.e., those that focus exclusively on adult populations), this system includes a considerable number of other internship opportunities that are appropriate for school psychology students. These opportunities include a limited number of school districts, consortiums between school districts and community agencies, child guidance centers, residential treatment centers for youths, children's medical centers, and some community mental health agencies that work extensively with schools and children. The advantage for students to securing internships through this established network is the all sites have agreed to provide training opportunities and appropriate supervision, areas that are sometimes problematic when a student develops his or her own internship.

Finding a good internship placement is a critically important element of becoming a successful school psychologist. A carefully planned and supervised internship experience will help a student move into the field appropriately prepared and well positioned for future success. Internships that do not meet one's expectations for training and supervision may prove to be disappointing and may even discourage a student from working in the field. As school psychology trainers, we have seen both results and much prefer the former outcome to the latter. With careful planning and a willingness to go where the best training opportunity is available, the positive outcome is more likely. Selection of the best internship site is dependent to some extent on whether a student is geographically mobile and thus able to go to where the better opportunities are. For students who are place-bound, opportunities must be secured within a limited locale, and in some cases the fewer choices involved in such situations means that extra planning and effort are required for a good internship experience. Almost all full-time internships in school psychology are paid experiences. Although accepting unpaid internships is sometimes a reality for students who are not willing or able to relocate to sites that offer paid opportunities, we do not encourage unpaid full-time internship situations and believe that some of these situations often border on exploitation. The rate of pay varies greatly by states and regions. It has been our experience that the lower-paid internships typically pay a student about half of what a fully credentialed beginning school psychologist would earn in that setting, although it is more typical for interns to earn five eighths to three fourths of the salary of a beginning credentialed professional in that setting. Some interns may even be able to negotiate for full salary, especially in districts in which interns are hired to fill vacant school psychologist positions rather than to fill position specifically allotted to interns. In addition to salary, it is important for interns to consider whether the district provides benefits, such as health care insurance. Particularly for interns with families, it may make monetary sense to take a lower-paying internship that comes with benefits rather than a higher-paying internship with no attached benefits. One's personal circumstances and needs will be important in determining how much the financial remuneration aspect of the internship will influence the selection of a training site.

## CREDENTIALING IN SCHOOL PSYCHOLOGY: CERTIFICATION AND LICENSURE

Completing the internship and receiving the graduate degree or completion certificate in a school psychology program is a necessary but insufficient step toward working as a school psychologist. To work as a practitioner in a public school or independent-practice setting, one must not only have the necessary academic preparation but must also possess an appropriate credential. In some cases, getting the necessary license or certificate credential following completion of the program and endorsement by the training program faculty is a formality—the training institution certifies that the individual who is applying for the credential has completed all essential program requirements, the applicant completes the paperwork process (including providing information for a criminal background check to be performed) and pays a fee, and the credential soon appears in the mail. However, in many cases, the process is more complex and in some instances downright intimidating, requiring a more lengthy application process, rigorous transcript evaluation, written exam, and in some cases an oral exam with licensing board members. This section provides a brief overview of the three most common credentialing processes that school psychologists are likely to encounter: state department of education certification/licensure, the Nationally Certified School Psychologist credential from NASP, and licensing for independent practice as a psychologist from state psychology licensing boards.

## State Department of Education Certification/Licensure

Each of the 50 U.S. states has particular processes in place for credentialing professional educators and related service professionals (e.g., school administrators, speech–language pathologists, school counselors, school psychologists) to work in the public school systems of that state. Prior to about the 1980s, this process was almost always referred to as *certification*, and it culminated in receipt of a certificate allowing one to work in public school settings. After some of the educational reform activities that were typical in U.S. states in the 1980s and 1990s, some states changed the title of the credential they awarded from certificate to *license*, but the intent and meaning was the same: to allow the holder of that credential to work within his or her specialty area within the public schools. The Canadian provinces have similar procedures for credentialing individuals to work as education professionals within public school systems. The purpose of state or provincial credentialing is quality control. The state legislature sets minimum preparation standards that must be attained for one to work as a teacher, counselor, school psychologist, and so forth, and then verifies that these standards have been met prior to issuing the practice credential.

The typical route to receiving a credential within the state in which one's training program is located is to obtain an endorsement from the training program, which is then accepted by the state or provincial department of education as evidence that the training criteria have been met. States may have additional requirements, such as evidence of satisfactory scores on general skills and communication tests (such as the National Teacher Exam Core Battery or the California Basic Skills Test) and specialty knowledge tests specific to school psychology (such as the Praxis II Educational Specialty Area Test for School Psychologists). Although some states have entered into reciprocal certification compacts with other states, for applicants who are applying for a state department of education credential following completing of a training program in another state or upon demonstrating that they are similarly credentialed in another state, the process may be more complicated. Because out-of-state institutions are not approved by that particular state department of education, a detailed transcript evaluation process may be required to ensure that the standards of the state have been met. In addition, the state credentialing body may require the applicant to demonstrate evidence of completion of their out-of-state training program through an additional endorsement process. As school psychology trainers, we have all had the experience of receiving such requests from graduates of our training programs, some of whom completed the program years before we were employed there. Because there is variability in the training and credentialing standards adopted by individual states and provinces, an individual may complete a training program in one state, obtain experience working as a school psychologist in that state, and still not meet the credentialing requirements of another state in which he or she is attempting to gain employment. In such instances, additional specific course work is sometimes necessary, although states may issue a temporary credential and allow the applicant a period of a year or two to show evidence of completing the additional requirements. Because credentialing requirements may vary considerably across states and provinces, we advise that individuals who are considering practicing in a state other than the one in which they were trained research carefully the specific requirements of that state and ensure that they complete the necessary expectations prior to completion of their training program, if possible.

## Nationally Certified School Psychologist Credential

In 1988, NASP established the National School Psychology Certification Board (NSPCB), which administers the process of awarding the Nationally Certified School Psychologist (NCSP) credential. The board and the NCSP credential were established for the purpose of providing a national standard that can be used as a measure of professionalism by interested agencies and individuals and to recognize school psychologists who meet this national standard. Additional purposes for establishing the NCSP program include the promotion of continuing professional development among school psychologists and a desire to foster cooperation and commonality among groups that recognize school psychologists. Among the circumstances surrounding the creation of the NCSP was the fact that so much variation exists across states with regard to the criteria for being considered for school psychology certification or licensure (Batsche & Curtis, 2003). Although NASP has made it clear that it is not the intent of the NSPCB to certify school psychologists for employment nor to impose personnel requirements on agencies and organizations (NASP, 2004), an implicit goal in the development of the NCSP is to promote the NASP standard of the 60-semester-hour specialist-level graduate training program, including a 1,200 hour internship, as the entry level for practice as a school psychologist.

Awarding of the NCSP requires the following:

- Completion of a minimum 60-semester-hour graduate level training program in school psychology
- Completion of an internship of at least 1,200 clock hours as part of the training program under the supervision of an appropriately credentialed school psychologist and including a minimum of 600 clock hours in a school setting
- Receipt of a passing score (currently 660) on the Praxis National School Psychology Examination administered by Educational Testing Service

Graduates of NASP-approved training programs automatically qualify to apply for the NCSP credential and to take the exam without a transcript review following completion of their graduate programs. However, the NCSP is not limited to graduates of NASP-approved programs. Individuals who graduate from any recognized school psychology graduate training program may be approved to take the national exam and ultimately receive the NCSP credential if they can demonstrate that their program included the appropriate amount and types of course work, practicum, and internship experiences. Course work requirements are explicit in the NCSP criteria, based on NASP standards, and include specific areas within the domains of psychological and educational foundations, interventions and problem solving, statistics and research methodologies, and professional school psychology. The process for making a determination of eligibility in such cases is the responsibility of the NSPCB.

According to Hunley (2004), the NCSP enjoyed an initial burst of popularity following its establishment in 1988, but interest appears to have leveled off, with only about half of NASP members currently possessing the credential; these members are disproportionately older than the NASP membership in general. Apparently, a majority of school psychologists who are relatively new to the field do not view the credential as something that is essential for them to pursue. Despite the less than universal interest in the NCSP, there are some practical reasons that recent graduates may wish to pursue the NCSP credential. It may be viewed favorably as an indication of one's commitment to professionalism when seeking employment or advancement in the field. Perhaps more important, the NCSP has slowly emerged as a standard for many state departments of education to accept when applicants from other states apply for a license or certificate to practice in that state. According to Hunley, 21 state departments of education currently accept the NCSP credential as evidence of meeting or exceeding their requirements for school psychology credentialing.

## State Board of Examiners in Psychology License

Obtaining licensure for the independent practice of psychology and for use of the term "psychologist" (not "school psychologist") requires that one have a doctoral degree in psychology and meet the specific application and approval requirements of a state board of examiners in psychology. Independent practice as a psychologist is sometimes confused with the term "private practice." Although it is true that psychologists in private practice settings are independently practicing as psychologists, independent practice is not limited to these. Psychologists who work in public and private hospitals, clinics, health-maintenance organizations, community mental health centers, college and university counseling centers, and various other settings are also engaging in the independent practice of psychology. That is, they are using the term "psychologist," offering psychological services to the public, and are not required to work under the supervision of another licensed mental health professional in order to engage in these activities. By contrast, the term "school psychologist" is recognized in the psychology licensing laws of most states as applying to those who have a state department of education credential in school psychology and whose practice is limited to school settings. These licensing and terminology differences have long been a point of contention between NASP (which advocates for specialist-level school psychologists being able to engage in independent practice) and APA (which advocates that independent practice be limited to those holding a doctoral degree).

It is important to understand that neither NASP nor APA "owns" or regulates the terms "school psychologist" or "psychologist," nor are there any federal laws dictating how these terms are to be used. Rather, legal regulation is the domain of states and provinces. Aside from contacting specific licensing boards, the best source for general information on state licensure for independent practice is the Association of State and Provincial Psychology Boards (ASPPB; P.O. Box 2125, Montgomery, AL 36124-1245; phone: 334-832-4580), an organization that coordinates and supports board licensing efforts among the states and provinces and that maintains an extensive website at www.asppb.org. Although there is some variation in the licensure requirements established by specific state boards, there are also many similarities. In most cases, being recognized as a licensed psychologist for independent practice requires:

- A doctoral degree in psychology
- Completion of at least 2 years of supervised (by a licensed psychologist) psychology practice experience, of which at least 1 of the years must be at the postdoctoral level
- A passing score on the Examination for Professional Practice in Psychology (there is no universal standard for passing scores—each state or province establishes its own criteria for passing)
- A passing score on a state or provincial jurisprudence (law and ethics) exam administered by the board and, in some cases, an oral exam or case presentation to the board

Despite the commonalities in requirements among state and provincial licensing boards, it is not a given that psychologists who are licensed in one state will automatically qualify for licensure elsewhere, and the process of obtaining licensure in a new area is sometimes complex and time-consuming. However, a recent effort of ASPPB has been to establish a procedure for making license reciprocity among states and mobility for psychologists easier than it has been in the past. This procedure involves registering one's credentials with ASPPB and obtaining their Certificate of Qualification in Professional Psychology.

Given the apparent complexity of obtaining licensure for independent practice as a psychologist, why would a doctoral-level school psychologist who already has a state department of education credential in school psychology want to go through this process? The major benefit is that an independent practice license allows school psychologists to practice in nontraditional settings (e.g., clinics, hospitals, community health centers, private practice groups) where their training in school psychology may allow them to provide unique services. Other benefits include the role expansion that such opportunities provide to school psychologists and the impact that school psychologists may be able to make in settings in which they may be the only professionals trained in their specialty.

## Specialty Credentialing

In addition to the basic licensure and certification types just described, various additional opportunities exist for school psychologists to receive recognition of their particular areas of competence, especially at the doctoral level of training. For example, the American Board of Professional Psychology (ABPP; see www.abpp.org for more information) has established processes for board certification in 13 different specialty areas of doctoral-level training, including school psychology. Some school psychologists with particular skills and interests in applied behavior analysis have obtained certification from the Behavior Analyst Certification Board (BACB; see www.bacb.com for more information), a credential that is available to master's- and specialist-level practitioners, as well as doctoral-level practitioners (and that includes fields other than psychology) and that requires specific course work and supervised experience in behavior analysis. Some school psychologists who have gone through training programs with a strong emphasis on counseling skills have earned the National Board Certified Counselor credential (NBCC; see www.nbcc.org for more information) in recognition of having developed specific expertise in the area of counseling. Other specialty credentials and recognition programs are also available. Specialty credentials are usually not required for specific employment, but they can serve as evidence to potential employers and the public that one has acquired specialized expertise.

## CONTINUING PROFESSIONAL DEVELOPMENT

Given the great effort required to get admitted to a graduate program in school psychology, to successfully complete the program, to complete a 1-year supervised internship, and to receive a certificate, license, or other credentials for the practice of school psychology and specialty areas, it is often surprising to new school psychologists that they are not really "done" with their training and professional development. On the contrary, continuing professional development is an important part of being a school psychologist. It is not only considered to be an important value within the profession but, in many cases, it is required for maintaining practice credentials. In thinking about the importance and necessity of continuing professional development, consider that new knowledge and techniques are constantly emerging in the field of school psychology and that what may have been best practice 10 or 20 years ago may currently be considered obsolete.

State boards of education vary in their specific requirements for renewal of school psychology certificates or licenses. These credentials are typically issued for a specified number of years—say 3–5—with the stipulation that the recipient must show evidence of meeting specified professional development requirements before the credential is renewed for another period of time. Some states require a minimum number of years of professional employment during the credential period for it to be renewed. Some states require completion of a specified minimum number of clock hours of approved continuing professional development activities (such as workshop or conference attendance). Some states have both experience and training requirements for credential renewal. NASP's NSPCB requires renewal of the NCSP certificate every 3 years, a process that requires documentation of 75 clock hours of continuing professional development activities during the 3-year time period. State and provincial psychology licensing boards vary somewhat in terms of their requirements for license renewal, but a typical approach is to require documentation of a minimum of 40 clock hours of approved professional training activities (e.g., graduate course work or approved professional training workshops) for every 2-year renewal cycle. In each of these instances, credential renewal requires not only documentation of the required activities but also completion of an application form and payment of a renewal fee, which in some instances can be over $100.

Continuing professional development activities can take a variety of forms, and each credentialing body has its own specific rules governing what activities are acceptable. The most common activities include attending professional workshops or taking graduate-level continuing education courses from school psychology programs or related professional training programs. The annual NASP and APA conventions provide a wealth of opportunities for professional training and development, as do most state affiliates of NASP and APA at their own annual or semiannual conferences. Many areas—particularly large metropolitan areas—have numerous opportunities available for attending privately sponsored professional training workshops in the education and mental health fields. In addition, independent study programs are available for continuing professional development from some national and state professional associations and from some of the same private organizations that sponsor professional training workshops.

## DISCUSSION QUESTIONS AND ACTIVITIES

1. If you are currently a graduate student in a school psychology training program and are using this text as part of an introductory school psychology course, discuss your own process of learning about the field and making the decision to apply to graduate training programs in the field. Why did you select school psychology over other areas of professional psychology (clinical or counseling) or over other professions within the field of education? Why did you choose to enter the particular graduate training program where you currently study?

2. Using the Internet, locate the standards for training programs in school psychology in the documents from APA and NASP that are referenced in this chapter. Review and evaluate the requirements for specific areas of course work and field experience for accredited programs. Do you consider these requirements to be sufficient? Do you think that the requirements should be more specific or more general than they are currently?

3. Although the debate regarding the appropriate entry level of training required to become a school psychologist (specialist level or doctoral level) has raged for years, there has not been a substantial increase in the percentage of doctoral-level school psychologists, who currently make up only about 25% of the professionals in the field. What are the issues and practical considerations that have resulted in little change in the entry-level debate or status of the field over the years?

4. Go to the APPIC website at www.appic.org or to recent issues of the NASP *Communiqué* or other professional newsletters and study the internship opportunities available to specialist-level and doctoral-level students in school psychology. What are the elemenostings that make them attractive or unattractive to potential applicants?

5. Increasingly, school psychologists are required to engage in specified continuing professional development activities to keep their practice credentials current. What are the advantages and disadvantages of typical methods of professional development training (e.g., attending workshops and conferences)? Are there possible alternative methods of continuing professional development for school psychologists that should be considered as evidence of meeting recredentialing requirements?

# 5

# Working as a School Psychologist

EMPLOYMENT TRENDS, OPPORTUNITIES, AND CHALLENGES

In the previous chapters we outlined general issues regarding what school psychologists do, the history of the field of school psychology and the broader field of education, and provided information on training to become a school psychologist. In this chapter, we focus more specifically on the job of a school psychologist and address the following questions: How does one obtain a job as a school psychologist? In what settings are school psychologists employed? What functions or roles do school psychologists serve? Who are school psychologists? And what is the job outlook in the field of school psychology? In our opinion there are some encouraging, as well as discouraging, trends in the field of school psychology. On the encouraging side, the job market in school psychology is quite favorable for those seeking employment in the field, and it is likely to remain so for the next several decades. A shortage of school psychologists became evident in the 1990s and shows no signs of remitting in the near future. Thus current students can be comfortable in the knowledge that there will be jobs for them (both in the practitioner sector and the academic sector) when they complete their graduate training. On the discouraging side are the data that indicate that changes in actual job functions of school psychologists are not keeping up with changing views of school psychology as a profession. Although leaders in the field of school psychology, the professional organizations that support school psychology, and many practicing school psychologists have been advocating for role expansion, the majority of school psychologists are still not engaged in comprehensive psychological services. Instead their roles—with some notable exceptions—are still primarily focused on the assessment aspect of service provision and likely still very much tied to the "sorter" or "gatekeeper" role of the school psychologist first discussed in Chapter 2. However, we continue to believe that role expansion is gradually occurring and that future school psychologists will be less tied to these roles than the school psychologists of today are.

## OBTAINING A JOB AS A SCHOOL PSYCHOLOGIST

Upon completion of graduate school, individuals with specialist-level degrees (including those with EdS degrees, as well as MA/MS/MEd degrees who have completed a 60-credit-hour program) and doctoral degrees are prepared to enter the workforce. (As noted in Chapter 1, some states may have lower entry-level requirements, but a 60-credit program as required by NASP is the most common standard.) Those with specialist-level degrees are most commonly employed in public school districts as school psychologists. Prior to obtaining a job as a school psychologist, an individual must obtain certification or educator licensure through the state's office of education (see Chapter 4 for more details on this process). The search for a job typically begins toward the end of a student's internship year. Many students may desire to continue to work in the districts in which they completed their internships. For such students, it should be easy to identify who to contact within the school district to inquire about job opportunities. For students wishing to find employment in a different district or to relocate to another state, the process of locating districts with open jobs and contact individuals within those districts can be somewhat daunting.

Unfortunately, there is no national posting of all jobs available in the field of school psychology. However, there are some resources students can use to attempt to locate districts with open positions. The NASP *Communiqué* (the official NASP newsletter), which is published 10 times per year, prints job announcements, and some school districts will advertise open positions in this publication. However, the number of open jobs listed in the *Communiqué* is very small, so students should not rely solely on this method to help them locate possible positions. NASP also maintains a career center as part of its website (www.naspcareer.org) on which employers can post jobs and job seekers can search the listed postings. However, as with the *Communiqué*, only a small number of jobs are actually posted on this website. In fact, in a recent search of this site, we found only 32 open positions listed, a figure that certainly represents only a small fraction of the total number of jobs available. Jobs may also be posted on the NASP members' electronic mailing list, as well as on websites of state school psychology organizations. In addition, school psychology program training directors are often sent job announcements to share with their students, and many of these announcements are also sent to college or university career planning centers. However, even taking into account all these different methods, it is likely that most jobs are secured through more informal avenues. Thus it is crucial that students be proactive in their job searches.

Most students locate open professional positions by contacting individuals in school districts in which they are interested in working and inquiring as to whether there are open positions within the district or whether it is anticipated that there may be open positions for the following school year. However, knowing who one should contact can be confusing and often varies by school district. In many school districts, it is the special education director or coordinator who will be able to provide this information. In other school districts, it may be someone in the human resources or personnel office. In still other districts, especially those that are quite small, it may be the superintendent or someone in the superintendent's office. If a prospective job applicant is unsure who the best person is to contact initially, a good course of action is to make contact with one of the district's school psychologists. This person can then (hopefully) direct the student to the appropriate person who will know about job openings.

Contacting current school psychologists also can be beneficial to applicants who are interested in obtaining more information regarding the practice of school psychology in a particular district. For example, applicants might ask about expected school loads, typical number of assessments completed, ability to engage in intervention and consultative services, and general work atmosphere of the district. Generally students can contact a district's school psychologists by calling the school district office. Some school psychologists may be housed in a central district office location. Others may have offices in their schools. Even for those with school-based offices, district office personnel should be able to provide information on how to best reach a school psychologist.

After finding the appropriate contact person in a school district, the applicant will likely be able to ask about the procedures involved in applying for a job in that district. Typically an application form must be completed. Along with this form, the applicant should provide a vita or resume, as well as names of references. School districts will often (although not always) desire formal letters of recommendation from individuals with whom the applicant has worked. In addition, some school districts have their own recommendation forms, which must be completed by the applicant's references. These recommendations should be completed by professional contacts who can attest to the applicant's skills and potential for excellence in school psychology. For individuals just out of graduate school, we recommend that the applicant seek one reference letter from his or her internship supervisor. Other recommendations will likely be obtained from graduate school instructors. If a recent graduate has formed a good working relationship with a school administrator at his or her internship site, such as a building principal, it may be useful to seek a letter of reference from that person as well.

In addition to the paper application and recommendations, school districts typically conduct interviews with job applicants. Applicants must treat these interviews seriously, arrive well prepared, and present themselves in a professional manner. In a pool of applicants in which many may be equal on paper, the interview can be the deciding factor in terms of who is offered the job. Interviews vary widely in terms of formality and questions asked. However, all applicants should be prepared to answer basic questions regarding their background in school psychology, perceived strengths and weaknesses, and their view of school psychology. Interviewers may ask applicants to respond to case scenarios. These can be intimidating for applicants, and, unfortunately, there is no specific way to prepare for such questions. By being familiar with best practices, applicants should be able to successfully answer questions of this nature.

In addition to the difficulty of knowing who to contact regarding job openings in a given school district, knowing when to look for jobs can also be a bit confusing. We recommend that individuals begin contacting school districts some time in late winter or early spring. However, many (if not most) school districts will be unsure of their funding situations and vacancy status at that time. Thus many school districts will not be in a position to make job offers until significantly later in the year. Many school districts will not even begin interviewing until later in the year; some may not begin the interview process until as late as May, when the school year is ending. Some districts may interview earlier in the year but then not make job offers for several months. Because this process is so variable by district, we recommend contacting districts earlier rather than later so applicants do not miss out on applying for a job simply because they did not get their application materials submitted early enough. That being said, applicants should not worry if they are told that a district is unsure of its ability to hire and will not know if there are open positions until later in the spring or even early summer. Although this type of response can be anxiety-provoking for students who want to know if they are going to be gainfully employed the following year, such a response is typical in many districts. As discussed later in this chapter, there is a nationwide shortage of school psychologists that is expected to continue for at least the next two decades. Given that shortage, it is highly likely that applicants who are not completely place-bound (i.e., in need of a job in one specific district) will be able to locate a job. In fact, our experience is that well-qualified, geographically mobile applicants often receive several job offers.

# OBTAINING A JOB IN A NON-SCHOOL SETTING

Individuals with doctoral degrees have more options than those with specialist-level degrees in terms of where they can find employment. Obviously, the K–12 schools are one common source of jobs for doctoral-level school psychologists, as well as specialist-level school psychologists. For doctoral-level school psychologists wishing to work in the schools, the process of locating a job is identical to that previously described for specialist-level graduates. In most school districts, there is no differentiation in the hiring process between those with PhDs and those with specialist-level degrees.

Other arenas in which doctoral-level psychologists may find employment include university training programs, medical centers or hospitals, and community mental health agencies. In addition, an individual with a doctoral degree may elect to pursue practice independently as a psychologist. Because most graduates of school psychology programs seek employment in public school settings, finding employment in each of these other areas is only briefly addressed.

## University Settings

The best places to look for postings of open faculty positions are in the APA *Monitor on Psychology* and the NASP *Communiqué*. In addition, prospective trainers would do well to stay in touch with their university training directors, as training directors often receive postings for academic positions from other programs and as job announcements are increasingly being sent via e-mail lists (e.g., the Trainers of School Psychologists mailing list). However, the majority of faculty positions in the United States and Canada, particularly those at research universities, are advertised in the APA *Monitor on Psychology*; thus this is the one best sources of information for such positions. Individuals interested in jobs in nonresearch universities may also find it helpful to look in the *Chronicle of Higher Education*. Unlike school-based positions, which often do not come open until later in the school year, university faculty positions are advertised early (generally in the fall and early winter of the year before the position is to begin). So, for an individual seeking a faculty position directly out of his or her doctoral program, the job search process begins almost immediately after beginning the internship year. Within each ad or announcement for a faculty position is a list of materials applicants must submit in order to apply for the position. Typically this includes a letter of application, curriculum vita, and three letters of recommendation. Universities may also want transcripts, copies of published articles, teaching evaluations, or other materials that demonstrate the potential for excellence as a faculty member. Applicants should mail copies of these materials and arrange for letters of recommendation to be sent to the address listed in the advertisement.

University positions typically involve a combination of research and teaching, but different universities place different weight on these activities. Typically, specialist-level programs place less emphasis on research than do doctoral-level programs. Due to the decreased emphasis on research, teaching loads in specialist-level programs may be higher than teaching loads in doctoral programs. Applicants should consider these differences and apply for positions that they believe are most suited to their interests and strengths.

Applicants for faculty positions should also keep in mind that "fit" (in terms of program philosophy and program needs) is an important quality in applying for academic jobs. It is important that applicants state clearly in their letters of application how they fit with the training program to which they are applying for a faculty position. Individuals should not apply for positions for which they perceive they are a poor fit. For example, if a job announcement indicates that the university is looking for a faculty member whose research involves behaviorally based interventions in the schools, it is unlikely that an individual whose research involves neuropsychological assessments for children with traumatic brain injury would be good fit for the program. It is important that applicants consider fit not just in terms of whether they would be competitive for the job but also in terms of whether they would enjoy the job. Teaching outside of one's area or working within a department in which the program philosophy differs substantially from one's own philosophy can make for a difficult job experience.

When evaluating academic positions, applicants should also seek to understand the supports available to them in the programs to which they are considering applying. As mentioned in Chapter 4, the demands on a university trainer can be many and are often not overtly rewarded. It is imperative that new faculty have good sources of support. This support may be partially provided by individuals outside of the university (e.g., a former graduate school advisor), but applicants for faculty positions should also assess support from within the program they are considering joining. For example, are colleagues friendly and easily accessible? Are administrative personnel (e.g., department head, dean) supportive of the program and its mission? Are new faculty assigned an experienced faculty mentor to help them navigate the complexities of academic life? Although these questions can be difficult to answer, taking time to investigate these supports can be invaluable to an applicant in choosing the position that is right for him or her.

## Clinical Settings

For individuals who desire to work in a clinical setting, such as a community mental health center, children's hospital, or specialty clinic, it may be important to first complete a postdoctoral fellowship. To practice independently in such settings, a license as a psychologist is necessary. This requires the completion of supervised postdoctoral hours; generally 2,000 hours are required. Thus individuals who have just graduated from a PhD program are not yet eligible for licensure. Some clinical settings may hire a person and provide the supervision necessary to obtain a license, but other settings will want applicants to have already achieved licensure. A postdoctoral fellowship is one way to obtain these hours and be eligible for licensure prior to applying for a full-time clinical position. Not only do postdoctoral positions allow individuals to accrue supervised hours toward licensure but such positions also allow individuals to obtain specialty training in certain areas (e.g., child neuropsychology, pediatric obesity). Although postdoctoral positions are by no means a required part of training, they do seem to be becoming more common in the applied fields of psychology, including school psychology.

Jobs in clinical settings, as well as postdoctoral positions, may be advertised in the APA *Monitor on Psychology* or NASP *Communiqué*, but, as with school-based positions, there is no one place in which individuals can find information on all such jobs. Informal networking (via faculty and internship mentors, as well as their contacts) may be needed to locate positions. Because clinical positions tend to be year-round jobs, there are no specific times of the year when most jobs are advertised. We recommend that individuals who desire a clinical position begin searching for these positions in the late winter or early spring of their internship years.

Although there are no specific qualifications (other than licensure) to work in most clinical settings, as with university positions, applicants should consider their "fit" with positions and how their prior training and interests match with the described job. For example, if applicants have no prior training working with children with autism, it is highly unlikely that they would be hired to fill a position in which this population was a large focus of the clinical work. Individuals should take care to the tailor their practicum, internship, and postdoctoral experiences (if any) so that they receive both the breadth and depth of experience that will prepare them for clinical jobs in their areas of interest following graduation.

## THE WORK SETTING

Although school psychologists, particularly those trained at the doctoral level, have the credentials to work in a number of different settings, the majority of school psychology graduates work in the public schools. According to data obtained from the 2002–2003 NASP membership survey, over three-quarters (77.1%) of school psychologists who are NASP members report working in public school settings. School psychologists not in the public schools report working in a variety of other settings, including: colleges or universities (5.4%), private practice (5.1%), private schools (2.4%), mental health agencies (1.2%), residential institutions (0.6%), and state departments of education (0.4%). A small number of individuals (7.9%) reported being employed in a setting other than one of these listed.

As would be expected given the employment settings of most school psychologists, the majority of these individuals report working as school psychologists. According to the NASP membership data of those school psychologists who reported their function, 78.5% reported working as school psychologists. The next most common function reported was that of an administrator; however, only 4.3% of individuals reported this as their function. Other functions endorsed included: trainer/educator (3.9%); clinical psychologist (2.3%); consultant (2.2%); supervisor (1.7%); counselor (1.2%); psychological examiner (1.2%); and educational diagnostician (0.8%). A small number of respondents (3.9%) indicated that their primary function was one "other" than those listed.

It should be acknowledged that these numbers likely underestimate the percentage of school psychologists working outside of school settings and those working in roles other than that of school psychologists, given that these numbers are based on responses to a NASP membership survey. It seems likely that individuals trained as school psychologists but no longer functioning in a school psychology–related role would be less likely to maintain their membership in NASP. However, it is clear from looking at this list of employment settings and roles that school psychologists are working in a number of areas in addition to the traditional school setting.

Even within the traditional school setting, a great deal of variability exists in the work settings (as well as the roles and functions, as will be discussed later) of school psychologists. For example, most school psychologists serve multiple schools. These school psychologists are frequently based out of a central district office (where they typically have their own office space) rather than having school-based offices. However, some school psychologists are school-based and serve just one school, allowing them to become a part of that school's daily workings and culture. In a recent survey of school psychologists across the country (Thomas, 2000c), school psychologists reported that on average (median) they served three schools. However, the medians by state ranged from one (in New York) to six (in Arkansas, Hawaii, Mississippi, North Dakota, and West Virginia), a very wide variation.

School psychologist-to-student ratios also vary considerably and will affect the services that a school psychologist is able to provide. Currently, NASP recommends a school psychologist-to-student ratio of 1:1,000. However, as Thomas (2000c) demonstrated, it is rare to find states that meet this recommended ratio. At a national level, the median school psychologist-to-student ratio is 1:1,500. Based on data from Thomas's survey, only five states met the recommended ratio based on their median reported ratios: Connecticut (1:700), Massachusetts (1:850), New Jersey (1:1,000), New Mexico (1:925), and New York (1:750).

## School Psychologists in Nontraditional Settings

As noted earlier, a small portion of individuals trained as school psychologists do not work in school settings or are not employed as school psychologists. However, it is almost impossible to obtain data specifically on what these individuals are doing given that most surveys of school psychologists are geared toward those working in more traditional settings and that most survey samples are drawn from NASP's membership list. As discussed in previous chapters and later in this chapter, increasing emphasis has been given to the expansion of the role of the school psychologist. With this role expansion, and as school psychologists become increasingly recognized as providers of comprehensive mental health and educational services rather than simply being psychometricians, it is likely that the number of school psychologists working in "nontraditional" (i.e., non-school) settings will expand. Obviously, this role expansion will also allow school psychologists to provide more comprehensive services within school settings. An example of this role expansion is the emergence of pediatric school psychology as a new subspecialty within the field of school psychology. Pediatric school psychologists specialize in meeting the needs of children with medical conditions, including collaborating with medical providers about optimal treatments and working with educators to meet the needs of individual children with health problems, as well as developing primary and secondary prevention programs to promote healthy behaviors (Power, DuPaul, Shapiro, & Parrish, 1995).

The likelihood of doctoral-level school psychologists working in non-school settings is probably, in part, related to the settings in which the individuals completed their predoctoral internships. It seems likely that school psychology students who complete their predoctoral internships in non-school settings will be more likely to choose such settings for their permanent employment. (Such individuals may also be more competitive for non-school positions than those who completed school-based internships.) How-ever, it can be difficult for school psychology students to obtain internships in non-school settings, as many non-school-based internship sites do not consider appli-cants from school psychology programs. According to a searchable internship directory available on the website of the Association of Psychology Postdoctoral and Internships Centers (APPIC; www.appic.org), 432 APA-accredited predoctoral internship sites (and 131 non-APA-accredited sites) consider applicants from clinical psychology programs, 404 accredited (and 123 nonaccredited) sites consider applicants from counseling psy-chology programs, and only 135 accredited and 54 nonaccredited sites consider appli-cants from school psychology programs. Although completing a school-based intern-ship is in no way a negative and we want to encourage school psychologists to seek internship and employment opportunities in the schools, the relative lack of alternative internship sites is concerning. It is likely that this furthers the perception that school psychologists predominately engage in assessment activities and are not prepared to undertake other types of activities more often associated with clinical and counseling psychologists.

A recent study provides support for the notion that school psychology students may have more difficulties locating non-school-based internships than students from clinical or counseling programs. Gayer, Brown, Gridley, and Treloar (2003) conducted an ana-logue study in which they sent internship training directors simulated internship appli-cation materials. The materials were identical, with the exception that one-third of the "applicants" were identified as being from clinical psychology programs, one-third were identified as students from counseling psychology programs, and one-third were identi-fied as school psychology program students. The internship training directors were asked to indicate whether they would accept, reject, or hold the student. Students identi-fied as clinical psychology students were most likely to be accepted, whereas students identified as school psychology students were most likely to be rejected. The acceptance rates were 66% for clinical, 48% for counseling, and 31% for school psychology. The rejection rates were 2% for clinical, 7% for counseling, and 40% for school psychology. Findings such as these support the notion that the opportunities for school psycholo-gists outside of the school setting may be more limited than for clinical and counseling psychologists. It is imperative that those within the field of school psychology increas-ingly advocate for themselves and their profession. We believe that schools and educa-tion should be the prominent focus within school psychology training programs, but at the same time, we advocate for school psychologists being able to work in a variety of other settings and decry stereotypes and biases against school psychology that limit such opportunities.

## Salaries and Time Spent Working

It is well known that school psychology is not the field to enter if one's sole desire is to become wealthy. That being said, salaries for school psychologists are not abysmal, and they compare favorably with those of other service-oriented professions, especially when one takes into account the fact that most school psychologists work on 9- or 10-month contracts. In a recent survey of NASP members, Thomas (2000a) reported that the mean national salary of school psychologists in the United States was $49,000, with the median salary being $48,000. Salaries varied considerably by state. School psy-chologists in the District of Columbia reported the highest salaries (mean of $60,777), followed by New Jersey ($60,217), California ($59,911), New York ($57,958), and Michigan ($56,082). The lowest salaries were reported by school psychologists in North Dakota ($37,907), Montana ($37,928), Louisiana ($38,752), Arkansas ($40,865), and Kansas ($40,983). It is important to keep in mind that these are average salaries across school psychologists with varying levels of experience and that starting salaries would typically be considerably lower than these figures. On average, but with exceptions in some regions, university trainers have slightly higher salaries that do practitioners ($52,271 for trainers, $49,089 for practitioners). However, practitioners' salaries vary based to some extent on the highest degree they have obtained, and the average salary for doctoral-level practitioners ($55,262) is slightly higher than that for university trainers (the vast majority of whom have earned a doctorate degree).

The average school psychologist works 9 to 10 months of the year. In a recent survey of school psychologists, practitioners reported working an average of 197 contract days a year (Thomas, 2000b). There was relatively little variability in this number by state. School psychologists in Mississippi reported working the most days ($n = 233$); however, this figure was based on only six responses. The next highest number was 216 days, worked by school psychologists in North Carolina and Virginia. School psychologists in Connecticut, Rhode Island, and Washington reported working the fewest days on average ($n = 185$). School psychologists reported that their average day was 7.3 hours, with the range being 6 for those in Rhode Island to 7.7 for those in California, Georgia, Iowa, Nebraska, Oregon, South Dakota, and Texas. Based on these data, school psychologists in Rhode Island earned the most per hour ($44), whereas school psychologists in Arkansas earn the least per hour ($26). The national average hourly salary for all school psychologists who responded to this survey was $35.40 (Thomas, 2000a).

# THE ROLE AND FUNCTION OF SCHOOL PSYCHOLOGISTS

In addition to variations in the work setting and environment from state to state, there are also likely to be differences in the role and function of the school psychologist from state to state and even from district to district within the same state. As discussed in Chapter 1, the definition of school psychology, as well as the role of the school psychologist, has changed over time. However, changes in practice may occur at varying paces and often lag behind philosophical changes regarding the practice of school psychology. The purpose of this section is to provide an overview of some of the stated roles and functions of school psychologists, as well as to provide some data on what school psychologists are actually doing.

School psychologists engage in a wide variety of activities; however, three activities are consistently identified as the main activities school psychologists perform. These include: (1) assessment, (2) consultation, and (3) intervention. School psychologists can also engage in a variety of other activities. In the NASP brochure titled *What Is a School Psychologist?* (available online at www.nasponline.org/about_nasp/whatisa.html), the following are identified as services school psychologists may provide: consultation, assessment, intervention, prevention, education, research and planning, and health care provision. Surveys of school psychologists, however, continue to identify assessment, consultation, and intervention as the three activities in which school psychologists most frequently engage. There are, of course, subcategories to each of these areas, as discussed in the following sections.

## Assessment

Assessment has long been identified as a function of school psychologists. Assessment became the primary function of many school psychologists following the passage of Public Law 94-142 in 1975. With the advent of this law, guidelines were put into place that required certain assessment procedures to be followed prior to placing children in special education programs. School psychologists provided these assessments, and quickly this function took over all other functions for many school psychologists. Because federal and state laws required assessments to be completed, when resources were scarce in districts school psychologists were often required to first complete these required activities before engaging in other activities. Unfortunately, school psychologists quickly began to be seen simply as psychometricians. In recent years, school psychologists, as well as school psychology training programs, have become more vocal regarding the fact that school psychologists are comprehensive mental health and education service providers working within the schools and that assessment is just one of the many functions that school psychologists perform. However, as is discussed later, many school psychologists still engage predominately in assessment activities.

It would be a mistake to assume that there is only one type of assessment. Although standardized intellectual ability testing (i.e., IQ assessment) is frequently conducted by school psychologists and although many think of this as the main assessment role of school psychologists, a variety of other assessment methods and procedures are employed by school psychologists. These are briefly discussed here, with more detail provided in Chapter 8. Ideally, assessment should be conceptualized not as one specific activity but as a problem-solving process. School psychologists receive referrals regarding children who are struggling academically, emotionally, or behaviorally. Prior to implementing an intervention, the school psychologist must conduct an assessment to determine what the problem is and what methods might be effective in remediating the problem. In some cases, this assessment may be done in part to determine whether a student is eligible for special education services. In other cases, the assessment may be conducted to identify the specific problems a child has in order to design an effective intervention program to target these difficulties. In addition to standardized assessments, school psychologists may conduct functional behavioral assessments and perform curriculum-based assessments. Assessment activities also include report writing and other related activities, such as records review and assessment planning.

Assessment is an extremely valuable task that school psychologists perform. Without an appropriate assessment, it is difficult to know what intervention to use and whether the implemented intervention is having the desired effect. However, far too many people (including many school psychologists) see assessment as simply the administration of a standardized measure or two and fail to see it as part of the broader problem-solving context. In our opinion, this is one reason that assessment is often seen as an undesirable activity. We believe it is imperative that school psychologists develop a broader view of assessment. As is discussed in much more detail in Chapter 7, school psychologists who engage in the problem-solving model of practice are continually using assessment in order to obtain the needed data to guide decision making at each stage of the problem-solving process. This type of assessment bears little resemblance to the standardized testing traditionally associated with school psychology. Assessment as part of the problem-solving process is key in guiding effective practice, and we encourage school psychologists to devote more of their overall assessment time to this type of assessment activity.

## Consultation

Consultation is usually conceptualized as a triadic relationship. The professional (in this case, the school psychologist) works with a third party in the interest of changing the behaviors of the targeted client (i.e., the child referred). Within the school setting, the third party is typically a teacher or parent. School psychologists engage in teacher consultation more frequently than in parent consultation—likely due in part to the fact that teachers are there at the schools and easier to access than parents. Consultative activities with teachers include assisting in the development of a classroom behavior management plan or helping develop an academic intervention for a student who is struggling in reading. Parent consultation may involve working with parents on issues related to effective parenting and assisting parents in setting up programs at home to reinforce homework completion.

Some school psychologists also conduct systems-level consultation. In this form of consultation, the school psychologist does not work with one individual to promote changes in one child but instead works to bring about broader change. For example, the school psychologist may assist the school district in developing a new prereferral intervention process. This type of consultation (discussed further in Chapter 11) has great potential to bring about changes that affect more than just one individual child. In addition, systems-level work is essential in developing prevention efforts that address the needs of all students at a universal level. Unfortunately, school psychologists have traditionally spent most of their time consulting with parents and teachers regarding the individual needs of students who are already experiencing difficulties. Although this level of consultation should not be ignored, we believe that school psychologists of the future will expand their role to consult at classwide, small-group, or schoolwide levels to address primary and secondary prevention needs in addition to tertiary prevention and intervention efforts.

## Intervention

Within the intervention domain, school psychologists may engage in indirect interventions or direct interventions, and these interventions may be conducted in group or individual settings. Indirect intervention is conducted via collaboration with important "others" in the child's life (e.g., parents, teachers), as we described in the previous paragraphs. For example, a school psychologist may run parenting groups concerning effective management of child behavior problems. School psychologists also may provide services directly to students. For example, a school psychologist may work one-on-one with a student to alleviate symptoms of depression that student is exhibiting. Another intervention activity may involve running a social skills group to increase appropriate social behaviors in a group of elementary school children.

As part of their intervention efforts, school psychologists may also engage in prevention activities. Obviously, it is better to prevent problems from occurring than to treat problems once they have occurred. Prevention efforts may include running groups for children identified as being "at risk" for emotional and behavioral problems, developing schoolwide programs to decrease problems such as bullying, and implementing early literacy programs. Although prevention activities are often conceptualized as occurring before any problems are noticed, prevention activities are probably most frequently put into place after problems are first identified but before they have reached a clinically significant level.

# CONFLICT BETWEEN IDEAL AND ACTUAL ROLE

Although school psychologists are trained to practice assessment, consultation, and intervention, as well as other activities such as research and program evaluation, there is a disparity between the amount of time school psychologists report engaging in these activities and the amount of time they would like to spend engaged in these activities. Although advocacy for role expansion is not new, on average school psychologists' workloads are still predominately focused on traditional assessment activities. In his recent survey of school psychologists, Thomas (2000c) reported that the median number of evaluations completed each year by school psychologists in the United States was 75. There was some variability in this number, with school psychologists in Connecticut completing the fewest evaluations ($n = 40$) and those in Alabama completing the most evaluations ($n = 138$). Given these numbers, it is not surprising that, in general, school psychologists report being involved in assessment activities at a much higher frequency than they would like.

As summarized later, a number of surveys have been conducted with school psychologists regarding their practice of school psychology. The findings from these surveys are, unfortunately, quite consistent. School psychologists tend to spend about half of their time in assessment-related activities, but they would ideally like to spend less time in assessment activities and more time in intervention and consultative activities. Despite this disparity between the ideal role and the actual role of the average school psychologist, most school psychologists report being generally satisfied with their jobs.

In a recent survey of approximately 400 school psychologists, assessment was the most commonly reported activity in which these school psychologists engaged. Results indicated that, on average, school psychologists spent 46% of their time in assessment-related activities. Consultation was reported to take 16% of their time, and intervention (including interventions, counseling, and parent training) was reported to take 22% of their time (Bramlett, Murphy, Johnson, Wallingsford, & Hall, 2002). The other 16% of their time was divided between conferencing (7%), supervision (3%), in-service activities (2%), research (1%), and other, unreported activities (3%). These findings are consistent with an earlier study (Reschly & Wilson, 1995) in which school psychologists reported that they spent most of their time in assessment-related activities. In this study, school psychologists reported spending an average of 22 hours a week (55% of their time) in assessment activities, 8.3 hours (21% of their time) in direct interventions, 8.8 hours (22% of their time) in consultative activities, and 0.8 hours (2% of their time) in research and program evaluation activities. However, in this same study, school psychologists reported that their preferred role would involve less assessment and more intervention work. The practitioners in this study indicated their preferred role breakdown would be to spend 12.9 hours a week (32% of their time) in assessment activities, 11.3 hours (28% of their time) in direct intervention activities, 13.1 hours (33% of their time) in consultative activities, and 2.7 hours (7% of their time) in research and program evaluation activities. Although practitioners in this study were not engaged in intervention and consultative activities to the extent they wished to be, they still reported a relatively high level of job satisfaction. However, it should be noted that respondents were most satisfied with their colleagues and were slightly less satisfied with other aspects of their jobs.

In a similar study, Hosp and Reschly (2002) examined actual and preferred roles of school psychologists across the United States. The findings from this study are consistent with those from Reschly and Wilson (1995). Overall, school psychologists reported spending 22.2 hours per week (55% of their time) in assessment activities but indicated that they would prefer to spend only 12.8 hours per week (32% of their time) in such activities. They indicated that they spent 7.6 hours a week (19% of their time) in intervention activities but would prefer to spend 11.4 hours (29% of their time) involved in intervention work. In terms of consultation, school psychologists reported spending 9.2 hours a week (23% of their time) but would prefer to spend 13.3 hours (33% of their time) in these activities. Overall, the school psychologists in this sample reported that they spent about 60% of their time in eligibility-related services (e.g., conducting evaluations, attending individualized education program team meetings).

In addition to looking at nationwide responses, Hosp and Reschly (2002) examined their data for differences based on geographic region. Although there was some variability in terms of actual and preferred role by geographic location, on average respondents from all areas of the United States indicated that they would prefer to engage in less assessment and more intervention and consultation. School psychologists in the Northeast (Connecticut, Massachusetts, Maine, New Hampshire, Rhode Island, Vermont), mid-Atlantic (New Jersey, New York, Pennsylvania), west south-central (Arkansas, Louisiana, Oklahoma, Texas), and mountain states (Arizona, Colorado, Idaho, Montana, New Mexico, Nevada, Utah, Wyoming) reported engaging in assessment activities 20 hours per week or less, whereas those in other regions reported engaging in assessment activities more than 20 hours per week, with those in the east south-central (Alabama, Kentucky, Mississippi, Tennessee) area reporting that they spend an average of 26.5 hours a week in assessment activities. School psychologists in all areas of the United States reported that at least half of their time was spent in eligibility-related activities.

With regard to job satisfaction, Hosp and Reschly (2002) obtained findings similar to those of Reschly and Wilson (1995). The school psychologists in Hosp and Reschly's study reported being at least moderately satisfied with their jobs, even given the disparity between their actual and preferred roles. On a scale of 1 to 5, with 5 indicating greater satisfaction, the respondents indicated that their satisfaction with colleagues was a 4.0 and their satisfaction with work duties was a 3.6. There were no differences in job satisfaction based on geographic region.

Not only do school psychologists report a disparity between what they would like to do and what they actually are doing, but school psychologists also face a problem with how others perceive the field of school psychology and the role of school psychologists. Perhaps in part because school psychologists do still predominately engage in traditional assessment activities, they are often perceived by others as primarily testers or sorters and not as providers of comprehensive mental health and education services. A recent article in the NASP *Communiqué* stresses the point that every school psychologist is a mental health provider (Dwyer, 2004), providing a full array of psychological services within the schools. However, this article also points out that sometimes even school psychologists themselves do not perceive that they have the skills to provide a full array of psychological services, and they may state that they cannot provide intervention services to children with emotional problems. This may occur for two reasons: (1) a school psychologist really may not have received training in his or her graduate program regarding interventions for mental health problems, and (2) a school psychologist may simply believe that providing mental health services is not appropriate within the schools. Both of these situations hinder the growth of our profession. Training programs must ensure that they are adequately preparing future school psychologists to provide a broad array of services, and school psychologists must view themselves as more than "sorters" and "placers."

In our opinion, school psychologists must continue to advocate for the expansion of their roles. Most school psychologists are trained to deliver comprehensive psychological services, and, based on surveys of practicing school psychologists, they clearly desire to provide more comprehensive services than they are currently doing. NASP guidelines for the provision of school psychological services (NASP, 2000a), as well as the standards for training and field placement (NASP, 2000b), clearly reflect the view that school psychologists should be providing a wide range of psychological and educational services within the school system. For example, the practice guidelines emphasize that school psychologists should use empirically supported problem-solving models in the context of assessment, intervention, and research and systems-level problems. The domains of school psychology practice that training programs must cover include data-based decision making; consultation and collaboration; and prevention, crisis intervention, and mental health. NASP has also developed several position statements (available online at www.nasponline.org/information/position_paper.html) that reflect the organization's view that school psychologists provide comprehensive service delivery in the schools and that school psychologists can provide a broad range of mental health services in the schools.

Although there is clearly a movement to highlight the multitude of skills that school psychologists possess, it nevertheless continues to be a struggle for school psychologists to apply all of their skills within the school-based context. As we pointed out in Chapter 2, the practice of school psychology has historically been tied to special education law. As special education law evolves, with, perhaps, less emphasis on traditional assessment (e.g., a move away from the discrepancy model for the identification of learning disabilities), there is hope that school psychologists will eventually be able to expand their roles so that they are providing truly comprehensive psychological and educational services. As Shapiro (2000) points out, we must move away from solving the little problems (assessing and intervening with one student at a time) to solving the big problems (addressing systemwide problems such as illiteracy). For this to occur, school psychologists must expand their roles and move away from activities that are so tied to traditional, norm-referenced, individual assessment.

# DEMOGRAPHIC CHARACTERISTICS OF SCHOOL PSYCHOLOGISTS

Now that we have considered what school psychologists do, we turn to the topic of who school psychologists are. The information presented here expands on sections of Chapter 4, in which the demographic characteristics of school psychology trainers and students were briefly discussed.

As discussed in Chapter 4, although the children and families served by school psychologists are an increasingly diverse group, school psychologists as a group are not very diverse. In general, school psychologists are predominately female and European American, and hold specialist-level degrees. School psychologists are also increasingly an aging population (on average), leading, in part, to shortages of school psychologists due to retirements.

## Gender

According to data from the 2002–2003 NASP membership survey, 72.6% of school psychologists who are NASP members are female. However, the gender ratio has not always been so lopsided. Reschly (2000) reported that the number of women in school psychology has gradually increased since the early 1970s, when the gender ratio was tipped toward men (about 60:40). By the mid-1970s the gender ratios were equal, and since the mid-1980s the field has become increasingly dominated by women. Current estimates are that approximately 80% of the graduate students in school psychology are female, whereas about 70% of practicing school psychologists are female (Reschly, 2000). Of course, over time, as current students enter the workforce, the practitioner population will become even more dominated by women unless there is a dramatic change in the student population, which seems unlikely. This trend is not unique to the field of school psychology but, rather, seems to be reflective of an increased feminization of the field of psychology in general. As reported in a recent article in the APA *Monitor on Psychology* (Bailey, 2004), approximately 67% of all psychology PhD graduates in 2002 were women (compared with 45% of all doctoral recipients).

Interestingly, the gender ratios are significantly different for university trainers of school psychologists, as compared with the general population of school psychologists. Although women are increasingly represented in faculty positions, women do not outnumber men in these positions as they do in practitioner positions. In the early 1970s fewer than 20% of school psychology faculty positions were filled by women. That percentage has changed over time so that, currently, slightly less than 50% of faculty positions are filled by women. Program directors, however, are still more likely to be male; only about 35% of program directors are female (Reschly, 2000). Although it is not clear why the gender ratios are so different for trainers versus students and practitioners, Reschly indicates that fewer women apply for academic positions than do men, with only about 40% of the applicants for faculty positions being female. It is unclear why women apply for faculty positions at a lower rate than do men, but research suggests that women are more likely than men to take time off from working as school psychologists or to work part time due to family responsibilities (Wilson & Reschly, 1995). It may be that more women than men perceive faculty positions to be too time-intensive or inflexible to fit in with the personal life they desire and thus choose not to pursue these positions.

## Age

The median age of school psychologists has been steadily increasing over the past two decades. The median age of practitioners increased from the late 1980s to the late 1990s, from the mid- to late 30s to the mid- to late 40s (Reschly, 2000.) Data presented by Curtis, Hunley, and Grier (2004) also support this trend and indicate that the percentage of school psychologists under 40 declined by about 15% from 1989–1990 to 1999–2000, whereas the percentage of school psychologists over 50 increased by about 14%. Curtis, Hunley, and Grier (2004) presented additional data demonstrating that the average number of years of experience of school psychologists has also increased from 1989–1990 to 1999–2000. In 1989–1990, only 23% of school psychologists had been practicing for more than 15 years. However, in 1999–2000, that percentage increased to 40%. As Curtis, Hunley, and Grier (2004) noted, and as discussed later in this chapter, this increase in median age has resulted in a shortage of school psychologists as older school psychologists retire and younger school psychologists are not available to step in and take their places.

## Ethnicity

Practitioners in school psychology tend to be overwhelmingly European American. According to the 2002–2003 NASP membership data, approximately 91.1% of NASP members are European American. This figure is consistent with findings from surveys of school psychologists that indicate that although the number of Latino/Latina school psychologists is increasing slightly (from 1.5% to 3.1% in a decade; Curtis, Hunley, & Grier, 2004), individuals from ethnic minority backgrounds are still substantially underrepresented in the field of school psychology. Minority representation does seem to be increasing somewhat in graduate programs (both in terms of students and faculty), where, according to Thomas (1998), 15% of faculty and 17% of students are nonwhite. However, these numbers are considerably lower than those of the general population, and clearly the field of school psychology must make more proactive efforts to recruit qualified, diverse individuals.

## Educational Level

Despite predictions that the field of school psychology would become increasingly populated with individuals with doctoral degrees, the specialist-level degree (EdS or a 60-credit master's degree or the equivalent) is still by far the most common highest degree that school psychologists report obtaining. According to the 2002–2003 NASP membership survey, 28% of NASP members have doctoral degrees. As Reschly (2000) points out, this percentage is unlikely to change significantly any time in the near future given that the majority of school psychology training programs do not grant doctoral degrees. Of graduate training programs in school psychology, only about 30% have programs at the doctoral level (Thomas, 1998). Thomas (1998) also reports that about 30% of school psychology graduate students are enrolled in doctoral programs. However, the graduation data for the 1996–1997 school year indicate that only about 17% of all school psychology graduates received doctoral degrees. Thus it seems likely that those prepared at the specialist level will continue to dominate the field of school psychology.

# JOB SUPPLY AND DEMAND

As mentioned earlier, a shortage of school psychologists has existed for a number of years, both of practitioners and of university faculty. Such a shortage also existed in the late 1980s; it seemed to briefly remit but began increasing again in the mid-1990s. It has shown no signs of remission since that time (Curtis, Grier, & Hunley, 2003; Curtis, Hunley, & Grier, 2004). Curtis and colleagues (2003, 2004) evaluated a variety of data and estimated based on these data, that the shortage of school psychologists will increase over the next several years and peak in about 2010. They also indicate that the shortage will be particularly acute for doctoral-level school psychologists and predict that there will be a large number of unfilled positions in university training programs.

These data are consistent with surveys that indicate that over the past several years one-quarter or more of school psychology training programs nationwide have had openings for faculty members (Demaray, Carlson, & Hodgson, 2003; Little & Akin-Little, 2004). Of course, some of these openings are created by individuals switching jobs but staying within the academic sector. As Little and Akin-Little (2004) point out, just because there are a large number of job openings does not necessary mean there is a shortage of trainers. However, both anecdotal data and formal survey data make it clear that not all of the advertised open positions have been filled. Of the training directors who responded to Demaray et al.'s (2003) survey, 75% reported that open positions within their programs had been filled. Thus it seems safe to conclude that there is currently a shortage of school psychology trainers.

The reasons for the shortage of trainers seem to involve several factors. Because of the rapid growth of the field in the 1970s and early 1980s, many of the faculty who have been with their programs since the programs' inceptions are of retirement age. Thus a number of individuals are leaving the field. However, Demaray et al. (2003) indicate that this is only part of the problem. In their survey, about one-third of the open positions were reportedly new positions. These positions may have been created as part of the increasing efforts of training programs to obtain NASP approval and/or APA accreditation (Little & Akin-Little, 2004). Another difficulty is that not all doctoral-level training programs focus on preparing students for possible academic careers. Of the 99 doctoral training programs identified by Little and Akin-Little (2004), 82 had at least one graduate in an academic position. However, since 1990 only 19 programs had more than one graduate in academic positions. Clearly, programs must do a better job of preparing and encouraging students to enter the academic world if the shortage of trainers is to remit. One difficulty that Little and Akin-Little (2004) hypothesize may influence the lack of interest in faculty positions is the perception that an academic job is much more difficult and demanding than a school-based job. Particularly when pay levels may not be all that different (and may, in fact, be higher for school-based professionals who have earned doctoral degrees), graduates of doctoral programs simply may not be interested in entering the academic world. Little and Akin-Little (2004) suggest that both adequate financial support in graduate school and increased mentoring may help create a more favorable outlook on academic jobs for potential future trainers.

The shortage of practitioners is likely tied, in part, to the shortage of university trainers. Without fully staffed programs, it becomes difficult for programs to maintain their student numbers, and increasing their numbers becomes even more difficult. Given the many impending retirements among practitioners, programs need to increase their numbers of graduates if there is to be any hope of filling the vacant positions created by these retirements. It seems unlikely that this will happen, which is one reason the school psychology shortage is projected to continue for a number of years. In a survey conducted by Thomas (1999), on average, school psychologists reported that they would retire within 14 years. In some states the reported average number of years until expected retirement was quite low (Mississippi = 5.3; Oklahoma = 8.6; Louisiana = 8.6; Alabama = 8.6), whereas in others the numbers were higher (Hawaii = 23.3; Nebraska = 18.3; Vermont = 19.8). Overall, 10% of the respondents indicated that they planned to retire within the next 3 years.

Curtis, Grier, and Hunley (2003) estimated that more than half of the individuals currently employed as school psychologists are expected to retire within the next 12 years and that those with doctoral degrees are expected to retire at a rate disproportionate to those with specialist-level degrees. In fact, they estimated that by 2020, 75% of doctoral-level school psychologists employed in 1999–2000 will be retired, compared with 52% with specialist degrees and 67% with master's degrees. Due largely to these retirements, Curtis et al. (2003) reported that there is likely to be a shortage of close to 9,000 school psychologists from 2000 to 2010. This projection then drops off to approximately 3,000 for the next decade. Although this shortage is likely to be a nationwide phenomenon, data suggest that different regions of the country will not be equally affected by the shortage. Historically, the mid-Atlantic and New England regions have had more consistency in the supply and demand for school psychologists, whereas the west south central region (Arkansas, Louisiana, Oklahoma, and Texas) has reported more shortages (Lund, Reschly, & Martin, 1998).

The shortage of school psychologists has not gone unnoticed by NASP or by Division 16 of APA. NASP has collected some anecdotal data on the shortage and has also begun efforts to address it. Examples of activities in which NASP has begun to attempt to increase the pool of school psychologists include coordinating with trainers and universities to expand school psychology programs, strengthening the Nationally Certified School Psychologist (NCSP) credential, communicating with Division 16 of APA to develop ideas to protect school psychology, and working for loan forgiveness programs through the federal government (Charvat, 2003). In addition, Division 16 of APA and NASP (as well as other school psychology organizations) held a Future of School Psychology Conference in November of 2002. One of the key areas of discussion at the conference was the shortage of school psychologists and how this shortage will affect service delivery to children, their families, and schools.

Two options for addressing the shortage of school psychologists are to retrain psychologists who were not initially trained as school psychologists and to allow licensed clinical and counseling psychologists to practice in the schools without obtaining their school credentials. These options are increasingly being seen as viable ones because of the continuing shortage of school psychologists, as well as what seems to be an oversupply of clinical psychologists. However, there is significant debate regarding how these options could be carried out. One possibility, would be to require clinical or counseling psychologists who wish to work in the schools to return to school for specific training in school-based issues. This retraining would include course work related to the climate of the school and education-specific issues (e.g., special education law, curriculum). The second possibility would allow licensed clinical or counseling psychologists to practice in the schools without becoming certified as school psychologists. They would be able to provide mental health services to children under their state psychologist licensure. Currently Division 16 of APA and NASP are working to develop a joint position statement regarding some of these issues (Tharinger & Palomares, 2004).

It remains to be seen what will happen with the school psychology shortage. It is likely that additional options for hiring school psychologists, as well as perhaps a change in the duties of school psychologists, will need to occur to deal with this ongoing problem. However, in the meantime, this shortage may be good news for students wondering about job possibilities. Given that shortages are expected to hit almost every region in the United States, students will likely be able to find jobs without significant difficulty and may be able to be choosy and select a job in which the role of the school psychologist matches their desired role.

## DISCUSSION QUESTIONS AND ACTIVITIES

1. Log onto the NASP Career Center (www.naspcareer.org) and search for school psychology jobs in your current state, as well as in states in which you may wish to work in the future. How many jobs are listed? What are the differences in jobs in terms of salaries, requirements, stated duties, and so forth?

2. Using the data obtained by Thomas (1999, 2000a, 2000b, 2000c) in his survey of school psychologists (available in the *Communiqué* archives on NASP's website: www.nasponline.org/publications/cqindexlist.htm), compare information about school psychologists in your state to that about school psychologists nationally or in other areas of the country. Based on your analysis of these data, do you think school psychologists in your state are in a good position? Why or why not?

3. What is your ideal breakdown of time for the different activities in which school psychologists engage? How does this fit with data presented in this chapter regarding what school psychologists actually spend their time doing?

4. As discussed in this chapter, school psychology is increasingly dominated by women. In your opinion, is this good, bad, or neutral? Why?

5. School psychology as a profession is dominated by European American individuals. How might this affect the provision of services to children in our public schools?

6. As discussed in this chapter, the current shortage of school psychologists is expected to continue for a number of years. Some possible solutions to this shortage, briefly mentioned in this chapter, include retraining of clinical and counseling psychologists and allowing clinical and counseling psychologists to work in the schools without obtaining their school psychology certification. What are some advantages and disadvantage to these solutions? How do you think these possible solutions would affect the field of school psychology as a whole?

# 6

# Legal and Ethical Issues in School Psychology

Numerous legal and ethical statutes guide the practice of school psychology. Within the legal area, federal legislation affects the provision of school psychology services at a national level. In addition, state legislation and case law based on rulings from civil lawsuits, which may eventually be codified into state law, impact the provision of services at the state level. Even services mandated by federal legislation can be delivered somewhat differently in different states because states have some flexibility in how they implement federally mandated services. For example, states can require that reevaluations for students in special education be conducted every 2 years, even though the federal guidelines indicate that they can be done every 3 years. However, states cannot be less restrictive than the federal law (so states could not require reevaluations to be completed every 4 years). Because of this flexibility, as well as the numerous laws that are made at the state level regarding the provision of educational and psychological services, there will always be some practice differences among states. Therefore, it is imperative that school psychologists become familiar with laws in the state in which they are employed. In particular, they should become familiar with their state's interpretation of federal special education legislation, as well as their state's statutes on the practice of psychology. At a federal level, school psychologists should be familiar with the laws that govern the provision of special education and other services within the schools, as well as those that cover general educational issues.

In addition to legal mandates, school psychologists must be familiar with ethical codes that apply to the practice of school psychology and of psychology in general. Ethical codes outline expected conduct in professional activities. Although ethical codes are not enforceable by law, ethical violations may result in dismissal from professional organizations or revocation of professional licensure and may be the basis for civil malpractice lawsuits.

This chapter provides an overview of the federal U.S. legislation, as well as of the ethical codes with which school psychologists practicing within the United States should be familiar. School psychologists practicing outside of the United States should take care to review the laws applicable in their countries. All school psychologists should recognize that laws frequently change and ethical codes are updated. Because of this, it is important that school psychologists engage in continuing education activities to ensure that they are familiar with the most recent laws and ethical guidelines and that they are practicing in a legal, ethically responsible manner.

# INDIVIDUALS WITH DISABILITIES EDUCATION ACT

The Individuals with Disabilities Education Act (IDEA) is the federal special education legislation that mandates the provision of free and appropriate public education services to students with disabilities. This law was originally passed as Public Law 94-142 in 1975 and was titled the Education for All Handicapped Children Act. Since that time the law has gone through several major reauthorizations, including one in 1990 in which the name of the law was changed to reflect its current title. In the following paragraphs we provide background information on the development of IDEA, as well as information on its current provisions. Table 6.1 provides a summary of the federal legislation discussed here. For those looking for a more comprehensive overview of some of these issues, Jacob and Hartshorne's (2003) *Ethics and Law for School Psychologists* is an excellent source.

## Background on Special Education Law

Under the U.S. Constitution, education is not a fundamental right of the citizens of the United States. However, the 10th Amendment to the Constitution provides that "powers not delegated to the United States by the Constitution, nor prohibited by it to the States, are reserved to the States." Thus the duty of education has been left to individual states, which provide education as an entitlement: All children have a right to an education provided by the state within which they reside. States must provide this education in a manner that is consistent with the principles outlined in the U.S. Constitution. In particular, the 14th Amendment to the U.S. Constitution provides for both equal protection (states cannot deny a person equal protection under state law) and due process (states cannot "deprive a person of life, liberty, or property, without due process of law") to all citizens. States may not enact laws that infringe on the rights of citizens, including their right to an education, which is considered a property right. Furthermore, if a state does intend to take away any rights, there must be a procedure in place to guarantee that the rights of the person are not being violated (a provision referred to as *due process*). However, historically (prior to the passage of Public Law 94-142), many students with disabilities were summarily excluded from public schools without any consideration of their rights. Children who were considered to be unable to benefit from a public education (including those with significant disabilities) were prevented from enrolling in school. Many of these children remained at home with their parents, others were institutionalized, and a small portion received education in a private school setting (Jacob & Hartshorne, 2003).

In 1954 the U.S. Supreme Court ruled in the landmark case of *Brown v. Board of Education* that separate educational facilities for racial minority children were "inherently unequal." The court ruled that state laws that required or permitted segregation of students in schools based on race were unconstitutional because they violated the equal protection clause of the 14th Amendment. Based on this ruling, states were

**TABLE 6.1. Timeline of Major Special Education and Related Legislation**

1965    Public Law 89-10    Elementary and Secondary Education Act (ESEA)

Under Title I of this Act, school districts were provided with federal financial assistance primarily intended to assist in the education of children who were economically disadvantaged. Four other Titles provided funding for other aspects of education, but children with handicaps were not specifically mentioned.

1965    Public Law 89-313    Elementary and Secondary Education Act Amendments of 1965

Established grant programs for state-run schools and institutions for children with disabilities.

1966    Public Law 89-750    Elementary and Secondary Education Act Amendments of 1966

Amended Public Law 89-10 to include a Title VI to assist states in developing programs for students with disabilities.

1970    Public Law 91-230    Education of the Handicapped Act (EHA)

Replaced Title VI of ESEA. Provided grant programs for states to provide services to children with disabilities.

1973    Public Law 93-112    Rehabilitation Act of 1973

Included Section 504, which prevents discrimination by public agencies based on a disability. Mandates that schools provide free, appropriate education to students with disabilities. No funding attached to this mandate.

1974    Public Law 93-380    The Education Amendments of 1974

Reauthorized ESEA and EHA. Increased financial assistance to states to provide services to children with disabilities. Federal aid for programs for students with disabilities was dependent on states enacting plans to educate students with disabilities.

1974    Public Law 93-380    Federal Educational Rights and Privacy Act (FERPA)

Protects the privacy of children's educational records. (Part of Education Amendments of 1974.)

1975    Public Law 94-142    The Education for All Handicapped Children Act

The landmark federal legislation that guaranteed children with disabilities the right to a free appropriate public education.

1986    Public Law 99-457    The Education of the Handicapped Act Amendments of 1986

Mandated special education services for children ages 3–5 with disabilities and provided financial incentives for states to provide services to children with disabilities ages birth–3.

1990    Public Law 101-476    Individuals with Disabilities Education Act (IDEA)

Amendment and reauthorization of EHA. Name changed to IDEA. Mandated transition services. Added autism and traumatic brain injury as disability conditions.

1990    Public Law 101-336    Americans with Disabilities Act (ADA)

Prohibited discrimination against individuals with disabilities by public and private organizations.

1997    Public Law 105-17    Individuals with Disabilities Education Act

Amendment and reauthorization of Public Law 101-476 (IDEA). Strengthened rights of parents.

(continued)

**TABLE 6.1.** (*continued*)

| | |
|---|---|
| 2001 | Public Law 107-110   No Child Left Behind Act |
| | Reauthorization of ESEA. Increased school accountability. |
| 2004 | Public Law 108-446   Individuals with Disabilities Education Improvement Act |
| | Amendment and reauthorization of IDEA. |

required not to limit access to particular schools based on race. Although this case did not mention students with disabilities, following the *Brown* ruling, parents of children with disabilities filed lawsuits using the same argument—that the denial of a public education to children with disabilities was a violation of the constitutional rights of these children based on the equal protection clause of the 14th Amendment.

Two important court cases, *Pennsylvania Association for Retarded Children (PARC) v. Commonwealth of Pennsylvania* (1971, 1972) and *Mills v. Board of Education of the District of Columbia* (1972) were key in the eventual granting of educational rights to all students regardless of their disability status. We briefly review these cases here.

In the *PARC* case, attorneys for the parents of 13 children with mental retardation who had been excluded from the public schools argued that the exclusion of these children violated their constitutional rights under the 14th Amendment. In a consent decree (i.e., the involved parties consented to a court-approved agreement), the Commonwealth of Pennsylvania agreed to provide "access to a free public program of education and training appropriate to his learning capacities" to every child between the ages of 6 and 21 with mental retardation. The state also agreed that school districts would provide services to children younger than age 6 if the district already provided preschool services to children without mental retardation. The consent decree also stated that a placement in the regular public classroom for children with mental retardation was preferable to a placement in any other setting (including a special classroom setting within the school). This decree further mandated that educational placements of and programs for children with mental retardation be reevaluated every 2 years.

The *Mills* case was filed by attorneys on behalf of seven students with varying disabilities (including mental retardation, behavior problems, and brain injuries). In the consent decree for this case, the court once again agreed that not providing these children with an appropriate education violated their constitutional rights. However, the District of Columbia failed to comply with the directives set forth in the consent decree, in part because it argued that the financial costs were prohibitive, and the case ended up back in court. In the *Mills* ruling, the District of Columbia was ordered to provide "each child of school age a free and suitable publicly supported education regardless of the degree of the child's mental, physical, or emotional disability or impairment. Furthermore, defendants shall not exclude any child resident in the District of Columbia from such publicly supported education on the basis of a claim of insufficient resources." The right of school districts to expel or suspend students with disabilities was also limited by the *Mills* case.

Following these rulings, as well a number of other, similar rulings, the momentum for a national special education law increased. Even prior to the *PARC* and *Mills* cases, there had been some federal legislation that assisted states in providing services to children with disabilities. In 1965, the Elementary and Secondary Education Act (ESEA;

Public Law 89-10) was signed into law. Title I of this legislation was intended to provide school districts with federal financial assistance to help meet the needs of students who were disadvantaged due primarily to economic circumstances. Four other titles provided funding for other aspects of education, but children with disabilities were not specifically mentioned. Later in 1965, this law was amended to include money for grant programs for state-run schools and institutions for children with disabilities. This law was amended again in 1966 and included a Title VI, which authorized funds to assist states in developing programs for students with disabilities. In 1970 a new law (Public Law 91-230; the Education of the Handicapped Act [EHA]) replaced Title VI of the ESEA and provided grant programs for states to provide services to children with disabilities. In 1974 amendments to ESEA and EHA were passed (Public Law 93-380) that increased financial assistance to states to provide services to children with disabilities. This law also included language that informed school districts that federal aid for programs for students with disabilities would be dependent on states developing plans for adequate services for children with disabilities. Finally, in 1975, the landmark Education of All Handicapped Children Act (EHA; Public Law 94-142) was passed. This law required that all students have access to a free and appropriate public education (FAPE) that is provided in the least restrictive environment (LRE).

Under Public Law 94-142, schools were required to provide services only for children of school age. In 1986, Public Law 99-457 (the Education of the Handicapped Act Amendments) was passed. This law mandated special education services for children ages 3–5 and provided financial incentives to states to provide services for children ages birth to 3. In 1990, EHA was amended and its name changed to the Individuals with Disabilities Education Act (IDEA; Public Law 101-476). In 1997 IDEA was amended and reauthorized (Public Law 105-17). This version of special education law is often referred to as IDEA-97. IDEA was recently reauthorized by Congress and was signed into law by President Bush on December 3, 2004, as the Individuals with Disabilities Education Improvement Act (Public Law 108-446). This new law was scheduled to take effect July 1, 2005. However, it is the U.S. Department of Education that will issue the final rules and regulations, which will guide practice, on compliance with the law. Once completed, these final regulations will be published in the *Federal Register*. It should be noted that there is often a significant lag time between final approval of the legislation (i.e., passage of the law) and the appearance of the regulations that guide the implementation of this law. For example, although IDEA-97 was signed into law in 1997, the regulations guiding the implementation of this law were not made available by the U.S. Department of Education until 1999. However, a specific notation in the IDEA-2004 law encourages the U.S. Department of Education to publish its rules and regulations within 1 year. Given this, hopefully these will be available by early 2006. Fortunately, many of the provisions in IDEA-97 remain unchanged in IDEA-2004—although there are some important changes, which we outline later in this chapter. First, though, we present a discussion of the provisions in IDEA-97.

## IDEA-97: Part B

There are four parts to IDEA-97: Part A, General Provisions; Part B, Assistance for Education of All Children with Disabilities; Part C, Infants and Toddlers with Disabilities; and Part D, National Activities to Improve Education of Children with Disabilities. Parts B and C are the key parts in terms of service provision to children with disabilities. Part

B is discussed in more detail in this section, and Part C services are discussed in a later section.

IDEA requires that each state have a policy to ensure that all children with disabilities between the ages of 3 and 21 have a right to a FAPE. The law specifies that services provided to children with disabilities must meet all of their special education needs, as well as related service needs, and that the services provided must be based on the individual needs of each child (34 C.F.R. § 300.300). Students with disabilities who have been suspended or expelled from school also have a right to a FAPE. Although all children have a right to a FAPE, students who are placed by their parents in private schools do not have "an individual right" to receive special education services (34 C.F.R. § 300.454). In these instances, who is provided with services as well as what services are provided is decided by the local educational agency (LEA) in collaboration with the private school. Children placed in a private school by their LEA (as opposed to parental placement) retain all of their rights under IDEA (34 C.F.R. §§ 300.401–300.402).

According to IDEA, a child with a disability is one who has been evaluated and determined to have one of 13 specific handicapping conditions. These, with brief definitions of each, are listed in Table 6.2. In addition to these specific disabilities, children between the ages of 3 and 9 can also be identified as developmentally delayed. To be classified as developmentally delayed, a child must exhibit delays in one or more of the following areas: physical development, cognitive development, communication development, social or emotional development, and adaptive development (34 C.F.R. § 300.7).

Not only are states required to provide services to all children with disabilities, but they must also proactively seek to find children who could benefit from special education services. The Child Find provision of IDEA (34 C.F.R. § 300.125) requires that states have a plan to ensure that all students with disabilities are "identified, located, and evaluated" to determine whether they are in need of special education services.

When children who may benefit from special education services are identified, states are required to complete a "full and individual evaluation," the purpose of which is to determine if the child qualifies for services and, if so, what educational needs the student has (34 C.F.R. § 300.320). Students must be reevaluated at least every 3 years (although this reevaluation does not necessarily need to involve complete retesting of the child; 34 C.F.R. §§ 300.321, 300.533). Evaluation procedures must be technically sound and nondiscriminatory and must be provided in the child's native language (or other mode of communication). The evaluation should be thorough enough to identify all of the student's special education and related needs (34 C.F.R. § 300.352).

The results of the evaluation are used to develop a written individualized education program (IEP) for each child with a disability. The IEP must be reviewed at least once a year by an IEP team that includes: the child's parents; at least one regular education teacher; at least one special education teacher; a representative of the public agency (e.g., school principal); an individual who can interpret the instructional implications of the evaluation results; other individuals deemed appropriate by the parents or school personnel; and the child, if appropriate (34 C.F.R. § 300.344). Parent participation in the IEP process is emphasized (34 C.F.R. § 300.345). Parents must be notified of an IEP meeting enough ahead of time so that they are able to attend, and the meeting must be scheduled at a time that is convenient for the parent(s). Schools may conduct IEP meetings without parents only if they have made multiple, documented attempts to try to secure the attendance of the parents.

The IEP must include the following information (34 C.F.R. § 300.347):

**TABLE 6.2. Definitions of Disabilities from IDEA-97 (34 C.F.R. § 300.7)**

**Autism**

A developmental disability significantly affecting verbal and nonverbal communication and social interaction, generally evident before age 3, that adversely affects a child's educational performance. Other characteristics often associated with autism are engagement in repetitive activities and stereotyped movements, resistance to environmental change or change in daily routines, and unusual responses to sensory experiences.

**Deaf-blindness**

Concomitant hearing and visual impairments, the combination of which causes such severe communication and other developmental and educational needs that they cannot be accommodated in special education programs solely for children with deafness or children with blindness.

**Deafness**

A hearing impairment that is so severe that the child is impaired in processing linguistic information through hearing, with or without amplification, that adversely affects a child's educational performance.

**Emotional disturbance**

(i) A condition exhibiting one or more of the following characteristics over a long period of time and to a marked degree that adversely affects a child's educational performance:
  (A) An inability to learn that cannot be explained by intellectual, sensory, or health factors.
  (B) An inability to build or maintain satisfactory interpersonal relationships with peers and teachers.
  (C) Inappropriate types of behavior or feelings under normal circumstances.
  (D) A general pervasive mood of unhappiness or depression.
  (E) A tendency to develop physical symptoms or fears associated with personal or school problems.
(ii) The term includes schizophrenia. The term does not apply to children who are socially maladjusted, unless it is determined that they have an emotional disturbance.

**Hearing impairment**

An impairment in hearing, whether permanent or fluctuating, that adversely affects a child's educational performance.

**Mental retardation**

Significantly subaverage general intellectual functioning, existing concurrently with deficits in adaptive behavior and manifested during the developmental period, that adversely affects a child's educational performance.

**Multiple disabilities**

Concomitant impairments (such as mental retardation-blindness, mental retardation-orthopedic impairment, etc.), the combination of which causes such severe educational needs that they cannot be accommodated in special education programs solely for one of the impairments.

**Orthopedic impairment**

A severe orthopedic impairment that adversely affects a child's educational performance. The term includes impairments caused by congenital anomaly (e.g., clubfoot, absence of some member, etc.), impairments caused by disease (e.g., poliomyelitis, bone tuberculosis, etc.), and impairments from other causes (e.g., cerebral palsy, amputations, and fractures or burns that cause contractures).

*(continued)*

**TABLE 6.2.** (*continued*)

### Other health impairment

Limited strength, vitality or alertness, including a heightened alertness to environmental stimuli, that results in limited alertness with respect to the educational environment, that—

   (i) Is due to chronic or acute health problems such as asthma, attention-deficit disorder or attention-deficit/hyperactivity disorder, diabetes, epilepsy, a heart condition, hemophilia, lead poisoning, leukemia, nephritis, rheumatic fever, and sickle cell anemia; and
   (ii) Adversely affects a child's educational performance.

### Specific learning disability

   (i) **General**. The term means a disorder in one or more of the basic psychological processes involved in understanding or in using language, spoken or written, that may manifest itself in an imperfect ability to listen, think, speak, read, write, spell, or to do mathematical calculations, including conditions such as perceptual disabilities, brain injury, minimal brain dysfunction, dyslexia, and developmental aphasia.
   (ii) **Disorders not included**. The term does not include learning problems that are primarily the result of visual, hearing, or motor disabilities, of mental retardation, of emotional disturbance, or of environmental, cultural, or economic disadvantage.

### Speech or language impairment

A communication disorder, such as stuttering, impaired articulation, a language impairment, or a voice impairment, that adversely affects a child's educational performance.

### Traumatic brain injury

An acquired injury to the brain caused by an external physical force, resulting in total or partial functional disability or psychosocial impairment, or both, that adversely affects a child's educational performance. The term applies to open or closed head injuries resulting in impairments in one or more areas, such as cognition; language; memory; attention; reasoning; abstract thinking; judgment; problem solving; sensory, perceptual, and motor abilities; psychosocial behavior; physical functions; information processing; and speech. The term does not apply to brain injuries that are congenital or degenerative, or to brain injuries induced by birth trauma.

### Visual impairment including blindness

An impairment in vision that, even with correction, adversely affects a child's educational performance. The term includes both partial sight and blindness.

   • A statement of the child's current educational performance and how the child's disability affects the child's involvement in the general curriculum
   • A statement of measurable annual goals, including benchmarks or short-term objectives
   • A statement of special education and related services and supplementary aids to be provided to the child, as well as a statement of program modifications or supports for the school personnel that will be provided to the child so that the child advances toward annual goals, is involved and progresses in the general curriculum as appropriate, and is educated with other children with and without disabilities
   • A explanation of the extent to which the child with a disability will *not* participate in educational activities with children without disabilities

- A statement of any modifications in state or districtwide testing that are needed for the child to participate in these assessments and, if the IEP team determines that the child will not participate in an assessment, an explanation of why the assessment is not appropriate and how the child will be assessed
- Dates services are to be provided, as well as the frequency, location, and duration of services
- A statement of how progress will be measured and how the child's parents will be informed of that progress
- Beginning at age 14, a statement of transition service needs that focuses on the student's course of study and, beginning at age 16, a statement of needed transition services

As indicated, the IEP must include information regarding involvement with children without disabilities. A key part of IDEA, dating back to the original legislation, is the provision of services within the least restrictive environment (LRE). As stated in IDEA, "to the maximum extent appropriate, children with disabilities, including children in public or private institutions or other care facilities, are educated with children who are nondisabled" (34 C.F.R. § 300.500). The law goes on to state that children can be removed from the regular education environment "only if the nature or severity of the disability is such that education in regular classes with the use of supplementary aids and services cannot be achieved satisfactorily" (34 C.F.R. § 300.500). Schools must provide a continuum of placements for students with disabilities so that the individual needs of each student can be met. This continuum includes regular classes at one end of the spectrum and special schools, institutions, or home instruction at the other end (34 C.F.R. § 300.551).

To ensure that each child is receiving a FAPE and that the rights of the child, as well as of his or her family, are not violated, IDEA also outlines *procedural safeguards*. These safeguards highlight the importance of involving parents in the special education process. Parents have a right to be present at all meetings in which educational placement decisions regarding their child are made (34 C.F.R. § 300.501). Parents also have a right to seek an independent evaluation of their child if they desire. If a parent requests such an evaluation, the school district may choose to hold a hearing to show that its evaluation was appropriate, or the district can simply agree to pay for the requested independent evaluation. If a hearing is held and the evaluation completed by the school district is determined to be appropriate, the parents can still seek an independent evaluation, but at their own expense (34 C.F.R. § 300.502). Before school district personnel can conduct an assessment, parents must provide consent for the evaluation to occur (34 C.F.R. § 300.505), and the parents must be given a copy of procedural safeguards that explain their rights in understandable language (34 C.F.R. § 300.504). In addition to requiring parental consent for testing, IDEA also requires consent for placement in special education programs (34 C.F.R. § 300.505). If a child's parents and the school district disagree on testing and/or placement issues, mediation can help resolve those differences. School districts must have a mediation process in place (34 C.F.R. § 300.506). However, if mediation does not resolve the differences, a due process hearing may occur. A due process hearing is conducted by an impartial hearing officer. If one party is dissatisfied with the outcome of the due process hearing, the next course of action is to file a civil law suit. If parents prevail in a lawsuit, they can be awarded attorney's fees (34 C.F.R. §§ 300.506–300.513).

Discipline procedures (34 C.F.R. §§ 300.519–300.529) are also an important topic addressed under procedural safeguards. School districts are allowed to suspend children with disabilities, as they would children without disabilities, for no more than 10 consecutive school days (or for no more than 10 total school days in a school year). A school district may also place a child in an interim alternative education setting (IAES) for up to 45 days if the child carries a weapon to school or possesses, uses, or sells illegal drugs while at school or at a school function. A hearing officer can also order a child to an IAES (for no longer than 45 days) if the officer considers the child to be a danger to him- or herself or others. However, removal for longer than 10 school days is considered to be a change in placement. For such children, an IEP meeting must be convened and the IEP reviewed. If no functional behavioral assessment had been completed prior to this time, and if there is no written behavioral intervention plan for the student, these must be completed. In addition, if the disciplinary action being considered is a result of a weapons or school code violation resulting in a recommended suspension of more than 10 school days, then a manifest determination review must be held. The point of this review is to determine whether the behavior in question was due to the child's disability. If the review finds that the behavior was *not* a manifestation of the student's disability, then the student can be subjected to the same disciplinary procedures as students without disabilities. However, the student must still be provided with a FAPE. In such case, a student could be suspended but would still need to be provided with educational services to allow the child to progress toward achieving his or her educational goals (34 C.F.R. § 300.121).

Since the inception of IDEA, numerous court cases have dealt with its implementation. We review some of the key cases in the following sections; however, these cases are too numerous to review in this chapter. Jacob and Hartshorne (2003), as well as Rothstein (2000) and Yell (1998), provide a more comprehensive overview of case law and IDEA.

## LRE and Court Cases

The idea of educating all children in the least restrictive environment (LRE) has been the subject of several court cases. In *Daniel R. R. v. State Board of Education* (1989) the parents of Daniel, a young child with Down syndrome, wanted him to be placed in a regular prekindergarten class. However, after a short time in such a class, the teacher reported concerns regarding Daniel's placement and believed that he was not able to benefit from being in the regular classroom. Daniel's placement was changed; however, his parents believed that his right to an education in the LRE had been violated. The hearing officer, as well as a district court, agreed that the school district had appropriately placed Daniel. In upholding the district court's ruling, the court of appeals proposed two criteria to evaluate the appropriateness of a child's educational placement: (1) whether education in the regular classroom, with the use of supplementary aids and services, can be achieved satisfactorily, and (2) if placement outside of a regular classroom is needed, whether the school has mainstreamed the child to the maximum extent possible.

A similar but expanded test of whether a placement is appropriate was created in a series of later cases. In the *Board of Education, Sacramento City Unified School District v. Holland* (1992), the parents of a 9-year-old girl with moderate mental retardation requested full-time placement in a regular education classroom, whereas the school district believed that half time in a regular classroom and half time in a special education classroom was the best placement. A hearing officer agreed with the parents, but the school district appealed this decision to the district court. The school district lost the case in district court but appealed. In the appeal decision, *Sacramento City School District v. Rachel H.* (1994), the court upheld the district court's decision and outlined a four-part test for whether the district had proposed an appropriate placement for Rachel:

1. The educational benefits to Rachel in a regular classroom, supplemented with appropriate aids and services, as compared with the educational benefits of a special education classroom
2. The nonacademic benefits of interaction with children who were not disabled
3. The effect of Rachel's presence on the teacher and other children in the classroom
4. The cost of mainstreaming Rachel in a regular classroom

Similarly, in *Oberti v. Board of Education of the Borough of Clementon School District* (1993), the court proposed that when deciding whether a child with disabilities can be educated in the regular classroom, the following should be considered:

1. Whether the school district has made reasonable efforts to accommodate the child in the regular classroom
2. The educational benefits available to the child in a regular class, with appropriate supplementary aids and services, as compared with the benefits provided in a special education class
3. The possible negative effects of the inclusion of the child on the education of other students in the class

In this case, the court ruled that the school district failed to comply with IDEA when they placed Rafael Oberti, a young child with Down syndrome, in a segregated special education classroom.

Based on these court cases, schools can place children in more restrictive settings. However, they must ensure that they have considered the appropriateness, including the benefits and possible negative outcomes, of both more restrictive and less restrictive settings prior to placing a child in the more restrictive setting.

## Appropriate Education and Court Cases

Although IDEA and its predecessors mandated that all children are entitled to a free and appropriate public education, the meaning of the term "appropriate" is not clearly defined. A number of court cases have attempted to provide clarity on this matter. The *Board of Education of the Hendrick Hudson Central School District v. Rowley* (1982) was the first case in which the U.S. Supreme Court addressed the issue of what constitutes an appropriate education. In this case, Amy Rowley, a deaf student with excellent lip-reading skills and some residual hearing, was placed in a regular kindergarten class and provided with an FM hearing-aid system. At the IEP meeting before her first-grade year, it was decided that Amy would remain in a regular class and continue to use the FM system. In addition, Amy was to receive instruction from a tutor for the deaf 1 hour a day and services from the speech–language pathologist for 3 hours per week. Amy's parents argued that she also needed an interpreter full time in the classroom. An interpreter had been provided on a trial basis for 2 weeks in her kindergarten class, but the interpreter reported that Amy did not need those services. In a hearing initiated by Amy's parents, the district's decision was upheld. Amy's parents then brought suit in a district-level court. The court ruled that Amy was not being provided with an appropriate education, and this ruling was upheld by a court of appeals. However, the U.S. Supreme Court ruled in favor of the school district and reversed the earlier rulings. In making their decision, the Supreme Court reviewed Public Law 94-142 and held that the IEP should be "reasonably calculated" to allow a child to progress; however, it does not require the state to "maximize the potential" of each student with a disability. Therefore, if the state has complied with special education law procedures and developed an IEP that is "reasonably calculated to enable the child to receive educational benefits," then the school district has met the requirements of the law.

Since the *Rowley* case, there have been a number of other court cases in which parents have argued that their children were not receiving an appropriate public education. Specific outcomes have varied, but in general the courts have ruled that schools must provide services that are likely to result in meaningful educational benefits to the child (e.g., *Polk v. Central Susquehanna Intermediate Unit 16*, 1988).

In a case dealing with needed related services (*Irving Independent School District v. Tatro*, 1984) the Supreme Court ruled that clean intermittent catheterization was a needed related service for an 8-year-old with spina bifida. The Court ruled that this service was needed to allow the child to stay in school during the day to benefit from her education. In a similar case, a school district was required to provide nursing care as a related service for a student who was wheelchair-bound and ventilator-dependent so that he could benefit from the educational environment (*Cedar Rapids Community School District v. Garrett F.*, 1999).

As a whole, these cases suggest that school districts should ensure that the services they provide allow children to benefit from their educational services. Services do not have to be the best available, but they do need to be adequate to allow children to access and benefit from their public educational experiences.

## IDEA-97: Part C

Part C of IDEA-97 contains the regulations applicable to early intervention programs for infants and toddlers from birth through age 3. Unlike Part B of IDEA, which requires a FAPE for all students, Part C provides grants to states to assist them in developing early intervention services for children up to age 3. However, states are not required to apply for funds to implement these programs (although all states are currently providing Part C services), and states can charge parents for a portion of the services provided under Part C. Part C regulations require that states identify a lead agency responsible for the provision of early intervention services (34 C.F.R. § 303.500). This lead agency then submits an application that outlines how early intervention services will be provided. In many states the lead agency is not the state's department of education but another state agency, such as the state's department of health. In addition to an identified lead agency, Part C regulations require that an interagency coordinating council be developed to assist the lead agency in the coordination and provision of services to children and their families (34 C.F.R. § 303.600).

Under Part C, children up to age 3 may be eligible for early intervention services if they have delays in one or more of the following areas: cognitive development, physical development (including vision and hearing), communication development, social and emotional development, and adaptive development. Children who have diagnosed physical or mental conditions that have a high probability of resulting in delays are also eligible for services. In addition, states can choose to provide services to children who are determined to be at risk for delays (34 C.F.R. § 303.16).

Children who receive Part C services are provided with a service coordinator. The coordinator's role is to help parents access and coordinate services for their children (34 C.F.R. § 303.23). Early intervention services are required to be provided in the "natural environment" to the extent that is appropriate. As stated in the regulations, this includes the home setting, as well as community settings in which children without disabilities also participate (34 C.F.R. § 303.12). A child receiving early intervention services is required to have an individualized family service plan (IFSP). This plan is essentially a downward extension of the IEP but should include more family-focused goals and objectives. IFSP meetings, as with IEP meetings, must include the parents of the child. The IFSP must be reviewed every 6 months (at a minimum), and annual meetings must occur to evaluate the IFSP.

In addition to having a Child Find program (as with Part B of IDEA), Part C requires that states have a public awareness program that focuses on the purpose of the early intervention program and how referrals can be made to it (34 C.F.R. § 303.320). After a child has been referred, the state has 45 days to complete the evaluation and develop an IFSP for the child (34 C.F.R. § 303.321). In the assessment and evaluation process, the inclusion of the family is emphasized. This process includes supports and services necessary to help the family meet the needs of the child (34 C.F.R. § 303.322). Under Part C, states may elect to impose a sliding-scale fee, requiring parents to pay a portion of the costs of providing the early intervention services (34 C.F.R. § 303.521). Procedural safeguards specified in Part C are much the same as those specified in Part B of IDEA.

## 2004 Reauthorization of IDEA

As noted, IDEA was reauthorized in December 2004, although the final rules and regulations (to be issued by the U.S. Department of Education) will likely not be available until sometime in 2006. Although many of the provisions of IDEA remained essentially unchanged, some changes are important to note. One of those that is likely to have a direct impact on the practice of school psychology relates to the identification of learning disabilities. IDEA-2004 indicates that school districts are not *required* to take into consideration whether a child has a severe discrepancy between his or her intellectual and achievement abilities. Instead, schools may use a process that evaluates whether a child responds to a research-based intervention in determining whether the child has a learning disability. Although the final law provides no specific guidance on how a response-to-intervention (RTI) approach might be used, separate reports issued by the House and Senate encourage research on these models so that local education agencies can make informed decisions regarding how to best identify individuals with learning disabilities. It is likely that some of the specifics regarding this part of the law will be addressed when the Department of Education issues its final rules and regulations.

Issues related to discipline and manifest determination were also sources of much discussion and controversy during the reauthorization process. Ultimately, much of the language in IDEA-97 was retained. Schools can now consider any unique circumstances on a case-by-case basis when making a decision regarding a change in placement. Children can still be removed to an alternative education setting for up to 10 school days without making a determination of whether the behavior in question was a manifestation of the child's disability. If a change in placement for longer than 10 school days is proposed, a manifest determination hearing must be held within 10 school days. The child's behavior is considered to be a manifestation of the child's disability if the behavior is determined to be caused by or had a direct and substantial relationship to the child's disability or if the behavior was the result of a failure to implement the IEP. If the behavior is determined to be a manifestation of the child's disability, the IEP team must conduct a functional assessment and implement a behavioral intervention plan (if it has not already done so) or review an existing plan and modify it to address the behavior of concern. In addition, the child should be returned to his or her educational placement unless the parents and LEA decide on a change of placement or unless the violation involves weapons, drugs, or serious bodily injury. Although the new law retains the provision that children can be removed to an IAES for up to 45 days in certain situations, the wording has changed to indicate that this can be for 45 *school* days rather than simply 45 days.

Some changes to the IEP were also made in the reauthorization of IDEA. Measurable, annual goals are still required, but short-term objectives and benchmarks no longer are (except for students with severe cognitive disabilities). The required age at which transition service needs must first be addressed on the IEP was changed from age 14 to age 16. The new law also makes some minor changes regarding holding IEP meetings and making changes to IEPs. Some members of the IEP team can now be excused from attending meetings if no modifications are being made to their area or if they provided input prior to the meeting. However, parents must agree to this. In addition, changes to the IEP can be made without holding a meeting if the school and parents agree. The new law also provides for a demonstration paper-work-reduction project which will allow 15 states to develop 3-year IEPs instead of yearly IEPs.

IDEA-97 requires reevaluations of students with disabilities at least once every 3 years. The new law has this same basic provision with some caveats. If the school and the parent agree that a reevaluation is not necessary, then one does not have to be conducted. In addition, the new law prohibits reevaluations more frequently than once a year (unless the school and parents agree differently).

The new law places greater emphasis on prereferral interventions by allowing local education agencies to spend up to 15% of their IDEA funds to assist students who are not yet identified with disabilities but who need additional academic and behavioral supports to be successful in the general education setting. Although these services can be provided to children in all grades, the focus is intended to be on children in grades K–3.

IDEA-2004 also contains a provision related to child medication. This provision states that school personnel cannot require a child to receive a prescription for medication as a condition for attending school or receiving an evaluation or services.

Very few changes were made to Part C services in the reauthorization of IDEA. One notable change is that states can opt to adopt policies that would allow parents of children receiving Part C services to continue to receive these services until the children are eligible to enter kindergarten (rather than being transitioned to Part B preschool special education services at age 3).

# SECTION 504 OF THE REHABILITATION ACT OF 1973 AND THE AMERICANS WITH DISABILITIES ACT

In addition to IDEA, the Rehabilitation Act of 1973 also promoted the development of services for children with disabilities. The Rehabilitation Act prevents discrimination on the basis of disability in programs that receive federal support. Section 504 of this act specifically states that

> no otherwise qualified individual with a disability . . . Shall, solely by reason of her or his disability, be excluded from the participation in, be denied the benefits of, or be subject to discrimination under any program or activity receiving Federal financial assistance. . . . (29 U.S.C. § 794).

Subpart D of Section 504 refers specifically to preschool, elementary, and secondary education. This subpart specifies that all children have a right to a FAPE.

Although many students with disabilities will be covered under IDEA, some students with disabilities may not be eligible for IDEA services but are still eligible for accommodations under Section 504. Section 504 is broader and less specific than IDEA. The definition of a "handicapped" person (and, therefore, one qualifying for services under Section 504) is "any person who (1) has a physical or mental impairment which substantially limits one or more major life activities; (2) has a record of such impairment; (3) is regarded as having such impairment." Physical or mental impairment is broadly defined, with no specific definitions of disability conditions as is found in IDEA. Children with medical conditions such as diabetes, as well as those with mental illnesses, are covered under Section 504.

Unfortunately, when the Rehabilitation Act was passed, it included no provisions for how the law should be implemented or enforced or how remedies should be decided upon in cases in which the law was violated. In 1976 a lawsuit (*Cherry v. Mathews*) resulted in a court order that the government create guidelines for the implementation of Section 504. In 1977, the first guidelines regarding Section 504 were issued (Jaeger & Bowman, 2002). Even following the issuance of Section 504 guidelines, schools were somewhat slow to respond to the mandates of this law. There were several reasons for this time lag, including confusion about who qualified for Section 504 services versus special education services. In addition, Section 504 has no funding attached to it as does IDEA. Although Section 504 lacks funding, school districts are required to comply with this law, and the Office of Civil Rights (OCR) is charged with investigating violations of Section 504 policy. If OCR finds that a school district is not compliant with Section 504, certain federal funds may be removed from the school district. In 1991 a memorandum from the U.S. Department of Education clarified school districts' responsibilities under Section 504 to children diagnosed with ADHD who did not qualify for special education services. (This memo also clarified how students with ADHD could be served under IDEA). It was after this that schools began to attend more closely to the appropriate development of 504 plans (Jacob & Hartshorne, 2003).

Under Section 504 schools must provide reasonable accommodations to students with disabilities. However, schools do not have to provide the best possible education—only one that is reasonably designed to meet the needs of the individual student. In order to comply with Section 504, school districts must appoint a 504 coordinator who ensures that students with disabilities (as defined under Section 504) are appropriately evaluated and that appropriate accommodations are made for students who have a need. Students receiving services under Section 504 should have written plans (similar to an IEP) that address the individual needs of the students (Jaeger & Bowman, 2002).

The Americans with Disabilities Act (ADA) of 1990 is similar in many ways to Section 504. However, whereas Section 504 applies only to organizations receiving federal assistance, ADA applies to employment and schooling organizations regardless of

whether they receive federal financial assistance. The definition of a person with a disability remains the same as the definition cited previously from Section 504. Because
elementary and secondary public schools, as entities that receive federal assistance,
were already required to comply with Section 504, ADA had minimal impact on services provided in preschool, elementary, and secondary schools (Jaeger & Bowman,
2002).

# OTHER IMPORTANT FEDERAL LEGISLATION

In addition to federal legislation (and related case law) dealing specifically with disability issues, there are pieces of legislation that deal with school-related issues in general.
These acts are important to understand for everyone involved in education, but because
they are less relevant to the day-to-day practice of school psychologists, we review them
only briefly.

## Family Educational Rights and Privacy Act

The Family Educational Rights and Privacy Act (FERPA) of 1974 protects the privacy of
students' educational records. Parents have a right to review the school records of their
children and request corrections to these records if they believe there are errors in the
records. This law also requires that parents provide consent in order for a school district
to release a child's educational records to a third party. There are certain exceptions to
this last provision. Schools may disclose information to other school personnel who
have a "legitimate interest" in knowing the information, as well as to a school to which a
child may be transferring. Other exceptions include health and safety issues and
requirements of law.

## No Child Left Behind

The most recent piece of legislation to receive considerable attention in the education
world is the reauthorization of the Elementary and Secondary Education Act in 2001.
This law, which was renamed No Child Left Behind (NCLB), was signed into law in
2002. At the heart of this law is greater accountability by school districts. As mandated
by NCLB, states must begin testing students in grades 3–8 in reading and math by the
2005–2006 school year, and by 2007–2008 schools must test students in science at least
once in elementary, middle, and high school. Schools must show progress on this
annual testing. NCLB requires that data from annual testing be reported by race, gender, and disability status. Within each of these groups, at least 95% of the children must
participate. Thus 95% of children with disabilities must take part in the annual testing.
However, 1% of all students can use scores on alternate achievement standards. So students with severe disabilities could be judged against standards other than schoolwide
standardized tests. (Schools can seek a waiver to this 1% cap.) According to the law, all
students must be "proficient" by 2013–2014. Prior to that, each school must meet "adequate yearly progress" goals. Schools that fail to make adequate progress for 2 years
must offer parents the option to transfer their children to another public school (unless
state law prohibits school choice). Schools that fail to make adequate progress 3 years in
a row must provide additional instructional services (e.g., tutoring, after-school classes).
If adequate progress is not made for 4 years in a row, corrective measures, such as

implementing a new curriculum or replacing staff, are required. If adequate progress is not made for 5 years in a row, then significant changes must be made. These could include a state takeover of the school, converting to a charter school, or hiring a private contract manager. In failing schools, parents may elect to have their children receive additional tutoring services or to use public funds to transport their children to another school. Schools are required to develop report cards showing how their test scores compare with local and state test scores. These report cards must show data by race, gender, and disability status. The law also specifies that by 2005–2006 all teachers be "highly qualified," generally meaning that they are certified and proficient in the subject matters they are teaching.

NCLB also provides individual school districts greater flexibility in spending their federal education monies. School districts can use up to 50% of their federal monies (except those designated for Title I services and excluding IDEA funds) to support any other educational program as long as student achievement improves.

Although greater accountability by schools may sound positive, the requirements of the NCLB act, particularly those regarding mandatory testing procedures and adequate yearly progress ratings, have generated significant controversy. There are numerous reasons for the controversy, including lack of adequate funding to implement assessment procedures and concerns regarding the use of test scores for students with disabilities, as well as students not proficient in English, to evaluate the overall performance of a school. Particularly because potential remedial actions for "failing" schools could be severe, schools serving large numbers of students who have limited proficiency in English and/or students with disabilities are concerned about the inclusion of these students in their school performance reports. However, some positive changes may result, including greater exposure to the regular education curriculum for students with disabilities and stronger links between students' IEP goals and the regular education curriculum (Council for Exceptional Children, 2004). Because NCLB is still in the beginning stages of implementation (and because the U.S. Department of Education is still issuing new policies regarding the implementation of NCLB), the true impact of this act remains to be seen.

## ETHICAL ISSUES

In addition to legal issues, school psychologists must be aware of ethical principles that guide the practice of school psychology and psychology in general. As indicated at the beginning of this chapter, ethical principles differ from legal mandates in that ethical codes are not enforceable by law. However, they are intended to guide the appropriate practice of psychology, and all psychologists should take these principles just as seriously as they do legal mandates.

Ethical codes provide a model for moral practice and are designed to help protect those whom a professional serves (e.g., children, in the case of school psychologists). In this context, morality involves an evaluation of professional actions based on some broader social or cultural context. Although they are not necessarily enforceable by law, ethical violations are taken seriously by professional organizations and licensing bodies. Individuals may have their memberships in organizations and/or their professional licenses revoked for serious ethical violations (Bersoff, 1995). However, individuals should not follow ethical guidelines simply out of fear of punishment. Individuals should follow ethical guidelines because they help us to best serve and protect our clients and their needs and interests. Both NASP and APA have developed ethical codes to help guide the professional practice of school psychology and psychology in general. However, it should be noted that simple knowledge of these codes is unlikely to be sufficient in helping individuals engage in ethical practice. Many ethical dilemmas faced by school psychologists do not involve violations of specific ethical principles but instead involve ethically challenging situations (Jacob-Timm, 1999). Partly because of this situation, there has been a focus in ethics education on teaching ethical decision making, in addition to covering the provisions of the appropriate ethical codes (e.g., Jacob & Hartshorne, 2003; Kenyon, 1999; Welfel, 2002). Although the models used to teach ethical decision making vary in their specific steps, they all involve some similar features, including: identification of the ethical dilemma, consideration of ethical guidelines, generation of possible resolutions to the ethical dilemma, evaluation of these possible resolutions and the effects certain actions would have on the involved individuals, and making a decision regarding which course of action to follow. As part of this process consultation with colleagues, reviews of ethics literature and of state laws and consideration of broad ethical values (e.g., respect for autonomy, fairness) are often considered.

As noted, many of the ethical dilemmas faced by school psychologists are not related to specific ethical violations but instead involve ethically problematic situations, thus emphasizing the need for broad ethical problem-solving education. In a survey of school psychologists regarding the ethical dilemmas they have faced, only a quarter of the respondents indicated that they had not faced an ethical dilemma over the past 2 years (Jacob-Timm, 1999). Of those who had faced ethical dilemmas, the most common incidents involved pressure from administrators to act in a way that was counter to the best interests of the child (e.g., pressure to tailor assessment findings to make or not make a child eligible for special education services or to fit with a certain special education classification; pressure to deliver services in a manner incompatible with ethical principles). Other common ethical problems encountered relate to assessment procedures (e.g., inappropriate use of tests), confidentiality (e.g., struggles with when to report suspected child abuse), and unsound educational practices (e.g., concerns about ineffective programs, discipline methods). Jacob-Timm (1999) argues that these findings support the idea that students must receive training in ethical decision making, in addition to being knowledgeable about specific ethical codes. We agree that school psychologists must be knowledge about the content of ethical codes governing our practice and that they must also have the ability to engage in problem-solving tactics when faced with an ethical dilemma.

The two primary codes of ethical conduct with which all school psychologists should be familiar are APA's *Ethical Principles of Psychologists and Code of Conduct* (2000a) and NASP's *Principles for Professional Ethics* published in NASP's Professional Conduct Manual (NASP, 2002a). The full text of these ethical codes can be found in Appendices A and B. In addition, NASP's conduct manual also contains *Guidelines for the Provision of School Psychological Services* (2000a), which contains NASP's views of best practices in school psychology. It is acknowledged that not all school psychologists will be able to meet every standard in these guidelines, but the document should serve as a guide for the practice of school psychology. The full text of this document is in Appendix B. Students and practicing school psychologists should read these codes and become very familiar with them. In addition, it is important to note that ethical codes are revised every decade or so, and it is important to keep up to date with changes in ethical codes.

The introduction to NASP's *Principles for Professional Ethics* states that the principles are based on two assumptions: "(1) school psychologists will act as advocates for their students/clients, and (2) at the very least, school psychologists will do no harm" (NASP, 2000a, p. 13). In addition, school psychologists are admonished to "provide only those services for which they have acquired an acknowledged level of experience, training, and competency" (NASP, 2000a, p. 13). APA's *Ethical Principles* has a similar introduction (preamble and general principles) in which psychologists are encouraged, among other things, to "benefit those with whom they work and take care to do no harm" (APA, 2002a, p. 3). Because there are a number of similarities between the ethical codes of NASP and APA, we have chosen to organize the following discussion of ethical principles around major ethical areas, highlighting both NASP's and APA's guidelines on these issues.

## Competence

Both the NASP and APA codes state that psychologists should engage in activities for which they are competent and qualified. Psychologists are to seek training, consultation, or supervision as needed to provide competent services. They are also encouraged to make referrals if they are not competent to handle a case. APA's ethical code does state that in an emergency situation, psychologists may provide services for which they are not trained to ensure that services are not denied; however, these services are to end as soon as the emergency ends or more appropriate services are available. Psychologists are also expected to engage in continuing professional development activities to develop and maintain their competence. Psychologists are to refrain from engaging in activities in which they have personal conflicts that would prevent them from providing competent services.

## Professional Relationships

Both NASP and APA address psychologists' relationships with others. In NASP's ethical principles, this is addressed under the heading of "Professional Relationships," and in APA's code, it is under the heading "Human Relations," as well as throughout other sections dealing with specific issues. Both codes discuss avoiding dual or multiple relationships. For example, a psychologist who is providing services to a family should not also be engaged in a business relationship with this family. However, APA's ethical code does state that "multiple relationships that would not reasonably be expected to cause impairment or risk exploitation or harm are not unethical" (§ 3.05, p. 6). NASP's ethical guidelines make no such provision and simply state that "dual relationships with clients are avoided" (§ III-A-6, p. 18). Both ethical codes specify that psychologists should engage in nondiscriminatory practice and not engage in harassment (including sexual harassment and harassment based on personal characteristics) or in exploitative relationships. Both ethical codes also emphasize working with other professionals to best serve their clients.

Both ethical codes address sexual relationships with clients. NASP states that "school psychologists do not engage in sexual relationships with their students, supervisees, trainees, or past or present clients" (§ III-A-6, p. 18). APA's ethical code prohibits sexual relationships with current clients and close relatives of current clients. In addition, psychologists are not to accept into therapy individuals with whom they have had sexual relationships. However, APA does indicate that psychologists could engage in sexual relations with former clients 2 years following termination of the professional relationship, but only under the "most unusual circumstances" (§ 10.08, p. 15). APA separately discusses sexual relations with students and supervisees and indicates that psychologists are not to engage in sexual relations with "students or supervisees who are in their department, agency, or training center or over whom psychologists have or are likely to have evaluative authority" (§ 7.07, p. 10).

In addition to general professional relationships, NASP's ethical guidelines address the school psychologist's professional relationships with specific individuals, including the child and family. School psychologists are expected to engage professionally with students and explain their role in the provision of services in a manner understandable to the child. Specific guidelines for relationships with parents and guardians include attempting to involve parents when working with their children, respecting the wishes of parents, and explaining all services and rights to parents in understandable terms.

APA specifically discusses the issue of informed consent, both in general and in relation to treatment and research. The APA guidelines specify that informed consent be obtained from the individual prior to engaging in research, therapy, assessment, and consulting activities. Assent should also be obtained when an individual is not able to give informed consent. Consent (and assent) must be documented by the psychologist.

## Privacy/Confidentiality

Both NASP and APA stress the importance of keeping information confidential. Information should be shared only after receiving informed consent from the client or parent or in situations in which it is required or permitted by law. APA specifies that the sharing of confidential information without consent may include instances in which information needs to be disclosed to "protect the client/patient, psychologist, or other from harm" (§  4.05, p. 8). Clients should be told about the limits to confidentiality prior to the initiation of services. APA specifies that, if the clients are being audiotaped or videotaped, permission specifically for these activities be given by the client (or the parents if the client is a child). If psychologists are presenting confidential information in a public presentation, they must either take steps to disguise the source of the information or obtain consent from the client for the presentation. APA also specifies that, if a psychologist consults with a colleague regarding a case, the psychologist not disclose confidential information (unless prior consent has been obtained) and that the psychologist disclose only enough information to meet the purpose of the consultation.

The NASP ethical guidelines state that records of students should not be transmitted electronically without a guarantee of privacy. Fax machines used to receive confidential information must be in a secure location, and e-mail messages must be encrypted or stripped of information that identifies the student/client.

## Professional Practice: Intervention and Assessment

The question of who the client is often arises when providing services to children: Is it the child, the family, the parent, or some combination? NASP directly addresses this issue and acknowledges that school psychologists do serve multiple clients; however, the child is considered the primary client if there is a conflict between clients. If school psychologists do provide services to different groups, they should inform all parties ahead of time of this arrangement to prevent misunderstandings. Although the APA ethical code does not address this issue as directly, it does specify that a therapist conducting group therapy or therapy with couples or families should clarify relationships with all involved parties at the beginning of therapy.

With regard to engaging in therapy activities, NASP specifies that school psychologists should use techniques that are research based and appropriate to the presenting problem. APA does not include this specification but does state that if therapy techniques being used have not been established psychologists must inform their clients of this, as well as of the potential risks associated with the treatment.

The ethical codes of NASP and APA have a number of similarities in their discussion of assessment-related issues. Both codes indicate that psychologists should be knowledgeable about the psychometric properties of instruments they use and should use instruments appropriate to the purpose of the evaluation. NASP also specifically states that school psychologists should use multiple assessment methods when completing an evaluation. The use of psychological assessment techniques by individuals who are not qualified to use such techniques is prohibited by both ethical codes. In addition, test security of all assessment instruments is to be maintained by the psychologist using these materials.

Interpretation of test results is also addressed in the ethical codes of both NASP and APA. APA refers to the use of automated scoring and interpretation programs and indicates that even when such programs are used psychologists must take into account the purpose of the assessment and individual characteristics of the client when interpreting results. The NASP ethical guidelines indicate that school psychologists should adequately interpret information and communicate findings in an understandable manner. These guidelines further state that written reports are prepared to be helpful and should emphasize recommendations and interpretations. The ethical guidelines point out that check-off or fill-in-the-blank reports or those that provide only scores and no recommendations are typically not useful. NASP also specifies that psychologists should be clear in their written documents regarding the source of information if more than one professional participated in the assessment process. NASP specifically states that it does not encourage inappropriate use of computer-generated test analyses or reports and that psychologists should not present such reports as their own. Both ethical codes indicate that psychologists should address limitations of interpretation or degree of confidence one has in the results of the assessment.

In addition to the discussion of general ethical principles of professional practice, NASP's ethical guidelines include a separate section on professional independent practice that addresses some of the issues faced by school psychologists who are employed by a school district and also have a private practice. In such situations, school psychologists are not to accept payment from clients who are entitled to receive their services within the school districts in which the psychologists are employed. In addition, school psychologists are to conduct their private practice business outside of school hours, and they should not use materials that belong to a public employer unless the employer approves of their use. The NASP guidelines also state that school psychologists in private practice have an obligation to inform parents of the services available through their school at no cost before providing services for payment.

## Research

Both NASP and APA discuss ethical principles as they relate to involvement in research. Both sets of ethical guidelines indicate that institutional approval should be obtained prior to beginning research, and NASP suggests that psychologists who are working in an agency without a research review board have their colleagues review the research prior to beginning the project. Both ethical codes specify that psychologists do not fabricate data, do not plagiarize, and do not publish the same finding twice. Both codes specify that steps should be taken to correct any errors discovered after publication of data. Both ethical codes indicate that authorship inclusion and order should be based on contributions to the project and that only those who have made substantial contributions should be included as authors. APA ethical codes further specify that, except under unusual circumstances, a student is listed as the first author when the manuscript is based significantly on the student's dissertation. Both ethical codes also specify that reviewers of manuscripts respect the confidentiality of these works.

APA's ethical code goes into more detail than does NASP's code on some of the specifics regarding conducting research. For example, it is specified that deception should not be used unless it is justified given the potential value of the study and the lack of suitable alternative methods. Psychologists are also instructed to not use deception when it is "reasonably expected to cause physical pain or severe emotional distress" (§ 8.07, p. 11). The APA ethical code also contains a section on ethics when using animals in research.

## Training and Supervision

Both sets of ethical guidelines cover issues in training or supervising psychology students, and although the ethical codes are somewhat similar, they address these issues from a slightly different perspective. APA specifies that training programs be designed to provide appropriate knowledge and expertise and that program descriptions be accurate and made available to those interested. APA further specifies that information presented in courses, syllabi, and other trainings be accurate. NASP's ethical principles specify that information presented in the context of teaching and training should be accurate and objective. Both ethical codes indicate that feedback should be provided to students and others being supervised and that this feedback should be fair. APA specifies that the feedback should be based on "actual performance on relevant and established program requirements" (§ 7.06, p. 10). The NASP ethical code specifies that school psychologists who supervise trainees or interns are responsible for the professional practice of those they supervise. NASP also specifies that interns and trainees should be clearly identified as such in reports and that supervisors must cosign all reports.

APA addresses disclosure of student personal information and therapy for students. The ethical guidelines state that psychologists cannot require students and others being supervised to disclose personal information—unless the program has clearly identified such information as a requirement of the program in its program materials, or unless the information is necessary to evaluate or obtain assistance for the student if problems could prevent the student from competently completing his or her training duties, or unless a threat is posed to others. APA specifies that if programs require student involvement in psychotherapy, the program faculty should allow students to select therapists not affiliated with the program. In addition, faculty who are responsible for evaluating the students should not provide the therapy.

## Advertising/Media Relations

Both NASP and APA specify that psychologists must provide accurate information in their announcements and advertisements. Both sets of guidelines also specify that psychologists should not directly solicit clients, and APA specifies that psychologists cannot solicit testimonials from former clients. Both ethical codes specify that psychologists do not compensate members of the media in return for publicity in a news item. Both ethical codes contain statements regarding presentations through mass media outlets and caution psychologists not to provide personal diagnosis or therapy (NASP) nor to indicate that a professional relationship has been established with an individual via this manner (APA).

## Record Keeping/Fees

APA's ethical code has a specific section on record keeping and fees. Likely because these issues are more relevant to psychologists in private practice than to those employed by a school district, the NASP guidelines say little about these issues. As has already been discussed in the confidentiality section, psychologists are expected to keep records confidential, and, if information is stored in a database, psychologists should code personal information so that individuals cannot be identified. Psychologists are not allowed to withhold records needed for a client's emergency treatment just because the client has not paid for services. Psychologists are to establish a fee agreement with their clients early in the therapy process. (NASP also specifies that school psychologists in private practice reach a fee agreement prior to providing services.) APA does indicate that psychologists may barter (accept goods, services, etc. in lieu of monetary payment) if this is not clinically contraindicated and if the arrangement is not exploitative.

## Ethical Decision Making

When ethical principles require a higher standard of conduct than what is set forth in the law, both NASP and APA indicate that ethical principles should be followed. In addition, when ethical behavior conflicts with policy or law, psychologists are expected to state their dilemma and commitment to their ethics and take steps to resolve this conflict. The APA ethical code does indicate that if the conflict cannot be resolved, psychologists can follow the law or regulation in question. If conflicts exist between ethical practice and the demands of an organization for which a psychologist works, APA's ethical code indicates that the psychologist must attempt to resolve the conflict in a manner that allows him or her to adhere to the ethical code. Both NASP and APA ethical codes indicate that if a psychologist becomes aware of a possible ethical violation on the part of another professional, an informal resolution should first be attempted by bringing the matter to the attention of the individual. If an informal resolution is not appropriate or, as APA specifies, if the violation is likely to cause substantial harm, the psychologist should contact appropriate organizations (e.g., professional organizations' ethics committees, state licensing boards). The filing of an ethics complaint that is frivolous or made without regard to the facts is itself an ethics violation.

# INTEGRATING ETHICAL PRINCIPLES AND THE LAW: LIMITS TO CONFIDENTIALITY

Several of the issues covered in the ethical guidelines of NASP and APA have also been the subject of case law. In particular, some of the issues related to confidentiality have been the subject of lawsuits that have brought about new laws in some states, as well as changes to ethical codes. Although both ethical codes are committed to confidentiality, this confidentiality has limits. The three main limits to confidentiality involve abuse of a minor child, threat of harm to another, and threat of harm to oneself. In cases in which these situations exist, psychologists have an ethical (and often legal) obligation to break confidentiality to ensure the safety of their clients and/or other individuals.

## Child Abuse and Neglect

All states have mandatory child abuse reporting laws that require certain individuals (e.g., physicians, mental health workers, teachers) to report suspected child abuse or neglect to the appropriate authorities (generally a state agency such as child protective services). The federal Child Abuse and Prevention Treatment Act as Amended by the Keeping Children and Families Safe Act of 2003 (Public Law 108-36) defines child abuse and neglect as "at a minimum any recent act or failure to act on the part of a parent or caregiver, which results in death, serious physical or emotional harm, sexual abuse or exploitation, or an act or failure to act which presents an imminent risk of serious harm." At a minimum, states must use this definition in terms of what they consider to be reportable abuse and neglect. However, states may add to this definition. Reporting laws are generally worded so that an individual does not need to be sure that abuse is occurring but have "reasonable cause" to believe that abuse has occurred.

## Duty to Protect

Duty-to-warn or duty-to-protect laws are also common, although not as universal as child abuse reporting laws, and there is no federal statute to guide state laws on this matter. These laws grew out of the *Tarasoff v. Regents of University of California* rulings in 1974 and 1976. In this case, Prosenjit Poddar had communicated to his psychologist (who was employed by Cowell Memorial Hospital at the University of California at Berkeley) his intention to kill Tatiana Tarasoff. Upon request of the psychologist, the police detained Poddar, but he was then released. Although the psychologist and two psychiatrists at Cowell agreed that Poddar should be committed, the chief of the department of psychiatry disagreed, and no action was taken. Two months later, Poddar murdered Tarasoff. Tarasoff's parents sued, arguing that Poddar should have been confined and that Tarasoff should have been warned of Poddar's threats. The case was initially dismissed, but in 1974 (*Tarasoff I*) the California Supreme Court ruled that therapists have a duty to warn a threatened person. The case was heard again in 1976 (*Tarasoff II*). In this ruling, the police were released from liability, but the court ruled that therapists have a duty to *protect* an intended victim:

> When a therapist determines . . . that his patient presents a serious danger of violence to another, he incurs an obligation to use reasonable care to protect the intended victim against such danger. This discharge of duty may require the therapist to take one or more of various steps . . . it may call for him to warn the intended victim or others likely to apprise the victim of the danger, to notify the police, or to take whatever other steps are reasonably necessary under the circumstances.

Thus, based on the second *Tarasoff* ruling, therapists have not simply a duty to warn an intended victim, but they must take steps to protect the intended victim.

Although most psychologists are likely familiar with the *Tarasoff* rulings, it should be noted that states differ in terms of their duty-to-protect requirements and that not all states have adopted laws that follow the *Tarasoff* ruling, which covered only the State of California. However, as noted, APA's ethical code indicates that confidential information should be disclosed, where permitted by law, to protect the client or another person. Thus, even if psychologists are not legally required to comply with a duty-to-protect law, they are ethically obligated to break confidentiality when the safety of an individual is in question.

### Privileged Communication

Whereas confidentiality is more of an ethical than a legal principle, "privileged communication" is a legal term that prevents the disclosure of information provided in confidence to certain individuals (with exceptions as mandated by law). Attorney–client privilege is the most well-known type of privilege, whereby information transmitted by a client to his or her attorney is considered private and cannot be revealed. In many states, psychologists are also granted privilege. However, school psychologists employed in schools are less commonly granted privilege. If a psychologist has privilege, he or she cannot be compelled to reveal communications with his or her client without the client waiving the right to privilege. If state laws do not consider psychologist–patient communications to be privileged, then the psychologist can likely be compelled to share communications in a court of law. However, even in states in which communication between a therapist and his or her client is considered privileged, the state may allow a judge to waive privilege.

## CONCLUSIONS

As should be clear from this chapter, legal and ethical issues are complex and multifaceted. They are also not static but change over time. Ethics are influenced by legal mandates, and legal mandates can be influenced by ethical principles. For example, prior to the *Tarasoff* rulings, the ethical code of APA stated confidentiality rights in more absolute terms than it does today. Much of what school psychologists do will be guided by both federal legislation and ethical principles. Given this, it is important that school psychologists stay up to date in both areas. Not only should school psychologists read texts such as this one, but they should also read professional newsletters and attend to announcements of changes in legislation so that they can receive current information on these important issues.

## DISCUSSION QUESTIONS AND ACTIVITIES

1. Search websites such as those of NASP (www.nasponline.org) and the Council for Exceptional Children (www.cec.sped.org) for information on the reauthorization of IDEA. If the final rules and regulations have been issued by the U.S. Department of Education, how are these different from the provisions in IDEA-97?

2. To school psychologists currently being trained, the requirement that all students (regardless of their disability status) be provided with a FAPE likely seems unquestionable. However, it was only 30 years ago that this requirement was put into place. Research, through readings or talking to educators and parents, what services for children with disabilities were like prior to the passage of Public Law 94-142.

3. IDEA is detailed in its requirements, but it can be overwhelming for parents to understand. Talk to parents of children with disabilities about their experience with the special education process: Have they understood their rights? Do they know what is in their child's IEP? Have they been satisfied with their child's experience? What suggestions do they have for improving the special education process?

4. Children with disabilities who do not qualify for special education services are eligible to receive accommodations under Section 504. However, the provision of these services is variable. What is your school district doing to comply with Section 504? How are students in need of accommodations identified? What accommodations are typically offered to these students?

5. Consider an ethical dilemma you have had or that you have heard about. Examine the NASP and APA ethical codes and list which guidelines apply to your dilemma and what the guidelines suggest in terms of resolving your ethical dilemma.

# 7

# Facilitating Change through Data-Driven Problem Solving

## A MODEL FOR SCHOOL PSYCHOLOGY PRACTICE

The first six chapters of this volume provided an overview and orientation to the field of school psychology, its historical context, and current trends and issues. With the chapters that follow, we shift our focus from issues of the "past and present" (i.e., history and current status of the field) to what we think is a more important purpose—mapping a vision for the "future" of the field. Although we acknowledge the fact that much of past and current school psychology practice has been dominated by traditional refer–test–place models wherein the school psychologist's role is largely that of "diagnostician" (Lentz & Shapiro, 1985) or "sorter" (Fagan, 1995), we are not bound by the notion that our past will necessarily dictate our future (Reschly & Ysseldyke, 2002). Instead, we believe a more promising future for school psychology lies in the data-oriented problem-solving role posited by Susan Gray in 1963 and currently advocated as "best practice" by many leading scholars in the field (e.g., Deno, 2002; Reschly & Ysseldyke, 2002; Shapiro, 2000; Tilly, 2002). This chapter begins by tracing the historical roots of this vision of school psychology as a problem-solving endeavor and contrasting it with traditional approaches. We argue the current need for adopting a data-based problem-solving approach in light of (1) growing concerns with inadequacies noted in traditional models that dominate current practice; (2) recognition of the critical need for reforms in our practices if we are to address the increasing numbers, complexity, and severity of educational and mental health problems facing our children and youth; and (3) increasing evidence of the utility of alternative approaches in improving educational outcomes for students. After establishing a history and rationale for a problem-solving approach to school psychology practice, we describe this approach, its processes, and the structures necessary to support its sustained use. In the chapters that follow, we expand on the areas of assessment (Chapter 8), intervention (Chapters 9–10), systems change (Chapter 11), and research (Chapter 12) within the context of a problem-solving model.

# TRADITIONAL AND ALTERNATIVE MODELS
# OF SCHOOL PSYCHOLOGY

As we have noted in previous chapters, the field of school psychology faces many challenges in the near future, one of which is a lack of clarity of purpose in our practice roles (Deno, 2002). Later in this chapter, we discuss the need to understand and define problems as discrepancies between "what is" and "what should be." Clearly, if we look at the field of school psychology from this perspective, we indeed have a *problem* with regard to our practice roles. As discussed in Chapter 4, disparity exists not only between actual and preferred roles but also between current and recommended best practices among leading scholars and professional organizations.

We believe that much of the existing struggle in moving forward and expanding our practice roles from "what is" in our current practice to "what should be" is a result of the difficulties we face as we try to step away from traditional roles that have now become institutionalized. In essence, what has traditionally or historically dominated our practice roles (i.e., traditional diagnostic and refer–test–place tasks) has become our *expected* role. Others (teachers, administrators, parents, etc.) have come to know the school psychologist as one whose primary and most visible function has been the psychoeducational assessment and diagnosis of children to determine their eligibility for special education and/or related services (Fagan, 1995; Lentz & Shapiro, 1985). Despite the fact that alternative models of school psychology as a problem-solving endeavor also have existed for many years (e.g., Baer & Bushell, 1981; Gray, 1963; Lentz & Shapiro, 1985), we have institutionalized the more traditional roles to the extent that others view us as "diagnosticians." Because of these traditional perceptions, policies and regulations have been put into place that in many instances mandate these roles.

It would be easy to continue to do what we have always done and what others have expected us to do, yet leaders in our field continue to challenge us to critically evaluate our current approaches to practice and, in light of what we find, to consider progressive alternatives (Deno, 2002; Reschly & Ysseldyke, 2002; Shapiro, 2000; Ysseldyke, 2000). In general, we are in agreement with individuals who argue for a fundamental shift away from our traditional practice roles. In order accomplish this objective, we believe it is essential that school psychologists: (1) critically examine current practice and recognize the need to move beyond our traditional roles (i.e., identify the gap between "what is" and "what should be" in our practice roles); (2) gain a thorough understanding of the shortcomings of the traditional model (understand why we need to try alternative approaches); (3) establish a clear vision of our role as a data-driven problem solver and implement this role in practice; and (4) carefully evaluate the utility of any alternative practice that we implement. As a first step, we believe it is important to have some historical awareness and consciousness of our field so that we have an understanding of how we got here in the first place.

## Historical Roots of Traditional and Alternative Models of School Psychology

In Chapter 2, we summarized six major historical dichotomies in psychology wherein tension and conflict have manifested in the field of school psychology (Chapter 2, pp. 35–37). We now add another, more specific dichotomy to our discussion as we contrast our vision of an alternative approach to school psychology as a data-driven problem-solving endeavor with the more traditional or refer–test–place models of school psychology practice. As aptly noted by Reschly and Ysseldyke (2002), this dichotomy has its historical and philosophical roots in the two approaches that have dominated the broader field of scientific psychology—namely, *correlational* and *experimental* psychology. In this section, we describe this dichotomy, place it in its historical context, and illustrate how it has manifested in our notions of traditional and alternative approaches to school psychology practice.

In his 1957 *American Psychologist* article, Cronbach commented that *experimental* psychology and *correlational* psychology were two *disciplines* that characterized the field of scientific psychology. According to Cronbach (1957), the task of a *science* is to "ask questions of nature," and "a *discipline* is a method of asking questions and of testing answers to determine whether they are sound" (p. 671). He noted that psychologists within the correlational discipline were "interested in the already existing variations between individuals, social groups, and species" (p. 671). They measured how these variations related to (correlated with) performance in other domains. With regard to intervention, for example, the correlational psychologist was concerned with predicting performance in treatment conditions based on naturally occurring variations across individuals. One early application of this approach that is relevant to school psychology was development of the Binet–Simon scales to identify children who were not likely to benefit from the general education curriculum. Performance on these tests was said to be positively correlated with school success. Children whose test scores indicated they were not likely to perform well in school settings were placed in alternative settings. Thus, within the correlational discipline, assessments were employed to determine placement based on individual differences, not unlike traditional diagnostic assessment for determining special education eligibility and placement. In contrast, psychologists within the experimental discipline were interested in controlling situational variables to permit "rigorous tests of hypotheses and confident statements about causation" (Cronbach, 1957, p. 672). Within the realm of intervention, the experimental psychologist was concerned with how different treatments resulted in the greatest average effects for individuals (single-subject designs) or groups of individuals (group comparisons). Great emphasis was placed on controlling for situational variations across treatment conditions in order to make valid comparisons of treatment effects. An example of this approach in school psychology is the study of instructional strategies for teaching reading. Within the experimental approach, individuals or groups of individuals would be exposed to different reading interventions to determine which approach resulted in the highest average performance on some reading outcome measure. Thus, whereas experimental psychologists focused on manipulating variables to cause differences (e.g., to determine which treatment condition produced the greatest effect), correlational psychologists focused on studying "what man has not learned to control or can never hope to control" (Cronbach, 1957, p. 672).

After contrasting the experimental and correlational approaches, Cronbach (1957) proposed a merger of these two opposing disciplines when he suggested the aptitude-by-treatment-interaction (ATI) method. He argued that psychologists should consider how aptitudes (naturally occurring or existing variations between individuals, social groups, and species) might interact with certain aspects of treatment to attenuate effects. The idea was that we should design treatments to fit individuals or groups of individuals with certain aptitudes or aptitude patterns. In this approach, what is meant by *aptitude* is "any characteristic of the person that affects his response to treatment" (Cronbach, 1975, p. 116). Some major assumptions behind ATI were as follows: "a person learns more easily from one method than another, and this best method differs from person to person, and that such between-treatments differences are correlated with tests of ability and personality" (Cronbach, 1957, p. 681).

This idea had intuitive appeal and was the focus of much attention in research and practice in psychology in the decades following Cronbach's proposal. Tests were developed to assess and classify students according to their preferred learning modalities or underlying processes (e.g., perceptual–motor, visual, auditory). In the field of special education, and learning disabilities in particular, many researchers set out to design instruction in accord with assessed patterns of modality strengths and weaknesses (e.g., Kirk, McCarthy, & Kirk, 1968). Despite the fact that research on the ATI model was in its infancy and evidence confirming its utility still pending, this approach enjoyed enormous attention from scholars who advocated its use:

> In some children information is absorbed more easily through auditory pathways; in others, learning is facilitated primarily by using visual channels. . . . We feel that exploration of modality strengths and weaknesses is of more than theoretical interest and should largely determine teaching methods. (deHirsch, Jansky, & Langford, 1966, pp. 80–83)

> The visual dyslexic rarely is able to learn by an ideo-visual approach since he cannot associate words with their meanings. He cannot retain the visual image of a whole word and consequently needs a more phonetic or elemental approach to reading. (Johnson & Myklebust, 1967, p. 156)

The school psychologists' role in this process was the careful assessment of processing and modality issues. With its intuitive appeal and widespread dissemination from educational leaders (e.g., Barbe & Milone, 1980; Dunn, 1979), this approach also pervaded special education practice. In one survey, for example, the overwhelming majority (i.e., 99%) of special education teachers reported that they believed a child's modality strengths and weaknesses should be a major instructional planning consideration (Arter & Jenkins, 1977). Although it is not surprising that this occurred, as we know that educational practice is not always driven by research (Carnine, 1997), the widespread adoption of ATI becomes problematic in light of mounting empirical evidence that failed to support the efficacy of this model.

During the decades following Cronbach's 1957 proposal of ATI, empirical investigations on the efficacy of this approach abounded. Contrary to the conventional wisdom that endorsed ATI, research syntheses did not substantiate its efficacy (e.g., Arter & Jenkins, 1979; Cronbach & Snow, 1977; Kampwirth & Bates, 1980; Kavale & Forness, 1987; Tarver & Dawson, 1978). In 1975, Cronbach reconsidered ATI in another *American Psychologist* paper. This time, he addressed ATI in light of its empirical evidence, commenting that as "important as ATIs are proving to be, the line of investigation I advocated in 1957 no longer seem sufficient" (Cronbach, 1975, p. 116). Cronbach was concerned with the inconsistency of findings across relatively similar studies (e.g., studies investigating the same treatment variables but finding different outcome-on-aptitude slopes), as only a fraction of these inconsistencies were due to statistical sampling error. He argued that these inconsistencies were evidence of unidentified interactions—complex interactions with other variables such as sex, ability, skill level, prior knowledge in the domain of interest, and so forth. In proposing the ATI model, Cronbach overlooked the possibility that the interactions he was interested in studying (i.e., aptitude × treatment interactions) might be moderated by other factors he had not considered. His original hypotheses were as follows: (1) when ATIs are present, generalizations about treatment effects are problematic because the effect will come and go (interact) across the kind of individuals who are treated; and (2) when ATIs are present, general predictions about treatment effects from aptitudes is uncertain because effects will vary depending on the selected treatment. After studying ATI, Cronbach realized the importance of other unforeseen interactions, noting that "interactions are not confined to the first order; the dimensions of the situation and of the person enter into complex interactions" (Cronbach, 1975, p. 116). He emphasized that "once we attend to interactions, we enter a hall of mirrors that extends to infinity" (p. 119) and "when we give proper weight to local conditions, any generalization is a working hypothesis, not a conclusion" (p. 125).

In light of the evidence derived from ATI research, Cronbach (1975) argued the need for applied psychology to embrace short-run empiricism and evaluation of interventions within local contexts. According to Cronbach (1975, p. 126), "short-run empiricism is 'response sensitive' . . . one monitors responses to the treatment and adjusts it, instead of prescribing a fixed treatment on the basis of a generalization from prior experience with other persons or in other locales." Later, Reschly and Ysseldyke (2002) drew parallels between Cronbach's suggested *short-run empiricism* and an alternative or *problem-solving approach* to school psychology practice. They comment that the majority of school psychology's practice (past and current) has been more consistent with the correlational and ATI approaches, as they urge us to consider the lack of evidence for traditional models and challenge us to consider the adoption of a problem-solving model of school psychology (Reschly & Ysseldyke, 2002). We also encourage school psychologists and school psychologists in training to consider the adoption of a data-driven problem-solving approach to school psychology. We ask them to do so in light of the history we have presented thus far and with consideration of other factors that we present in the next section.

## RATIONALE FOR ADOPTING A PROBLEM-SOLVING APPROACH

As we have noted in the preceding section, the philosophical assumptions driving traditional practice have not been substantiated empirically. Despite this fact, these approaches continue to monopolize the majority of school psychologists' professional practices. Why would school psychologists and educators in general continue to engage in practices that have been deemed questionable? One plausible explanation can be found in commentaries positing that education (Carnine, 1999) and within education, school psychology (Tilly, 2002), are relatively immature professions that do not necessarily rely on the scientific method to determine the efficacy of their respective practices. According to Carnine (1999, p. 2), "an immature profession is characterized by (a) expertise based on the subjective judgments of the individual professional, (b) trust based on personal contact rather than on quantification, and (c) autonomy allowed by reliance on perceived expertise and trust that staves off standardized procedures based on experimental research findings." He comments that the field of education fits these criteria. Similarly, Tilly (2002) argued that school psychology is currently evolving, as do all sciences, from a philosophically based system to a scientifically based system. In a philosophically based system, reasoning occurs "from premise to conclusions: *If this is true, then that would be true*" (Tilly, 2002, p. 21). Within school psychology, for example, this logic is seen in traditional diagnostic work. The premise that assessment based on form and structure of symptoms leads to diagnosis and that, in turn, *diagnosis informs treatment* is presumed to be "true." Thus the focus of practice becomes systematic assessment (e.g., diagnostic testing) to determine the presence of a disability (diagnosis). And the practice of diagnostic assessment is deemed an important endeavor because it presumably leads to a diagnosis that will inform treatment.

As professions mature, however, they reach "a point in their development where philosophical reasoning, assumptions, and practice no longer sufficiently addressed problems at hand" (Tilly, 2002, p. 21). When faced with sufficient practice "failures," practitioners begin to question the premises and conclusions of their current practices. At this point, reasoning begins to shift and becomes more scientifically based, by which observation leads to a tentative hypothesis that is subsequently evaluated. Carnine (1999, p. 2) claims that maturation of a profession is triggered by "pressures from groups that are adversely affected by the poor quality of service provided by a profession." When this occurs, there is: "(a) a shift from judgments of individual experts to judgments constrained by quantified data that can be inspected by a broad audience, (b) less emphasis on personal trust and more emphasis on objectivity, and (c) diminished autonomy by experts and a greater role for standardized measures and procedures informed by scientific investigation" (Carnine, 1999, p. 3). Tilly states that school psychologists and educators in general have amassed a significant enough number of "failures" resulting from current assumptions and practices to warrant movement from a philosophically based system to a scientifically based system.

Individuals who are currently practicing, in training for, or simply considering a career in school psychology will no doubt encounter differing opinions and controversy regarding traditional and alternative professional practice roles. We are hopeful that, as they are faced with choices regarding how they approach their professional practice, they do so in a very conscious and informed manner. Further, and in keeping with the problem-solving approach we are advocating, we hope that school psychologists carefully evaluate the practices they choose and make adjustments as necessary. In this section we provide a rationale for selection of the data-oriented problem-solving approach to school psychology practice, namely, (1) a lack of empirical support for the philosophical underpinnings of the traditional model and evidence that the current (i.e., traditional) systems are not working; (2) information suggesting the urgency of the need for a change; and (3) evidence supportive of the problem-solving approach to professional school psychology practice.

## Evidence That Current Systems Are Not Working

Within the literature, there are many criticisms suggesting that what we are currently doing is not working. First and foremost, foundational assumptions underlying much of current school psychology practice have been challenged. For example, extensive efforts to document the efficacy of assessing processing strengths or learning modalities and matching these to instructional strategies to capitalize on strengths have failed to produce intended results (e.g., Kavale & Forness, 1987). In her critique of this approach as it applies to reading, Snider (1992) eloquently illustrated the logical fallacy behind this approach as she considered the application of modality instruction or learning styles interventions to the nonacademic skill of basketball. She supposed that a physical education teacher gives a learning styles inventory to her class and discovers that her students were auditory/analytical learners who had weaknesses in tactile/kinesthetic areas. She imagined further that the teacher attempts to match basketball instruction to the students' learning styles through auditory means (e.g., having them listen to tapes) and analytic means (e.g., analyze plays, engage in group discussions).

Snider asked, "Why do some educators reject the notion that students can learn to play basketball by only thinking and talking about it, but embrace the idea that students can learn to read by only global and visual or tactile/kinesthetic methods?" (p. 15). Further, she wondered why this approach to instruction considers *who* and *how* to teach but ignores *what* is to be learned. The "what" of beginning reading involves certain analytical and phonological skills, whereas the "what" of basketball requires certain tactile and kinesthetic skills. She cautioned the use of any process that disregards this part of the teaching equation.

In addition to criticisms of the theoretical basis for our current practices, the methodological soundness (i.e., reliability and validity) of current diagnostic approaches, particularly with regard to learning disabilities, has been questioned. Typically, a diagnosis of a learning disability (LD) involves assessment of a discrepancy between a child's ability (via IQ tests) and achievement (via norm-referenced achievement tests). Alarmingly (but not surprising to any current practitioner), evidence indicates that practitioners do not diagnose LD consistently across students or districts (Epps, Ysseldyke, & McGue, 1984; Ysseldyke, Algozzine, & Epps, 1983). In addition to problems noted in the reliability of the assessment process across practitioners, other methodological issues surround traditional assessment processes. The ability–achievement discrepancy model, for example, is "fraught with measurement error," yet significant decisions are made on the basis of a few ability–achievement discrepancy points (Reschly & Ysseldyke, 2002, p. 9). Further, when the model is applied to students with low reading performance, results do not support the validity of differential diagnosis based on an ability–achievement discrepancy as compared with assessment based simply on low achievement in reading (Fletcher et al., 1994). More specifically, differences are large when children with low reading performance are compared with children who do not have reading difficulties, but differences are small or insignificant between children with low reading performance who met the ability–achievement discrepancy and those who did not (Fletcher et al., 1994). Finally, concerns have been raised about delays in service delivery that result when children who are initially referred for reading problems in the early grades and do not qualify for services (i.e., do not meet the ability–achievement discrepancy) are referred again in later grades, when their achievement levels fall far enough behind to qualify for the ability–achievement discrepancy (Fletcher et al., 1998). This practice is quite concerning when evidence suggests that there is a critical and short period in which we can alter reading trajectories (Simmons & Kame'enui, 1998).

Within the current system, one assumed benefit of traditional assessment is that diagnosis leads to treatment via access to special education placement and/or related services and, more important, that special education and related services benefit students. Given the amount of time and resources devoted to diagnostic and classification activities, some researchers have attempted to evaluate the degree to which diagnostic assessments actually inform treatments, as well as the degree to which students who are diagnosed and receiving services actually benefit from those services. Early studies failed to demonstrate the efficacy of special education placement (e.g., Carlberg & Kavale, 1980; Glass, 1983). Further, some studies indicated that students identified through the assessment process were not necessarily receiving instruction that differed from instruction provided to their peers without disabilities, thus calling into question the differential service delivery assumption behind diagnostic assessments (e.g., Thurlow & Ysseldyke, 1982) and special education placements (e.g., Ysseldyke, Christenson, Thurlow, & Bakewell, 1989; Ysseldyke & Thurlow, 1984). Because students with and without disabilities are not randomly assigned to various educational services, one cannot conduct true experimental studies in this area, so studies must rely on outcomes for individual students. This is also a difficult process because students with disabilities are often exempted from state- and district-level assessments. With recent movements toward accountability within systems, these data are becoming more available, yet the evidence does not systematically demonstrate benefits for students with disabilities. In fact, "when performance over time is tracked, the gap in performance of students in general and special education gets wider every year, with a continual decline in the performance of the group of students assigned to special education" (Reschly & Ysseldyke, 2002, p. 7). Clearly, more research is needed in this area, as preliminary evaluations have failed to demonstrate the effectiveness or efficiency of special education placement alone as an intervention (Reschly & Ysseldyke, 2002).

On a final note, criticisms of the traditional role of the school psychologist have been long-standing:

> The school psychologist is not a well man. His malady, while not particularly acute, is nonetheless a chronic one, endemic to his profession. The patient often presents such symptoms as distention of the referral . . . rupture of the arteries of communication . . . atrophied recommendations . . . and accumulation of jargon deposits in the report. . . . The syndrome might best be described as a "paralysis of the analysis." (Forness, 1970, p. 96, as cited in Ninness & Glenn, 1988, p. 6)

Despite early awareness of the potential shortcomings of our practices, the current system continues to be deficit-focused, and often the school psychologists' role in that system is to respond after problems are apparent and to search for pathology (e.g., Alessi, 1988). This practice is troublesome when one considers the stigma associated with many diagnostic or categorical labels, their typical lack of treatment utility, and the need for a preventative focus to comprehensively address student needs and to consider *all* students, not just those who are experiencing difficulties or eligible for special services (e.g., Hoagwood & Johnson, 2003; Hunter, 2003; Power, 2003; Shapiro, 2000; Strein, Hoagwood, & Cohn, 2003). "The search for pathology dominates eligibility evaluations and confers an overall, often implicit, obsession with deficits that deflects attention from effective treatment and the explicit pursuit of goals related to adult social roles" (Reschly & Ysseldyke, 2002, p. 7).

### Urgency of the Need for Change in Current Practices

As we noted in Chapters 2 and 3, schools are currently faced with many challenges, such as rising numbers and diversity of students; complexity and severity of student behavior and learning needs; the need to prepare students for the ever-changing workforce; and increasing accountability requirements. Further, educators are often expected to address these issues in the face of decreasing resources or support. According to Carnine (1999, p. 3) "because educational performance determines economic well-being for individuals and society as a whole, widespread underachievement is detrimental and unacceptable to the public as well as to government and to business." He argues that when conditions become unacceptable to the public, this serves as a catalyst for systemic changes in practice. Currently, we are facing such a crisis. For some students, for example, learning or behavior problems are often chronic and associated with significant later life difficulties that are quite costly to society (Adams, 1994; Walker, Colvin, & Ramsey, 1995). To efficiently address these growing concerns, research indicates that schools need to adopt a systemic approach with a focus on preventative and early intervention (e.g., Hoagwood & Johnson, 2003; Hunter, 2003; Strein et al., 2003). For example, some pivotal skills such as reading present a critical and short period in which we can alter developmental trajectories (Simmons & Kame'enui, 1998). Similarly, research suggests the importance of prevention and early intervention if the development of severe behavior problems is to be curtailed (Biglan, Mrazek, Carnine, & Flay, 2003). In the face of these concerns and of failures of current practices to address these issues with demonstrated efficacy, scholars in school psychology urge us to consider the "big picture" and to solve the "big instructional problems" that our schools are facing (Shapiro, 2000; Ysseldyke, 2000). Further, they argue that our traditional approaches are insufficient in doing so.

## Growing Evidence Supportive of an Alternative (Problem-Solving) Approach

Within the literature, support for the data-oriented problem-solving approach to school psychology is growing. Some developments in this area have their history embedded in the problem-solving approach posited by Susan Gray in 1963, and others developed in response to frustrations with traditional approaches. A few noteworthy examples include the development of assessment tools for direct measurement of academic and behavioral outcomes, advances in problem-solving approaches for linking assessment to intervention, expanding knowledge on effective instruction and interventions, improved methods for data-based decision making, and the development of alternative service delivery systems that are noncategorical in nature.

Tools for direct measurement of academic learning outcomes have been developed and show great promise in assessing student progress in the curriculum. Curriculum-based assessment (CBA; e.g., Shapiro, 1996, 2004), curriculum-based measurement (CBM; e.g., Deno, 1985; Shinn, 1989, 1998), curriculum-based evaluation (e.g., Howell & Nolet, 2000), and Dynamic Indicators of Basic Early Literacy Skills (DIBELS; e.g., Good, Gruba, & Kaminski, 2002) are examples of assessment methods that focus on assessing learning outcomes rather than learning modalities or processes. These tools have demonstrated efficacy for direct assessment and monitoring of student academic performance within the curriculum. They provide an alternative to traditional norm-referenced assessment practices and have the advantage of being more closely tied to the curriculum, they are of shorter duration, they are sensitive to incremental changes, and they can be used repeatedly to monitor growth formatively. Further, these tools have been embedded within school psychology practice and are considered acceptable by practitioners (e.g., Eckert, Shapiro, & Lutz, 1995; Shapiro & Eckert, 1993, 1994). Advances in this area have led scholars to argue for the use of these tools in tackling screening and monitoring of student progress to identify students at risk for school failure and to promote early intervention and prevention efforts (e.g., Good et al., 2002; Shapiro, 2000; Simmons, Kuykendall, King, Cornachione, & Kame'enui, 2000).

In addition to alternative assessment tools that lend themselves to direct measurement of student progress, school-based technologies for linking assessment to intervention have proven useful for problem solving in school settings (e.g., Gresham & Noell, 1999; O'Neill et al., 1997; Witt, Daly, & Noell, 2000). Functional behavioral assessment (FBA) is a process that focuses on collecting information pertaining to relations between *behaviors* (e.g., aggression, work completion), their *antecedents* (i.e., environmental factors that tend to precede and possibly predict them, such as a teacher prompt to begin reading), *consequences* (i.e., environmental factors that tend to follow and possibly maintain them, such as escape from a task, access to a preferred object or activity, or social attention), relevant *setting events* (i.e., distal antecedents, such as an argument with a parent or sibling before school, that may play a role in exacerbating problem behavior) and *establishing operations* (i.e., conditions of satiation or deprivation, such as hunger, that tend to alter the reinforcing value of certain stimuli, such as preference for food). Information on behavior–environment relations is then considered in the development of interventions. For example, if data suggest that a student's disruptive behavior (e.g., calling out in class) is *functionally* related to access to teacher attention, then an intervention is built around this hypothesis (e.g., the student could be taught to use a different and more appropriate means of accessing teacher attention, such as raising his or her hand; or the teacher could provide attention only when the student is not being disruptive). Alternatively, if data suggest that a student's disruptive behavior is functionally related to escape from task (e.g., reading group), a quite different intervention strategy might be used. Thus functional assessment helps the problem solver to consider not just the "what" (i.e., form or structure) of behavior but also the "why" or "what for" of behavior (i.e., function). Preliminary empirical evidence indicates that functional assessment has shown promise in school settings and is an integral part of a movement toward a more data-driven, problem-solving orientation to the field (e.g., Gresham & Noell, 1999).

Advances in instructional and intervention technologies and data-based decision-making methods have helped to enhance the utility of curriculum-based and functional assessment tools. We have accumulated a wealth of information regarding effective intervention strategies for a wide range of presenting problems (e.g., Lloyd, Forness, & Kavale, 1998; MTA Cooperative Group, 1999a, 1999b; Quinn & McDougal, 1998; Rathvon, 1999; Shinn, Walker, & Stoner, 2002; Stoner, Shinn, & Walker, 1991; Swanson, 1999). "Evidence-based practice" (EBP) is a term that has received a great deal of attention in recent literature. It refers to "a body of scientific knowledge defined usually by reference to research methods or designs, about a range of service practices (e.g., referral, assessment, case management, therapies, or support services)" (Hoagwood & Johnson, 2003, p. 5) in the fields of medicine, psychology, and education. Strategies for evaluating and selecting evidence-based practices also are being articulated within the field of school psychology (e.g., Kratochwill & Shernoff, 2004; Kratochwill & Stoiber, 2000a, 2000b, 2002). These efforts are promising, as EBPs offer a useful place to start when selecting interventions. Equally important, however, is the need to carefully evaluate EBPs, as we cannot assume that interventions with demonstrated efficacy in one setting or with one population will result in similar effects with a different population or in different contexts (Campbell, 1988; Cronbach, 1975). Thus improvements in intervention technologies are useful when paired with concomitant advances in alternative assessment tools (e.g., CBA/CBM, FBA) and careful attention to monitoring and evaluation of learning outcomes.

In addition to evidence suggesting the utility of practices related to a data-driven problem-solving orientation to school psychology, efforts have been made to develop and implement administrative and policy alternatives to traditional categorical service delivery systems (e.g., Reschly, Tilly, & Grimes, 1999). Unlike many current systems that search for pathology and produce labels that may be stigmatizing, "non-categorical approaches facilitate placing more emphasis on gathering assessment information related to designing interventions that enhance competencies" and are permitted under U.S. federal law (Reschly & Ysseldyke, 2002, p. 7). The noncategorical approach to special education eligibility assessment has been used successfully for several years now in certain area education agencies in the State of Iowa, and in other educational systems as well. We believe that the emerging noncategorical approach movement is an interesting and worthwhile endeavor and that the idea has several positive aspects.

Some scholars have made compelling arguments for maintaining certain aspects of current categorical systems but augmenting them with functional approaches to assessment when moving to treatment planning (Scotti, Morris, McNeil, & Hawkins, 1996). Scotti and colleagues (1996) acknowledge the fact that categorical systems that are limited to structural assessment of problems based on form have their limitations, but they also make compelling arguments for the value of certain diagnostic systems as they assist us in delineating the typical duration and developmental course of certain clusters of covarying behaviors. For example, if we know that a child meets diagnostic criteria for certain disorders (e.g., attention-deficit/hyperactivity disorder [ADHD] and oppositional defiant disorder [ODD]), we know that they are at a higher risk than the general population for the development of other problems (e.g., conduct disorder [CD]). This information can help guide the assessment process toward the identification of protective and risk factors that might be important to target for treatment. According to Scotti et al. (1996), assessment could take the form of a funnel approach that begins with a more traditional, structural assessment and moves to a more functional process as treatment planning becomes the focus.

Whether these systems offer a worthwhile alternative to current categorically based systems remains an empirical question worthy of further investigation. From a problem-solving standpoint, we believe these systems are worth our exploration and careful evaluation prior to wholesale endorsement. It is likely that school psychologists who are just entering the field will encounter one or more of these alternative service delivery systems in their practice.

## OVERVIEW OF THE DATA-DRIVEN PROBLEM-SOLVING MODEL

According to Deno (2002), the purpose of schooling is to foster the cognitive, affective, social, and physical developmental outcomes of students. Viewed in this light, Deno argues that school itself is an intervention that we as a society have deemed important to implement on a universal level. In other words, *all* children who participate in schooling are part of this widespread intervention designed to alter their development from its "natural" (i.e., unschooled) course. Within this context, it follows that the purpose of problem solving is to "eliminate the difference between 'what is' and 'what should be' with respect to student development" (Deno, 2002, p. 38). Thus, at a universal or schoolwide level, the problem-solving process begins with determination of the discrepancy between where students are with regard to their skill levels in various developmental domains when they enter school and where we would like them to be when they graduate. Schools establish a general scope and sequence of competencies that students should master along the way (i.e., benchmarks or indices of progress), and instruction is focused on moving students forward through the various curricula toward the desired goal at graduation.

Movement along this continuum of curricular materials and mastery of desired skills and outcomes does not occur at the same pace for all students, nor does it occur evenly across domains for individual students (Deno, 2002). Within a second-grade classroom, for example, the range of skills in the domain of reading may vary widely across students, with some students reading at targeted benchmarks and others reading slightly or significantly behind desired levels. Teachers must employ a problem-solving process and adapt instruction to address the varying instructional needs of all students within a particular instructional domain (e.g., reading). Similarly, at the individual student level, teachers will need to address varying student needs across domains. For example, an individual child may be viewed as not making adequate progress in a particular domain, such as reading, when his or her level of performance is not at the level expected along the continuum set by the school; yet the same student may be viewed as on target across other domains of functioning (e.g., social, mathematics, writing). Thus, even for children who are making adequate progress within the general education curriculum, problem solving is needed to address various instructional needs as they move along all the continua of development.

The problem-solving model so construed is *outcome-focused* and *context-specific*. Emphasis is placed on measuring discrepancies between current and expected performance on important domains of functioning, and problem solving focuses on the development of interventions to reduce this discrepancy (outcome). All of this (assessment of the discrepancy, intervention development, and evaluation) occurs within the context (setting and activity) in which the problem occurs. This focus directs the problem-solving agent (e.g., the school psychologist) toward solutions (e.g., instructional modifications) that fit the problem context (e.g., independent seatwork during math class). When school problems are viewed from this perspective, one might argue that "failure to profit from general education is relatively common and results to some extent from idiosyncratic, inappropriately arranged environmental events" (Lentz & Shapiro, 1985, p. 199). Further, school psychology within a problem-solving system might be viewed as "a system of service provision designed to help remediate school-based problems of children [that is] preventative [and] incorporates explicit efforts to resolve problems before child placement in special education is required" (Baer & Bushell, 1981, p. 192). This perspective, though not new, is very different from the reactive focus of traditional diagnostic assessment that dominates current practice. The problem-solving model is focused on gathering information about the problem (i.e., quantifying discrepancies) and the problem context to develop working hypotheses about why problems are occurring and what solutions might work. These hypotheses are then evaluated within the natural context. In contrast, the traditional model is focused on gathering information about presumed underlying learning processes and individual differences that might lead to diagnoses with the assumption that the diagnosis will inform treatment. *Thus the problem-solving model uses the scientific method to determine what works, whereas the traditional model is more likely to produce recommendations based on diagnosis.*

Problems that present themselves in school settings can vary on many dimensions (e.g., intensity, frequency, duration, severity, magnitude, complexity, resistance to intervention). Thus, the intensity of problem solving exists along a continuum and can be varied to match the presenting problem. For example, for some students, the discrepancy between actual and desired performance may be quite small, and problem resolution may be achieved with relatively minor adjustments (e.g., increased practice, corrective feedback, prompting) to instruction that could be managed by the classroom teacher within the general education curriculum. Other students, whose presenting problems are of a higher level of intensity, severity, or complexity, may require additional problem-solving efforts (e.g., consultation between the teacher and a special education teacher or school psychologist) and perhaps more intensive instructional supports to resolve their presenting concerns and to curtail the development of more significant problems. For a smaller percentage of students, current functioning in some domain(s) may occur at levels that are severely discrepant from expected levels or that are extremely complex, intense, or resistant to intervention. These students might require ongoing problem solving to systematically address their needs and prevent exacerbation of existing problems. Finally, when a child's problem becomes pronounced (e.g., the discrepancy between a child's current rate of acquisition and retention occurs at a level that is significantly behind his or her peers), it may be necessary to provide instructional supports beyond what would typically be delivered in general education.

As noted, the problem-solving approach can be applied along the continuum of student needs to address the wide range of problems presented by students within school settings. At each level of intensity, problem solving also may vary in intensity, yet it will always follow a consistent process (i.e., series of steps). Many models of problem-solving appear within the literature (e.g., Bergan & Kratochwill, 1990; Kratochwill & Bergan, 1990; Witt et al., 2000). Across these models, Tilly (2002) notes that "four thematic questions guide practitioner thinking: What is the problem? Why is it occurring? What should be done about it? Did it work?" (p. 27). This same line of questioning is used not only to guide problem solving along the continuum of student needs but also to address problems at small-group and schoolwide levels. In this next section, we summarize the line of questioning and the steps involved in the problem-solving process (see Figure 7.1). We end with a description of how this process might be embedded and sustained within the school context to address the needs of *all* students from a preventative stance.

### Step 1: What Is the Problem? (Problem Identification and Validation)

The initial step in solving any presenting problem is, first, recognizing and confirming its existence as a problem and, second, determining that it is in fact a problem worth solving. As we noted earlier in this chapter, in a data-oriented problem-solving model, problems are defined as discrepancies between "what is" (current performance/outcome) and "what should be" (expected/desired performance) on some domain of functioning (e.g., reading). For example, when there is a discrepancy between a student's *current* and *expected* reading performance, in some circumstances this discrepancy may be viewed as a *problem*. In order for this step to occur, someone (e.g., a teacher or parent) must first notice the problem (i.e., discrepancy). This recognition requires some monitoring of or experience with the student's current reading performance, as well as experience and/or information pertaining to expected reading performance (e.g., relative to same-age peers or some other criterion). Further, in order to gain a clear understanding of the problem, it is important to use objective means to measure the discrepancy and confirm its existence.

Selecting standards for comparison to determine expected levels of performance (e.g., professional experience, teacher preference, parental expectations, developmental norms, medical standards, template matching, curriculum standards, local norms, national norms, and classroom peer performance) is not always an easy task. It requires professional judgment and some understanding of measurement issues. In Chapter 8, we discuss a variety of assessment tools that are used in school psychology practice, and in Chapter 12 we cover important measurement issues relevant to this process. Within a problem-solving framework it is important that selected assessment tools and measurement techniques help to clearly define the problem in objective,

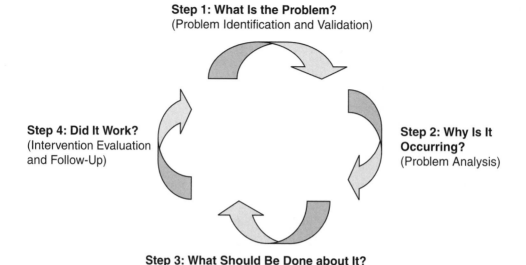

**Step 1: What Is the Problem?**
(Problem Identification and Validation)

**Step 4: Did It Work?**
(Intervention Evaluation
and Follow-Up)

**Step 2: Why Is It
Occurring?**
(Problem Analysis)

**Step 3: What Should Be Done about It?**
(Intervention Development and Implementation)

**FIGURE 7.1.** Questions and steps involved in a data-driven problem-solving process.

observable, and measurable terms. In addition, we need to consider direct measurement of problems within the context in which they occur. Precision is extremely important at this stage of the problem-solving process, and quantifying the problem as "discrepancy or difference score causes problem solvers to be objective about the problem" (Tilly, 2002, p. 29). The question becomes, How wide is the gap between actual and desired performance in this particular domain of functioning? To quantify discrepancies it is important to think in terms of measurement categories (e.g., frequency, duration, latency, magnitude).

This careful measurement process helps to formalize goals for students (i.e., a reduction in the discrepancy). When the discrepancy is large, it is sometimes necessary to consider short- and long-term goals. For example, a student who is reading at a level that is significantly below his or her peers (e.g., a discrepancy of three grade levels) is not likely to catch up in a short period (e.g., a year). Instead, a more reasonable goal might be set and progress monitored along the way (formative assessment). Direct and frequent measurement is helpful in identifying problems, promoting agreement across stakeholders (e.g., parents, administrators, and teachers) about what the problem is, and, once an intervention is in place, determining whether or not it is improving. Further, with discrepancy scores, one can discern magnitude or problem severity in an objective fashion, and this can be helpful when prioritizing problems within and across students. Of course, there are certain practical constraints to measuring discrepancies in applied settings (e.g., time, resources, and skills). Thus skillful practitioners will need to consider the precision, objectivity, practicality, and social validity of various measurement options when engaging in this first step of the problem-solving process. The problem-identification phase of the problem-solving process does not end until the problem is defined and validated as a quantifiable discrepancy between current and desired performance.

## Step 2: Why Is It Occurring? (Problem Analysis)

Once we have established that a problem exists and is worth our time and effort to solve, we move to the next stage in the problem-solving process. In this stage, we gather information about the problem and ask the question, Why is this problem occurring? In a problem-solving approach to school psychology, emphasis is placed on linking assessment to treatment and evaluation (Lentz & Shapiro, 1985). In this stage of the process, "instead of measuring student performance to find disabilities, our purpose is to diagnose the conditions under which students' learning is *enabled*" (Tilly, 2002, p. 29). To do this, we need to conduct an analysis of the problem context and function. One important question to answer in this phase of the process is whether the problem is a *skill* (can't do) or *performance* (won't do) problem (for more information on this process, see Witt et al., 2000). More specifically, if the issue is a behavioral deficit (i.e., the student's actual performance level is less than what is expected), is the reason for this deficit that (1) the student does not want to perform the task or activity, (2) the student gets something (e.g., attention, access to a preferred activity or object, sensory stimulation) as a result of not performing the task, (3) the work is being presented at a level that is too difficult for the student, (4) the student has not been provided enough assistance to acquire the skill, (5) the student has not been given sufficient time or practice with the skills to do it fluently, or (6) the work is being presented in a way that is different from the way the student has usually done the work?

This phase of the problem-solving process is focused on gathering information to answer questions such as those just posed in order to gain an understanding of why the problem exists and to use this information to generate hypotheses about what might be done differently to enable learning to occur. For example, if we suspect that the student's reading problem is related to the fact that the student has not been provided enough assistance to acquire the skill (i.e., the student has an acquisition problem), then our hypothesized intervention strategy might focus on providing instructional assistance directed toward skill development in reading (e.g., cueing, prompting, corrective feedback). Alternatively, if we suspect that the student's reading problem is due to the fact that the student has not had enough time to practice the skill (i.e., a fluency issue), then our hypothesized intervention strategy might focus on increasing opportunities to read (e.g., paired reading, reading at home). If we are concerned that the student's reading problem is not related to a skill deficit but is instead a performance (won't do) problem—a way of escaping the task—then our hypothesized intervention strategy will focus on addressing this problem. For example, we might make the task less aversive (e.g., considering the use of interesting reading materials or choice of materials), teach the student a different and more appropriate way to let us know that the task is aversive (e.g., asking for a break), and/or allow escape from the task contingent on some criterion of performance (e.g., allowing brief breaks from reading for appropriate performance for a certain number of minutes). In each of these scenarios, the problem is the same (i.e., a discrepancy between actual and desired reading performance), but the solutions are very different.

During the problem-analysis phase, information may be gathered from a variety of sources (e.g., student, teacher, parent, peers, administrator) via a variety of assessment tools (e.g., formal and informal direct observational methods, semistructured and unstructured interviews, anecdotal reports, rating scales, review of records, curriculum-based assessment of skills) to answer the preceding questions. The purpose is to understand why (under what conditions) problems are more pronounced and to identify patterns and factors that contribute to the problem. We focus on directly measuring when, where, with whom, and during which activities the problem is more or less likely to occur or become exacerbated. Given the assumption that many, if not most, student problems are a result of inappropriately arranged classroom and instructional events, attempts are made to examine potential contributing factors (e.g., materials, instructional strategies) that can be easily altered. Of course, factors that are outside of the school's control (e.g., allergies, illness, divorce) may play a role in the development or maintenance of the presenting problem. Yet, when developing interventions, it is important to focus on what we can change to enable learning and reduce the discrepancy. For example, knowing that a student has a significant visual impairment is important for instructional planning, but it is unlikely that the cause of the visual impairment will be the focus of the intervention for school personnel. Instead, it is likely that the school will consider instructional accommodations (e.g., modified materials, vocal cues) to enable the student to benefit from instruction, despite the visual impairment. This phase of the process ends with the development of hypotheses regarding why the problem is occurring (under what conditions, etc.) and, based on this information, of hypotheses about what intervention strategies are likely to be effective.

## Step 3: What Should Be Done about It?
## (Intervention Development and Implementation)

When we conceptualize problems as discrepancies between "what is" and "what should be," we are driven by the need to identify a solution that will reduce this discrepancy. It is at this stage of the problem-solving process that we use the information gathered thus far and decide what should be done about the problem. In addition to developing hypotheses about why the problem is occurring and linking this information to the selection of intervention strategies (contextual fit), one should consider interventions that have demonstrated empirical validity (see Chapters 9 and 10 for more discussion). Thus, in a problem-solving approach, an intervention strategy is selected based on its functional relevance to the problem, contextual fit, and likelihood of success. After identifying an appropriate intervention strategy, it is important to specify the intervention tactics that will be used. For example, when deciding what we should do about a problem, we need to clarify the intervention steps, roles, and responsibilities, as well as monitoring and evaluation techniques. In addition, it is important to determine the adequacy of existing resources and the need for additional resources in plan development. Further, timelines for implementing objectives and achieving desired goals should be specified. A clearly delineated intervention plan is the outcome of this phase in the process.

## Step 4: Did It Work? (Intervention Evaluation and Follow-Up)

As indicated previously, the goal of the problem-solving process is to resolve the discrepancy between "what is" and "what should be." Thus the process does not simply end with a thorough description or analysis of the problem. Nor does it end with a careful description of a potential solution or solutions to the problem. In order for the process to be completed, the problem should be resolved. Collecting ongoing information regarding the discrepancy between desired and actual performance is the best way to determine whether or not the intervention is effective. Thus continuous monitoring and evaluation are essential parts of an effective problem-solving process.

At this stage, objective evidence should be gathered to determine whether plans are effective (i.e., change behavior in the direction of the goal), practical (i.e., relatively easy to implement with integrity), and acceptable. To ensure that the intervention and not some other factor was responsible for problem resolution, it is important to compare the extent of a problem (discrepancy) during intervention and its extent when the intervention was not in place. Single-subject design methods (discussed in detail in Chapter 12) are useful for evaluating the effects of treatments for individual students. Information gathered during this phase of the process is analyzed, and, if necessary, intervention plans are revised and/or goals are adjusted accordingly.

## Summary of the Critical Features of a Data-Driven Problem-Solving Model

The data-driven problem-solving model is *outcome-focused*, *data-driven*, integrally *linked to intervention* and *context-specific*. One of the most important features of this approach is the emphasis on measurement to guide decision making throughout each phase of the process. In fact, if we were asked to identify the most important feature of this process, it would be *its focus on data*. Consistent with an empirically or scientifically based approach to practice, this model depends less on subjective judgment than on quantifiable feedback provided from the information collected throughout the process. An important feature of the type of information used in this process is that it is objective, observable, and measurable. The focus is on learning outcomes rather than internal processes. In addition, data collection emphasizes direct over indirect methods, as well as methods that are repeatable and lend themselves to formative assessment of learning outcomes. At all stages of the process, attempts are made to use tools and procedures that do not require significant levels of inference (Tilly, 2002). Similarly, the problem-solving process is context-specific, and disabilities are viewed as problems only if they result in a functional impairment within a particular context. This viewpoint keeps the focus on aspects of the problem situation that are modifiable (i.e., what we can change) and reduces the interpretive leap necessary to move to intervention.

## Systems to Support Sustained Use of Problem Solving

As with any shift in practice, one must consider how new practices fit within the existing school context in order to ensure their sustained use. As we noted in Chapters 2 and 3, school contexts are quite complex systems. They serve a diverse student population with a continuum of learning and social-behavioral needs. Concern with ever-increasing numbers, diversity, and severity of student needs urges us to examine our practices and, in light of evidence suggesting that what we are currently doing is not working, to explore alternatives. Further, recognized leaders in school psychology have promoted the adoption of evidence-based practices and data-oriented problem solving (e.g., Deno, 2002; Reschly & Ysseldyke, 2002; Shapiro, 2000; Tilly, 2002; Ysseldyke, 2000). Despite advocacy for this approach and despite advances in alternative assessment techniques, problem-solving methodologies, and interventions, schools do not readily adopt evidence-based practices (e.g., Abbott, Walton, Tapia, & Greenwood, 1999; Carnine, 1997, 1999; Forness, 2003a; Friedman, 2003; Gersten, Vaughn, Deshler, & Schiller, 1997; Hunter, 2003). When external supports are provided to schools to facilitate the adoption of evidence-based, problem-solving approaches, these endeavors have demonstrated improved outcomes for students, yet schools fail to sustain these practices when external supports are subsequently removed (e.g., Fuchs, Fuchs, Harris, & Roberts,

1996; McDougal, Clonan, & Martens, 2000). These failures have led researchers to consider that an important but often neglected aspect of translating research into effective school-based practices is careful consideration of the "fit between empirically validated interventions and organizational structures" (Hoagwood & Johnson, 2003, p. 5). In order to facilitate lasting change, we need to consider systems and organization structures of school systems and to work directly with stakeholders and policy makers (e.g., Curtis & Stollar, 2002; Grimes & Tilly, 1996).

In recent years, efforts to promote adoption of evidence-based, problem-solving approaches to addressing literacy (e.g., Simmons et al., 2000; Simmons et al., 2002) and behavior (e.g., Sugai & Horner, 2002a, 2002b; Sugai et al., 2000) have emphasized the need to address organizational issues and contextual fit to promote successful adoption and sustained use of data-based decision making. On a larger scale, the State of Iowa has focused on combining many aspects of general and special education services to meet the needs of all students through the adoption of a "problem-solving orientation to assessment, intervention design, data-based decision making, and outcome orientation" (Grimes & Tilly, 1996, p. 466). Many of these efforts have focused on schoolwide, districtwide, and/or statewide applications of data-driven problem-solving and evidence-based practices to address the needs of *all* students in the system in a proactive and preventative manner. Systems-level challenges that arise when attempting to build capacity for schools to adopt such approaches are discussed in detail in Chapter 11, but it is important to note here that consideration of these issues is paramount to successful adoption of a data-oriented problem-solving approach to school psychology.

## A Focus on Prevention

In addition to organizational and systems issues, in order for the data-driven problem-solving model to successfully address the learning, social, and behavioral needs facing today's youths, a prevention focus is critical. The following quote aptly illustrates this point:

> Communities cannot afford, and I mean this in hard economic terms as well as in humanitarian terms, to invest only in repair services. . . . To illustrate the point there is a fable concerning three people who were having a picnic beside the river. As they were enjoying their lunch in the sunshine, one looked up to see a child floating down the river. Immediately he leaped in and brought the child ashore. As he did so, his companions saw two more children helplessly bobbing in the water. Upon diving in to bring them out, they were dismayed to find still three more children in the river. Very quickly, they realized that the river was alive with struggling children in need of rescue. As they frantically worked to save as many as possible, one of the three suddenly left the water and began to run upstream along the bank. Seeing this, the others shouted after him in alarm, "Where are you going? Come back, we must help these children!" Continuing to run, he yelled, "You do the best you can there, I'm going up the river to try to stop them from falling in!" (Kisler, 1967, as cited in Drum & Figler, 1973, p. 13)

To date, school psychologists have invested much in "repair services." The children we typically serve are referred to us because they are already experiencing difficulties of some sort. Using the preceding analogy, one could argue that school psychologists spend a great deal of their time attempting to "pull kids from the river" or, if we are unable to pull them out, throwing them supports so they can stay afloat. Within the mental health literature, the work that we do falls into the category of *tertiary prevention*

(Walker et al., 1996). In tertiary prevention, emphasis is placed on reducing the intensity, severity, and complications of chronic cases. This is accomplished through the
delivery of specialized and individual interventions. Whether this occurs through traditional diagnostic approaches or through a problem-solving orientation, the focus is on
addressing student needs on a case-by-case basis (i.e., one child at a time) in a reactive
manner (i.e., after problems are noted). Problems are noticed, students are referred to
us, we assess the issue using traditional or alternative means, and from this information
interventions are determined, implemented, and, hopefully, evaluated. Given the
ever-increasing number of students in need of such services, tertiary prevention efforts
are essential.

Unfortunately, and as the preceding parable indicates, a focus on repair services
alone takes great effort and still may not be successful due to the increasing numbers,
severity, and complexity of problems that we face. We know, for example, that by late
elementary school, learning and behavior disorders are often chronic, resistant to intervention, and associated with negative long-term outcomes and costs to the individual
and to society (e.g., Adams, 1994; Biglan et al., 2003; Hunter, 2003; Walker, Colvin, &
Ramsey, 1995). Without early intervention services, the stability of learning and behavior problems is alarming. In contrast, with proactive services, prevention, and early
intervention, prognosis is much more promising (e.g., Biglan et al., 2003; Simmons &
Kame'enui, 1998). Further, comprehensive prevention and intervention efforts that
focus on building competencies and resiliency characteristics on a schoolwide level
seem to be the most promising from a public health standpoint (e.g., Biglan et al., 2003;
Hunter, 2003; Shapiro, 2000).

Several scholars in school psychology have argued for the adoption of a public
health model of school psychology (e.g., Hoagwood & Johnson, 2003; Power, 2003;
Strein et al., 2003). We agree with this perspective. As Figure 7.2 illustrates (OSEP Center on Positive Behavioral Interventions and Supports, 2000; Walker et al., 1996), public
health models focus on comprehensive service delivery at three levels of prevention for:

1. Students who currently are not experiencing learning and/or social-behavioral
   difficulties (primary prevention).
2. Students determined to be at risk for the development of learning and/or
   social-behavioral difficulties (secondary prevention).
3. Students who currently are experiencing significant learning and/or social-
   behavioral difficulties (tertiary prevention).

The triangle in Figure 7.2 represents all students within a school setting, the majority of
whom are not experiencing difficulties (i.e., the bottom portion of the triangle), some
of whom are at risk to develop significant problems (i.e., the middle portion), and an
even smaller percentage who are currently experiencing significant difficulties (i.e., the
top portion). Using the river analogy, children who are already "in the river" are like
those at the top of the triangle who are currently experiencing learning and or
social-behavioral difficulties. School psychologists currently spend the majority of their
time and effort providing tertiary prevention (i.e., individualized assessment and intervention services) to these students on a case-by-case basis. These students make up the
smallest percentage of the school population, but because of the significance of their
problems, they often require the majority of time and resources from school personnel
(Walker et al., 1996).

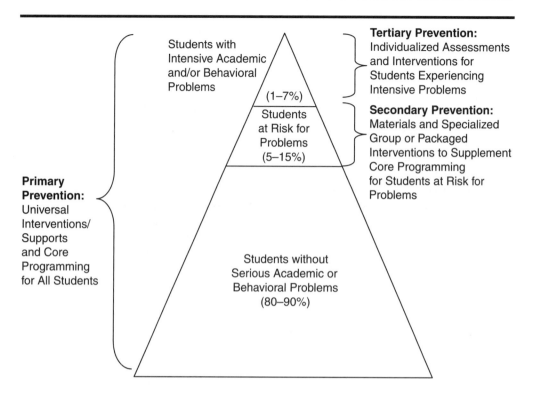

**FIGURE 7.2.** Triangle of support for the prevention of academic and behavioral problems.

Shifting to a prevention model requires that we take a step back and look at the "big picture" by considering the needs of *all* students, not just those who are referred to us because they are experiencing difficulties (Shapiro, 2000). The foundation of a prevention approach is the use of universal interventions (i.e., *primary prevention*) designed to enhance the delivery of effective instruction and improved school climate designed to promote academic, social, and behavioral resilience of *all* students in the school. The idea is that we send some folks "up river" to attend to students by implementing practices that are likely to enable them to remain on safe ground. More specifically, *primary prevention* for students who are not currently experiencing learning and/or social-behavioral difficulties is accomplished through schoolwide reform that involves the consistent use of research-based effective teaching and behavior management practices, ongoing monitoring of these practices and student outcomes, staff training and professional development, and systems-level decision making. The goal of primary prevention is to create school and classroom environments that promote student learning and decrease the number of students at risk for learning and/or social-behavioral problems.

We also know, however, that not all students respond similarly to prevention and intervention efforts. Thus it is important to monitor student progress and to assess whether students are at risk (i.e., in need of secondary prevention efforts) or experiencing significant learning and/or social-behavioral difficulties (i.e., are in need of tertiary prevention efforts). In other words, the people who are working to keep students on safe ground should monitor students to determine those who are at risk for falling in the river. Identifying students at risk of learning and/or social-behavioral difficulties is an important aspect of comprehensive prevention efforts. For students identified as at risk and in need of *secondary prevention* efforts, the focus is on the delivery of specialized interventions (often at a small-group level) to prevent the exacerbation of problems and to prevent the development of more significant concerns. In contrast to traditional diagnostic approaches, wherein students may actually "wait" to meet criteria for a disability prior to receiving services, in a prevention model, efforts are made to identify at-risk students early and to provide immediate services. The focus on early identification and early intervention is important. With regard to reading problems, for example, current evidence suggests that there is a critical and short period in which we can alter reading trajectories (Simmons & Kame'enui, 1998). In addition, if low-achieving students can be brought up to grade level within the first 3 years of school, their reading performance tends to stay at grade level (Adams, 1994). Thus, if we focus on early prevention and intervention services, our impact is likely to be greater.

### The School Psychologist's Role

With a data-oriented problem-solving approach, we believe the school psychologist can make significant contributions at all levels of prevention noted in the triangle in Figure 7.2. The same problem-solving process (i.e., What is the problem? Why is it occurring? What can be done about it? Is it working?) can be applied at the school, classroom, and individual levels. One key to success in this model is the use of quantifiable, objective data to guide decision making. Thus school psychologists are in a unique position to make significant contributions to prevention and intervention efforts given their knowledge and skills in the use of alternative assessment tools (CBA/CBM, FBA) useful for frequent and formative monitoring of student progress along expected continua of development, of proactive screening of students at risk, and of intervention evaluation purposes. Overall, we believe the school psychologist of the future has much to offer in a preventative data-oriented problem-solving system.

## DISCUSSION QUESTIONS AND ACTIVITIES

1. Visit the library and consult the early issues (i.e., prior to 1980) of *School Psychology Review*. See if you can find at least one example of an article that espouses a traditional (i.e., correlational or ATI) approach and one example of an article that espouses a problem-solving (i.e., experimental) approach.

2. Interview parents, teachers, administrators, and school psychologists regarding their perceptions of the current and their ideal/preferred role of the school psychologist. If differences between current and ideal/preferred roles are expressed, ask what barriers the individual thinks are getting in the way of the ideal/preferred role. Were there differences between perceptions of current and ideal/preferred roles? Were perceptions of the school psychologists' *current* role more consistent with a traditional (diagnostic) or an alternative (problem-solving) approach? What about perceptions of the ideal/preferred role?

3. Despite evidence that was unsupportive of the ATI approach (i.e., Cronbach, 1975), in a 1977 teacher survey, the overwhelming majority of special education teachers reported that they believed a child's modality strengths and weaknesses should be a

major instructional planning consideration. Interview 10 special education teachers and 10 school psychologists to discover if this view is still held today.

4. Interview a school psychologist about the typical process (steps) she or he follows when working with an individual referral. Is the process more consistent with a traditional or with problem-solving approach? Do they define problems as discrepancies? Is measurement an integral part of the process? What type of information is collected to inform treatment? Is evaluation of the treatment part of the process, or does this process end with assessment and recommendations?

5. Search the literature for problem-solving formats that were developed for use in school settings. From the information you collect, examine the forms and create your own version of a line of questioning that helps guide the process.

# 8

# The School Psychologist's Role in Assessment

MODELS, METHODS, AND TRENDS IN GATHERING, ORGANIZING, AND ANALYZING DATA

Assessment is one of the more controversial topics in school psychology. If one were to interview 10 school psychologists on their views of assessment and what constitutes an appropriate evaluation, there would likely be significant disagreement. School psychologists have, traditionally, been very tied to assessment in terms of their job function (as discussed in Chapters 2 and 5). However, more recently somewhat of a backlash has occurred against the role of evaluator, and many school psychologists are attempting to move away from this role. Although we strongly endorse the idea of school psychologists as comprehensive educational and mental health providers, we also believe that assessment plays an important role in the provision of comprehensive services. Assessment is necessary to ensure that children's difficulties are adequately identified and that interventions are developed that are appropriate for the problems a child is experiencing and the context in which the problems occur. In traditional views of school psychology, assessment is often thought of as standardized testing, particularly using standardized measures of intellectual ability and achievement for the purpose of determining diagnosis and/or eligibility for special education services. However, when assessment is viewed in the context of the problem-solving process (as outlined in Chapter 7), it can become much more than this limited view indicates. In fact, assessment is an important part of the problem-solving process, as this process should be guided by information (data). In our view, assessment should be primarily used to facilitate the problem-solving process.

A helpful distinction between traditional assessment and problem-solving assessment is made by Howell and Nolet (2000), who differentiate between evaluations conducted for purposes outside the classroom and those conducted for purposes inside the classroom. Evaluations conducted for outside purposes include those typically conducted by school psychologists to determine whether a child meets criteria for a certain disability category. Evaluations conducted for inside purposes are those intended to obtain data to identify students who need specific skills, to inform intervention decisions, and to monitor implemented interventions. At a broader program evaluation level, inside assessments may be conducted to determine whether educational programs are having the intended positive effect. Evaluations with an inside purpose facilitate the problem-solving process in which information is gathered to help answer the questions that guide the process (i.e., What is the problem? Why is it occurring? What can we do about it? Did it work?) in an objective manner. This type of assessment is formative in nature; it is conducted in an ongoing fashion to guide decision making at all levels of problem solving (individual child, classroom, school, district, etc.).

In our opinion, the most important goal of an evaluation should be to develop recommendations that will guide the implementation of effective interventions for the child's problems and, subsequently, to determine whether or not those interventions resulted in positive outcomes for the child. Thus, even if there is an outside purpose to the evaluation (e.g., a disability label is needed in order for a student to access certain services), we believe the inside purpose should also be addressed. In our opinion, many school psychologists engage in too much outside assessment and not enough inside, intervention-focused assessment. We acknowledge the fact that standardized norm-referenced assessment practices are useful for some evaluation purposes (e.g., comparisons of performance across schools, comparison of a student's performance with that of a large normative sample). However, we also believe such assessments are overutilized and that alternative assessment methods (e.g., CBA, FBA) are underutilized. In addition, standardized norm-referenced measures are typically less useful in facilitating the selection of interventions and in evaluating interventions formatively (i.e., on an ongoing basis) than are alternative assessment methods. In this chapter we outline some of the common assessment techniques utilized in school psychology practice. We include assessments that are used for a variety of evaluation purposes and give an overview of standardized, norm-referenced measures, as well as alternative methods of assessment. We conclude this chapter with an integrated view of assessment and the problem-solving process.

# ASSESSMENT STANDARDS AND PSYCHOMETRIC PROPERTIES

Before discussing specific assessment techniques, we need to provide some background regarding assessment standards and psychometric issues. Understanding the reliability and validity of instruments is a key part of evaluating the usefulness and appropriateness of assessment measures. Although a complete overview of these important psychometric properties is beyond the scope of this chapter, we briefly review these concepts and urge readers to familiarize themselves with these issues.

## Assessment Standards

Most ethical codes address assessment standards in some manner. For example, as noted in Chapter 6, the ethical codes of both NASP and APA require that psychologists be knowledgeable about the psychometric properties of instruments and use instruments appropriate to the purpose of the evaluation. In addition to the assessment standards mentioned in specific ethical codes, the *Standards for Educational and Psychological Testing* were published in a joint effort of the American Educational Research Association, the American Psychological Association, and the National Council on Measurement in Education (1999). As stated in the introduction to these standards, their purpose is to "promote the sound and ethical use of tests and to provide a basis for evaluating the quality of testing practices" (p. 1). These standards are divided into three parts: test construction, evaluation, and documentation (including standards related to reliability and validity); fairness in testing; and testing applications. These standards are quite numerous and lengthy, covering everything from the importance of using reliable and valid measures to best practices in assessing individuals of diverse linguistic backgrounds to standards relating to the use of tests in specific applied settings (e.g., educational testing, employment). Related specifically to assessment in educational settings, the Joint Committee on Testing Practices (JCTP) has published the *Code of Fair Testing Practices in Education* (available online at http://www.apa.org/science/jctpweb.html), which provides guidance for both test developers and test users in four different areas: developing and selecting appropriate tests, administering and scoring tests, reporting and interpreting test results, and informing test takers. These guidelines are intended to help professionals develop and use tests that are fair to all individuals. Readers are encouraged to familiarize themselves with these various standards and general best practices in assessment.

## Reliability

The reliability of a measure refers to the *extent to which the measure is consistent*. This consistency can be shown across the items within the measure (internal consistency reliability), over time (test–retest reliability), across respondents or raters (interrater reliability), and across different forms of the same measure (alternate-form reliability). Reliability coefficients are expressed as correlation coefficients ranging from .00 (no association, meaning no reliability) to 1.00 (perfect reliability). An important related concept is the *standard error of measurement*, which is the amount of error associated with a score. The lower the reliability of a measure, the larger the standard error of measurement associated with the measure. The standard error of measurement can then be used to form confidence intervals, or ranges of scores that are likely to contain an individual's "true" score (Sattler, 2001). It is important to note that not all forms of reliability should be expected to be high. For example, interrater reliability between parents and teachers on behavior rating scales is typically quite low. This does not necessarily indicate that the test is unreliable—simply that parents and teachers may observe different behaviors in different settings.

## Validity

Validity is a somewhat more complex concept than reliability. Validity refers to *the extent to which a test measures what it is intended to measure*. Given this, validity must be considered in the context of the purpose of the test. Although validity is generally viewed as a unitary construct, there are various ways of determining validity. Traditionally, the three main forms of validity are *content*, *criterion*, and *construct*. Content validity refers to whether the items on the test are representative of the domain they are intended to evaluate (e.g., do items on a depression inventory actually measure depression, or do they represent another, perhaps related, construct, such as anxiety?). Criterion validity has to do with the relationship between the score on the measure and an outcome, such as a classification. There are two types of criterion validity: concurrent validity (which examines the test score as it relates to some currently available outcome) and predictive validity (which examines the test score as it relates to future performance). Construct validity is considered to be the overarching or superordinate form of validity. This notion refers to whether the test measures the particular construct it is intended to measure. When evaluating construct validity, both convergent validity (whether the test correlates with other, similar measures) and discriminant validity (whether the test does not correlate with measures of unlike constructs) are evaluated (Sattler, 2001).

Although validity is often thought of as relating specifically to the technical adequacy of a measure, Messick (1995) argues that one must also consider the "social consequences of test interpretation and use" (p. 744). As such, Messick refers to both evidential bases of validity (the psychometric/technical adequacy of a measure) and consequential bases of validity (the appropriateness of a test's use in terms of social consequences). The consequential basis of validity is an "appraisal of the value implications of score meaning" (p. 748), which relate to labels and actions generated as a result of testing. Thus Messick argues that we should evaluate tests based not only on their psychometric grounds but also on their ethical grounds.

Clearly, both reliability and validity are important in helping us evaluate whether we should use a certain test for a given purpose. Although test developers should attend to these issues when developing new assessment instruments, it is imperative that test users also attend to these issues—especially to issues related to validity, as the documentation of a test's validity tends to be an ongoing process and not limited to studies conducted prior to a test's publication.

## INTELLECTUAL ASSESSMENT

As discussed in Chapter 5, school psychologists spend about half of their time in assessment-related activities. In terms of actual assessment measures, administered, standardized measures of intellectual ability (IQ tests) are some of the most commonly used, with the Wechsler intelligence scales (Wechsler, 1997, 2002, 2003) consistently being the most widely used of the intellectual measures. Wilson and Reschly (1996) surveyed school psychologists in 1991–1992 and compared school psychologists' use of certain assessment instruments in that year to their use in 1986. The Wechsler scales were the most commonly administered measures at both times (although observation was the most commonly used assessment method in 1991–1992). Almost all school psychologists in 1991–1992 reported that they used the Wechsler scales, with the average use being about 9 times per month. Other measures of intelligence were used, but their use was reported by less than half of the school psychologists. In a more recent survey, school psychologists reported that intellectual measures, behavior rating scales, and projective measures were the most commonly used assessment techniques (Hosp & Reschly, 2002). School psychologists in this survey reported giving an average of 15 intellectual measures a month (these were not broken down by specific measures).

Although measures of intellectual ability are commonly used, their use is certainly not without controversy. A complete discussion of the controversy surrounding IQ instruments is well beyond the scope of this chapter. Numerous books, chapters, journal articles, and scholarly talks have been devoted to these issues. We attempt to outline briefly some of the main issues involved in this controversy, but we encourage readers to seek additional information. Although a significant focus of past debates regarding IQ tests centered on whether these measures are biased against certain populations of individuals, current debate is more focused on the utility of these measures, although it should be noted that the issue of potential bias has not been resolved. Questions such as the following are being asked and debated with increasing frequency (e.g., Kaufman, Lichtenberger, & Naglieri, 1999; Reschly, 1997): What theoretical constructs are measured by these instruments? Is interpretation of subtest scores valid? Do results from IQ measures assist in planning interventions?

The question of what is being assessed via IQ measures is theoretically complex. A number of different theories of intelligence have been developed over the years. In general, these theories can be placed into two different categories: (1) those that focus on intelligence involving a *general factor* (generally referred to as *g*) and (2) those that subscribe to the notion that intelligence has *multiple factors*. Even most professionals who subscribe to the notion of a general factor of intelligence agree that there are a variety of specific skills that contribute to a person's overall level of intelligence. However, those who subscribe to a multiple factor theory of intelligence believe that these different facets of intelligence are distinct and cannot be simply combined to obtain one general intelligence factor (Sattler, 2001). Just as there are many theories of intelligence, there are many definitions of intelligence. In reviewing these definitions, Sattler (2001) suggested that all "definitions of intelligence emphasize the ability to adjust or adapt to the environment, the ability to learn, or the ability to perform abstract thinking" (p. 135).

The issue of whether IQ measures have treatment validity has been an increased focus of attention in school psychology as researchers and practitioners are increasingly advocating for a more direct link between assessment and intervention. If the goal of assessment is to guide treatment planning, how do results from traditional IQ tests fit in with this goal? It is clear that IQ measures do have moderate predictive validity; children with higher scores are more likely to perform well in school than those with lower scores, with the correlation between IQ scores and grades being about .50 (Neisser et al., 1996). However, as Reschly (1997) noted, IQ measures "are rarely used as predictors of how well children will perform in an academic setting. Rather such tests are used *after* children have performed poorly" (p. 238). Reschly further stated that the concerns for these children have more to do with identifying "goals and instructional methodologies that will result in improve academic performance" (p. 238) than with identifying whether there is a difference between a referred child's current abilities and those of his or her peers.

Historically, the use of intellectual measures has been necessary in schools to help determine whether a child qualified for special education services. The IDEA-97 definitions of learning disabilities (LD) and mental retardation (MR) both mention intellectual ability. According to the definition of LD in IDEA-97, to be classified as having a learning disability, a person must evidence a "severe discrepancy between achievement and intellectual ability" (34 C.F.R. § 300.541). Mental retardation involves "significantly subaverage intellectual functioning, existing concurrently with deficits in adaptive behavior" (34 C.F.R. § 300.7). Given that the definitions of these disabilities have been directly tied to intellectual measures, it has been difficult for school psychologists to get away from performing IQ tests, even if such assessments do not seem to be necessary to develop an appropriate treatment plan for a child. However, given the changes to the definition of an LD in the recent reauthorization of IDEA (discussed in Chapter 6) that eliminate the requirement that students have a severe discrepancy between their intellectual and achievement abilities to be classified as having an LD, it will be interesting to see what happens with the standardized-assessment focus of school psychologists. Will school psychologists continue to evaluate intellectual ability in children referred for learning problems? Or will they decide that the use of such measures is not needed and rely more heavily on the response to intervention mentioned in the current version of IDEA?

Although there is certainly much controversy surrounding the use of IQ measures, we believe that these measures, when used appropriately, have their place in the assessment of *some* children (although in far fewer children than are currently administered IQ tests on a routine basis). Assuming the IQ measure was validly administered, the obtained IQ score can have *implications* for interventions for the child, even if knowing the child's IQ does not lead *directly* to an intervention. For example, reading interventions for a second-grade child who is struggling because of an ability problem (i.e., a child who cannot do the work) may need to focus on basic literacy and prereading skills, whereas a child who is struggling with reading because of a motivation problem may show an improvement in reading if incentives for reading grade-level material are provided.

For intellectual measures to be used responsibly, it is important that users of these measures understand what these measures are and what they are not. IQ measures provide an estimate of *current* intellectual functioning. Although IQ scores are relatively stable in most individuals by the early elementary school years, variation in scores may occur across testing times. This may have to do with measurement error and the circumstances surrounding the assessment, but it is also likely that there may be some change in the individual and/or his or her environment (Reschly & Grimes, 2002). It is important that users and consumers of IQ measures understand that these measures do not assess only some "innate" intellectual ability. Although genetics and biology obviously play an important role in the development of intellectual ability, environmental factors such as early exposure to reading and quality of environment in the infancy and preschool years are also important (Neisser, 1996). We also need to understand that the scores obtained from IQ measures are *estimates* of a person's true abilities. Confidence intervals are increasingly being emphasized in interpreting the limits or realistic ranges of test scores. We believe that their use is very important in demonstrating that the obtained IQ score is not the specific IQ but rather our best estimate of a person's current intellectual ability.

Before deciding to use an IQ measure, we must determine whether it is needed and justified for the decision that is to be made based on the evaluation. Using a measure just because it is typically what is administered or because "that's just the way it is done" is not good practice and has likely served to contribute to some of the negative perceptions of IQ measures. It is also important to choose a measure that will provide valid information. School psychologists must remember that just because an instrument has adequate psychometric properties, it is not necessarily valid for the purpose for which it is being used or the populations with which it is being used. For example, an IQ measure may be a valid measure of current intellectual functioning; but it is not a valid measure of whether a child has impairments in reading. An intelligence test normed on an American, English-speaking population may be a valid measure of current intellectual functioning for a child who is a U.S. citizen and a native English speaker. It is likely not a valid measure of current intellectual functioning for a child who recently emigrated from Mexico and speaks little English. When interpreting results, remember also that no decisions should be made on the basis of one data point (e.g., one test score) alone.

Results from the assessment must be interpreted within the context of other information. For example, how the child approached the task is important to consider: Did the child rush through items and complain about being there, or was the child focused and on task? Are there other pieces of information that may argue against a certain conclusion? For example, perhaps a child scored poorly on an IQ measure but has always obtained adequate grades in school and complained of receiving little sleep the night before the test. In this case, it seems likely that the results from the IQ measure may underestimate the child's true abilities—perhaps due to extreme fatigue.

Historically, school psychologists have had little choice when selecting an IQ measure, but an increasing number of such measures are being developed, and many of the newer tests bear little resemblance to the traditional IQ measures. Even with the increasing availability of measures, the Wechsler Intelligence Scale for Children, now in its fourth edition (WISC-IV; Wechsler, 2003), remains the measure with which most clinicians are familiar. Parallel measures for young children (Wechsler Preschool and Primary Scales of Intelligence–Third Edition [WPPSI-III], Wechsler, 2002) and adults (Wechsler Adult Intelligence Scale–Third Edition [WAIS-III], Wechsler, 1997) are also commonly used, although less so in schools due to the age of the school clientele. The WISC-IV has undergone some significant revisions from its earlier versions in terms of its factor structure. On the current version of the WISC, a full-scale IQ score is obtained, as well as index scores in four areas: Verbal Comprehension, Perceptual Reasoning, Working Memory, and Processing Speed. The WISC-IV contains 15 individual subtests, 10 of which contribute to the overall or full-scale IQ score. Although the WISC-IV manual cites extensive evidence of its psychometric properties, because it has been so recently revised, no published independent evaluations of its psychometric properties are currently available.

Another popular IQ measure with a long history is the Stanford–Binet, recently published in its fifth version (SB-V; Roid, 2003). Like the WISC-IV, the Stanford–Binet has a full-scale IQ score, as well as a several composite scores (Fluid Reasoning, Knowledge, Quantitative Reasoning, Visual Spatial Processing, and Working Memory). Verbal and nonverbal IQ scores can also be obtained. The popular Kaufman Assessment Battery for Children has also recently been published in a new edition (K-ABC-II; Kaufman & Kaufman, 2004a). The K-ABC-II provides users with two theoretical models (the Luria neuropsychological model and Cattell–Horn–Carroll theory) that can be used to interpret the results of this measure. The K-ABC-II is purported by the authors to be more culturally fair than other traditional measures of IQ; it attempts to achieve this fairness by limiting verbal instructions and responses, as well as using items with limited cultural content. As with the WISC-IV and SB-V, the newness of this instrument means that independent evaluations of its reliability and validity have yet to be done. The Woodcock–Johnson Tests of Cognitive Abilities (WJ-III-Cog; Woodcock, McGrew, & Mather, 2001b) is another recently revised intellectual measure and was conormed with the Woodcock–Johnson Tests of Achievement (Woodcock, McGrew, & Mather, 2001a). The WJ-III-Cog is based on the Cattell–Horn–Carroll (CHC) theory of intelligence, with subtests designed to target factors of intelligence as outlined in this theory (McGrew & Woodcock, 2001). Based on anecdotal data from individuals employed in school districts, the WJ-III-Cog seems to be increasing in use. The Differential Ability Scales (DAS; Elliot, 1990) is another standardized measure of intellectual ability that is used with some frequency.

In addition to these more traditional measures of IQ, which tend to have a significant verbal component to them, are newer, "nonverbal" measures of intelligence, which are designed to rely less heavily on verbal skills. Some of these measures include the Universal Nonverbal Intelligence Test (UNIT; Bracken & McCallum, 1998), the Leiter International Performance Scale–Revised (Leiter-R; Roid & Miller, 1997), and the Comprehensive Test of Nonverbal Intelligence (CTONI; Hammill, Pearson, & Weiderholt, 1997). These non-verbal tests have gained in popularity as our school's populations have become more diverse, with larger non-English-speaking populations. Nonverbal tests can also be helpful when evaluating children with limited language abilities due to disabilities. Although non-verbal measures of intelligence correlate substantially with more traditional measures of intelligence and thus appear to be still measuring the theoretical construct of general intelligence, significant variability still exists in the psychometric properties of nonverbal measures. Users should be cautious when selecting nonverbal tests and ensure that the test they choose has been adequately standardized and normed and has strong psychometric properties (Bracken & Naglieri, 2003).

## ASSESSMENT OF ACADEMIC SKILLS

In contrast to the assessment of intellectual abilities, relatively less controversy surrounds achievement testing. This situation likely occurs in part because achievement tests are considered to have more "face validity" than IQ measures. They are intended to measure current academic performance, and the subtests on these measures clearly involve basic academic skills such as reading, math, and writing. However, in recent years, discussion of how to best evaluate academic skills has grown. Traditionally, these skills were evaluated via standardized, norm-referenced measures of achievement. Increasingly, though, psychologists are turning to alternative methods of assessment for academic problems that are tied more directly to a student's current curriculum. In particular, CBA methods have been noted as being valuable methods of assessing a child's academic performance within the context of his or her curriculum.

It is interesting to note that although texts such as the most recent editions of *Best Practices in School Psychology* (Thomas & Grimes, 2002) and *The Handbook of School Psychology* (Reynolds & Gutkin, 1999) include specific chapters on intellectual assessment, they contain no general chapters on the assessment of academic skills, only chapters on the use of curriculum-based measurement. Although this may be taken as a good sign that school psychologists are increasingly using alternative assessment methods to identify learning problems, surveys of school psychologists indicate that they still frequently use standardized, norm-referenced instruments for this purpose. School psychologists who responded to Wilson and Reschly's (1996) survey indicated that they were using standardized achievement tests much more frequently than they were using CBA methods. In this survey, the three most commonly used achievement measures were used, on average, approximately eight times per month, and CBA methods were used only once per month. Even in a more recent survey, school psychologists reported using standardized achievement tests more often than CBA methods (Chafouleas, Riley-Tillman, & Eckert, 2003). However, the use of CBA methods is clearly increasing. A recent survey (Shapiro, Angello, & Eckert, 2004) indicated that more school psychologists reported using curriculum-based methods in 2000 (54%) than in 1990 (46%). In addition, school psychologists who had recently completed their graduate training were much more likely to have received training in CBA methods than were those who had been in the workforce for some time. Shapiro et al. (2004) reported that of school psychologists who have been working 1–3 years, 90% had received training in CBA during their graduate education, whereas less than 20% of those in the workforce 13 years or longer had received training in CBA in their graduate programs. Training in CBA and use of CBA methods have been noted to be significantly correlated, and school psychologists do rate CBA methods as acceptable—in fact, these methods have been rated as more acceptable than norm-referenced measures of achievement (Chafouleas et al., 2003). Given that school psychologists seem open to the use of CBA methods and that they are increasingly receiving training in these methods, it seems likely that CBA methods will continue to increase in use over time.

In the following sections we discuss the use of both standardized, norm-referenced measures of academic skills and CBA. We believe that school psychologists should be familiar with both types of these assessment techniques. It seems likely that CBA procedures will continue to gain in popularity, but it is also likely that many school psychologists will still administer and/or interpret standardized, norm-referenced measures of achievement on a regular basis. Although school psychologists should be familiar with these assessment techniques, it should be noted that in many school districts it is not the school psychologist who is responsible for assessing a child's academic achievement; instead, it is the special education teacher or an educational diagnostician. However, even in such districts, school psychologists will need to be familiar with these measures to aid in the interpretation and intervention planning.

## Standardized, Norm-Referenced Achievement Tests

As noted, although CBA methods appear to be gaining in use, standardized, norm-referenced achievement tests are still more frequently used by school psychologists to evaluate academic skills. Some of the more common measures include the Woodcock-Johnson Tests of Achievement—Third Edition (WJ-III; Woodcock, McGrew, & Mather, 2001a), the Wechsler Individual Achievement Test—Second Edition (WIAT-II; Wechsler, 2001), the Wide Range Achievement Test—Third Edition (WRAT-3; Wilkinson, 1993), the Peabody Individual Achievement Test—Revised (PIAT-R; Markwardt, 1989, 1997), and the Kaufman Test of Educational Achievement—Second Edition (K-TEA-II; Kaufman & Kaufman, 2004b). These measures all include subtests intended to assess a variety of achievement abilities (e.g., reading, math, written language, oral language). In addition to these broad measures of academic achievement are measures that assess academic ability in one specific area. Examples of such instruments include KeyMath—Revised (Connolly, 1988, 1997), Woodcock Reading Mastery Tests—Revised (WRMT-R; Woodcock, 1987, 1998), and the Gray Oral Reading Test—Fourth Edition (GORT-4; Wiederholt & Bryant, 2001). These single-subject tests are used less frequently than the multiple-subject tests and are typically used to follow up on problems noted when using a comprehensive achievement measure. Obviously, the advantage to using a comprehensive test is that one can obtain information on a student's abilities in a variety of academic areas with the use of a single assessment instrument. However, a single-subject test might be used when the referral question relates directly to a specific problem or when more in-depth information is needed in a certain area (Stetson, Stetson, & Sattler, 2001).

Two trends in the development of comprehensive achievement tests have become evident over the past several years. One is that achievement tests are increasingly being developed to match specific IDEA categories of learning disabilities (oral expression, listening comprehension, written expression, basic reading skills, reading comprehension, mathematics calculation, and mathematics reasoning). The other trend is that achievement tests are increasingly being conormed with parallel IQ tests, theoretically for a more accurate comparison of whether there is a significant discrepancy between a student's intellectual ability and achievement performance. For example, the K-TEA-II, WJ-III, and WIAT-II all have subtests that match the seven areas of learning disabilities identified in IDEA-97. Each of these tests is also linked to an IQ test, either through conorming (as was done with the K-TEA-II and K-ABC-II and the WJ-III tests of achievement and cognitive ability) or via administering intelligence tests to a subset of those in the achievement test sample (as was done with the WIAT-II and associated Wechsler intelligence scales). Both the PIAT-R and WRAT-3 are more limited in scope than these newer measures of academic achievement. Most notably, neither has a subtest that assesses oral language. The WRAT-3, for example, contains only three subtests measuring reading, spelling, and arithmetic, and it is considered more of a screener than a comprehensive test of achievement (Hendry, 2003).

A complete review of the available tests of achievement is beyond the scope of this chapter. However, it should be noted that each of the comprehensive multiple-subject tests of achievement described in this chapter has adequate psychometric properties. Which of these measures one ends up using (if a standardized, norm-referenced test is being used at all) may depend in part on personal preference. Many of these instruments have recently been updated, and independent evaluations of their psychometric properties are not yet available. Thus school psychologists should look to future literature in this area so that they can make informed decisions about which of these instruments may be most appropriate for their use.

## Curriculum-Based Assessment/Measurement

As noted, CBA methods are increasingly being touted as alternatives to standardized, norm-referenced achievement testing. These methods have in common that they use materials adapted from actual classroom materials—for example, assessing a child's reading skills by using a passage from a text the child is reading in class. Curriculum-based *measurement* (CBM) is a specific type of curriculum-based assessment. CBM involves a set of specific procedures that are technically adequate, that include standardized measurement tasks, and that have specific administration and scoring guidelines (Deno, 2003). CBM methods are intended to be time efficient and generally consist of probes that last a maximum of several minutes in duration. For example, the most commonly used CBM probe for reading involves having the child read aloud from a text for 1 minute. The total number of words read correctly is calculated by the observer/test administrator (Deno, 2003).

Shinn (2002) specified that CBM techniques are to be used by teachers to evaluate the effects of their instruction. He specifically stated that "CBM is not a tool to be used on a daily basis by school psychologists as part of their assessment activities" (p. 671). However, Shinn strongly advocates for the use of CBM to develop better IEP goals for children, to link assessment and intervention more directly, and, in the process, to improve the special education outcomes for students. According to Deno (2003), an increasingly common use of CBM procedures is to evaluate students who are academically at risk. Local norms may be developed for this purpose with those children who perform toward the bottom, being considered to be at risk for academic difficulties. In fact, CBM methods have been proposed as an alternative to standardized norm-referenced tests for the identification of children in need of special education services. Fuchs, Fuchs, and their colleagues (e.g., Fuchs & Fuchs, 1998; Fuchs, Fuchs, & Speece, 2002) have proposed a treatment-validity approach to the identification of children with learning disabilities. Within such an approach, they specify that the assessment system must document that the regular classroom is producing acceptable growth (in general, that children in the classroom are learning); that there are discrepancies between the target child's academic performance and that of his or her peers, as well as between the child's academic growth rate and that of his or her peers; that the child cannot learn adequately in the regular classroom even with modifications; and that special education can improve the child's academic growth. They suggested that CBM procedures can provide the information needed to address each one of these points. In 2002, the final report from the President's Commission on Excellence in Special Education recommended that the methods of identifying children with learning disabilities, as outlined in IDEA-97, be simplified and that response to intervention be a key component of the identification process. Although the commission did not refer to CBM specifically, clearly these procedures would fit in with their recommendations. As noted in Chapter 6, the new revisions to IDEA have incorporated this suggestion by eliminating the requirement for an achievement–intellectual discrepancy in the identification of children with learning disabilities and specifying that a response-to-intervention approach can be used.

One example of a measurement system that makes significant use of CBM methods is the Dynamic Indicators of Basic Early Literacy Skills (DIBELS) system developed by researchers at the University of Oregon (Official DIBELS Homepage, dibels.uoregon.edu for more information). DIBELS is intended to be used to assess several of the "big ideas" in basic literacy skills, including phonological awareness (the ability to hear and manipulate sounds into words), alphabetic principle (the ability to link letters to sounds and to form words), and fluency with connected text (the ability to effortlessly read words in context). The DIBELS system includes brief measures that address each of these areas. The measures are standardized and can be used over time to help monitor the reading progress of students (Good et al., 2002; Official DIBELS Homepage). Five main measures are used in the DIBELS system. These include two that measure phonological awareness: Initial Sounds Fluency (in which the child is asked to identify out of four pictures one that begins with a certain letter) and Phoneme Segmentation Fluency (in which the student is asked to verbally break words into their individual phonemes). Nonsense Word Fluency is a measure of alphabetic principle and requires students to read nonsense words presented on paper or verbally produce the letter sounds in the nonsense word. Oral Reading Fluency is a measure of fluency with connected text in which students are required to read passages aloud. Letter Naming Fluency, in which students are asked to name letters presented on paper, is intended to provide a measure of risk for early literacy problems (Official DIBELS Homepage). The DIBELS system is intended to be used with children in kindergarten through third grade. The system contains benchmark goals for the beginning, middle, and end of the year to help determine whether students are achieving at an adequate level. Students considered to be at risk would be provided with instructional support to attempt to increase their literacy skills (Good et al., 2002; Official DIBELS Homepage).

Given the significant research regarding CBM procedures over the past quarter century and the strong advocates for the use of CBM procedures in the evaluation of student performance and the link to academic interventions, it seems likely that this momentum will continue and that CBM will increasingly be used as a means of assessing academic achievement and, more important, of students' responses to intervention. This method, which is viewed as highly acceptable by most school psychologists, more clearly ties assessment to intervention than do most other methods of assessing academic skills.

## Functional Assessment

Although functional assessment methods have historically been tied more to behavior problems than to academic problems (and are discussed in more detail later in this chapter), this methodology has also been used to address academic issues. Daly, Witt, Martens, and Dool (1997) describe a functional approach to understanding academic failure as one that relates "academic performance to aspects of the classroom instruction that precede and follow student performance" (p. 555). They argue that because aspects of the classroom are external to the child, viewing academic difficulties from this perspective allows one to identify areas for instructional intervention. Daly et al. (1997) discuss five "reasonable hypotheses" about why students perform poorly from a functional perspective. These include: (1) the student does not want to do the work, (2) the student has not spent enough time on the work, (3) the student has not had enough help to successfully complete the work, (4) the student has not previously had to do the work in the requested manner, and (5) the work is too hard for the student. If the function of the difficulty is identified, interventions can be developed that match (e.g., if the student does not want or is not motivated to do the work, provide incentives for completion of the work). When using a functional approach, hypotheses regarding the function of the academic problem are formed and are then evaluated using miniexperiments. CBA techniques are integral to this process, as the evaluator must be able to make quick, repeated assessments of a child's performance under different conditions. For example, a student's reading level may be assessed under several different academic interventions, each tied to a functional hypothesis (e.g., with a reinforcer for completing work; with repeated practice with correction).

Functional approaches to academic problems have much merit and clearly fit within the problem-solving model. However, as Daly et al. (1997) note, the process can be time-consuming, and school psychologists have not historically received training in this method. As functional methods become more commonplace in schools in general, it is our hope that they will be used as part of the problem-solving assessment process for children with academic difficulties, as well as for those with behavior problems.

# ASSESSMENT OF SOCIAL–EMOTIONAL AND BEHAVIORAL FUNCTIONING

The assessment of social–emotional and behavioral problems has typically not generated as much attention within the field of school psychology as has the assessment of intellectual ability and academic achievement. Likely this gap has to do with the fewer number of children being served under the IDEA-97 category of emotional disturbance (8.2% of all children in special education in 2000–2001; U.S. Department of Education, 2002) compared with the number of children being served under the category of learning disabilities (50% of all children in special education in 2000–2001; U.S. Department of Education, 2002). However, there are signs that attention to this topic is picking up. This trend is likely due to several factors, including an increased recognition that school psychologists have expertise in mental health issues, as well as academic issues. In addition, the number of children identified as having attention-deficit/hyperactivity disorder (ADHD)—a disorder that requires an assessment of behavior—is increasing. Although there are no exact numbers on school-based evaluations for ADHD, many children with ADHD who are eligible for special education services receive services under the "other health impaired" category, and the number of children being served in this category rose almost 400% from 1991–1992 to 2000–2001, with 5.1% of all students in special education now receiving services under this category (U.S. Department of Education, 2002).

As with the other areas of assessment, some controversy exists regarding the utility of certain measures in this area. Much of the controversy centers around the use of projective assessment techniques (which almost always have significant problems with test–retest reliability and construct validity; see Merrell, 2003, for a discussion of this issue) versus the use of other techniques considered by many to be reliable and valid measures of emotional and behavioral functioning (e.g., observations, rating scales, functional assessment methods). Although earlier surveys of school psychologists' assessment practices indicated that behavioral rating scales were used less frequently than projective measures (e.g., Wilson & Reschly, 1996), this trend seems to be reversing. Hosp and Reschly (2002) reported that school psychologists administer slightly more behavior rating scales per month (17.2) than projective measures (15.2), and Shapiro and Heick (2004) reported that behavior rating scales were the most common assessment method used in cases involving a referral for emotional or behavioral problems.

In addition to behavior rating scales and projective measures, numerous other procedures can be used in the assessment of emotional and behavioral problems. These include interviews (with parents, teachers, and the child), observations (which may be either informal or formal), and self-report measures. In addition, FBA methods have been gaining in popularity over the past 5–10 years and are currently seen as key in linking assessment to intervention in the area of emotional and behavioral problems. Each of these methods is described briefly here. However, as with the discussion of intellectual and achievement measures, this discussion is not intended to be a comprehensive overview of these methods but instead to provide an introduction to these methods. School psychologists should consult other sources (e.g., Merrell, 2003; Shapiro & Kratochwill, 2000, 2002) for more detailed information.

## Projective Techniques

We discuss projective assessment techniques first because they have the longest history in the assessment of emotional and behavioral problems. Their use dates back to at least the early 1920s, and, by some accounts, projective drawing techniques were used as long ago as the 1890s (Merrell, 2003). Projective techniques include drawing techniques (e.g., Draw-a-Person, House–Tree–Person, Kinetic Family Drawing), thematic techniques (e.g., Children's Apperception Test, Bellak & Bellak, 1949; Roberts Apperception Test for Children, McArthur & Roberts, 1982), and sentence completion techniques. These methods are all based on the assumption that, when presented with ambiguous stimuli, children will "project" their own feelings, thoughts, and emotional conflicts onto these stimuli. As noted, the use of projective techniques by school psychologists has historically been very common. In Wilson and Reschly's (1996) survey, the Draw-a-Person test was the fourth most commonly used measure *overall* (not just for evaluating children referred for emotional and behavioral problems); House–Tree–Person was sixth; and Kinetic Family Drawing was eighth. In a more recent survey (Hosp &

Reschly, 2002), projective methods were the second most common assessment procedure used overall—just behind rating scales and ahead of IQ measures. Shapiro and
Heick (2004) indicate that about one-third of school psychologists regularly use projective methods for children referred for emotional and behavioral problems and that
about one-third never use projective methods.

Although projective methods continue to be commonly used by many school psychology practitioners, they are certainly not without controversy. In fact, other than IQ
measures, projective measures have likely created the most controversy within the field
of psychology (although, unlike with IQ measures, there has been a lack of controversy
regarding the use of these methods among nonpsychologists). The controversy regarding these methods stems from questions regarding the validity of these techniques: Do
they really measure what they say they measure? Most projective measures lack adequate psychometric properties, and many professionals argue that such measures do
not reflect internalized feelings but are simply a sample of overt behavior. Others argue
that at least some of the projective techniques have changed considerably over time (the
Rorschach with its more objective scoring system being the prime example) and that
one should not dismiss all projective measures simply because the measures as a group
lack adequate data to support their use (Prevatt, 1999). However, given the dramatically
poor validity of many projective measures and the wide availability of other measures
with superior psychometric properties, we do not believe that projective measures
should be routinely used in the schools. They provide little useful information in terms
of either diagnostic decision making or treatment planning. They may be helpful in
building rapport with a child (they are typically nonthreatening to a student, and are
sometimes perceived as fun) and may help generate hypotheses for further evaluation
with measures with adequate psychometric properties. However, when used in this fashion, these measures cease to be truly assessment measures. Therefore, in our opinion,
the use of projective measures is outdated and provides little to no useful information,
either in terms of identifying problem areas or linking assessment to intervention.

## Behavior Rating Scales

Although behavior rating scales have become increasingly popular (and psychometrically sound) over the past several decades, their use also dates back to at least the
early part of the 1900s. Wickman (1928) discussed behavior problems as rated by children's teachers and divided problems into "attacking" traits and "withdrawing" traits,
which are similar to our conceptualization of externalizing and internalizing problems
today. However, it was not until much more recently that behavior rating scales became
the well-standardized and normed tests that they are today. In 1973 Spivak and Swift
reviewed the available behavior rating scales and found that, although there were 19
such measures, only three had norms and reliability information. Today there are
numerous behavior rating scales that are well normed, are based on large standardization samples, and have extensive reliability and validity information.

Behavior rating scales are generally divided into two categories: broad-band and
narrow-band. Broad-band measures, such as the Child Behavior Checklist (CBCL;
Achenbach & Rescorla, 2001) and Behavioral Assessment System for Children (BASC;
Reynolds & Kamphaus, 2004) measure behaviors in a variety of domains and include
subscales that evaluate both externalizing (e.g., aggression) and internalizing (e.g., anxiety, depression) problems. Narrow-band measures assess functioning in just one
domain (e.g., attention-deficit/hyperactivity disorder, autism). Broad-band measures

are particularly useful in gathering a significant amount of information in a relatively short period of time. However, because broad-band scales do not provide detailed information on specific areas, narrow-band scales are typically used to obtain more information on problems noted on broad-band scales.

Rating scales are considered to be objective measures, given that the assessor does not interpret responses to individual items nor insert his or her potential bias in the rating process. However, it should be noted that rating scales provide the point of view of the person completing the scale and that different informants often do not agree on the severity (or even the presence) of behaviors. Thus, although it is an advantage that rating scales can be used to gather information from multiple sources and that many rating scales have parallel parent and teacher versions, it is left up to the evaluator to integrate the findings from the scales.

As noted, behavior rating scales are the most common assessment method that school psychologists currently report using for children referred for emotional and behavioral problems (Shapiro & Heick, 2004). This finding is encouraging given the positive qualities that behavior rating scales have. However, school psychologists must ensure that they are using measures with adequate psychometric properties and that are germane to the referral question. In addition, it is all too easy with behavior rating scales to say "Levi scored high on measures of ADHD so he must have ADHD." School psychologists must remember that scores do not dictate diagnoses. Scores on behavior rating scales provide data that can help in the diagnostic process, but these scores must be considered in the larger context (e.g., Are the symptoms impairing? Have they been present for a significant amount of time and since early childhood? Can the symptoms be better accounted for by something other than ADHD?). In addition, behavior rating scales do not provide information that is directly linked to interventions. Behavior rating scales are more helpful in assessing the severity of a problem (e.g., Does Levi have more symptoms of ADHD than his peers?) but are less useful in providing direction on what to do about those problems.

## Interviews

Interviews are a commonly used method of obtaining information related to a child's social–emotional functioning, with informal clinical interviews being the most common interview method. Clinical interviews involve the practitioner asking the interviewee (child, parent, teacher, etc.) a series of questions regarding symptom presentation and background information in order both to obtain more information on the referral problem and to put this information in a broader context. In addition to the commonly used clinical interviews, there are also structured and semistructured interviews. Structured interviews are highly scripted and typically involve the interviewer asking a series of yes/no questions regarding the presence of symptoms. Although such interviews are relatively common in research, they are rarely used in clinical practice. Semistructured interviews allow the interviewer slightly more leeway in questioning and typically consist of open-ended as well as structured questions (Merrell, 2003).

Clinical interviews are useful for several reasons. They allow the clinician to obtain a large amount of information on a wide variety of topics at one time in a flexible format. The flexible format of the clinical interview allows the clinician to build rapport with the interviewee. This is one reason interviews are typically conducted as the first step in the assessment process. Interviews can also be used to obtain information from different sources and to informally compare the perceptions of the problems, as well as to clarify issues. As is discussed in more detail later in this chapter, interviews can also be used to help conduct a functional assessment through asking questions about antecedents and consequences of behaviors. Although interviews have numerous advantages, as with all assessment methods, they also have disadvantages. Clearly, with informal clinical interviews, there is no way to evaluate their psychometric properties, and it is likely that different interviewers will obtain somewhat different information from the same respondent due to differences in questioning style, rapport built, and so forth. It is also possible that interviewers will have some biases that will color their interpretation of the information presented. For example, if the interviewer has already formed an impression about the child, he or she may ask questions that are geared toward supporting this impression. With young children in particular, interviews can be difficult. Children may have difficulties verbalizing thoughts and feelings, and young children can easily become confused regarding temporal aspects of events. It is very important when interviewing not to ask leading questions but instead to make questions open-ended (e.g., instead of saying "You like school, don't you?" say "Tell me what you think about school"; Hughes & Baker, 1990).

Although interviews are standard practice when conducting evaluations in clinical settings and are used frequently by school psychologists, we believe they are underutilized in school psychology. Shapiro and Heick (2004) indicated that only about one-third of school psychologists regularly use interviews with parents and teachers for children referred for emotional and behavioral problems and that about 20% do not use interviews at all. Involving parents and teachers in the assessment process is critically important, and interviews are an easy method to solicit this involvement, as well as to obtain significant background information on the child. In fact, given the many assessment advantages of interviewing, we think that the use of this method among school psychologists should be standard practice.

## Observations

Observations are another commonly used assessment procedure. Shapiro and Heick (2004) reported that school psychologists complete observations on most of the students they evaluate for emotional and behavioral problems. Observations are typically done in a child's classroom and often involve the assessment of several key behaviors of concern. Observations provide the assessor with a direct picture of a child's problems (as well as positive behaviors). In addition, the observer is able to see the child's behaviors in the context in which they naturally occur. This ecological–contextual information may be particularly helpful when conducting a functional assessment. Not only can the observer obtain information on the child's behavior, but information on the context in which the behavior occurs, as well as the antecedents and consequences of the behavior, can also be obtained.

Although observations have clear advantages and we believe they are an important part of the assessment process, they are also relatively time-consuming, and they can require extensive training. It is impossible to obtain data on many behaviors at once with observational techniques, as can be done with interviews and behavior rating scales. In addition, although, theoretically, observations are objective (the observer directly sees the behavior), the observer can bias the observation results by focusing on negative (or positive) behaviors. It is generally best to observe several behaviors and to include at least one positive behavior. It is also important to observe comparison peers to help determine whether the observed behavior of the child is unusual in the context of the child's classroom and peers (Merrell, 2003).

## Self-Report Measures

Self-report measures include both rating-scale-type measures (e.g., the Youth Self-Report [Achenbach & Rescorla, 2001], which is the parallel self-report measure to the CBCL), as well as measures of "personality." The rating-scale-type measures are similar to those completed by parents and teachers, and most broad-band parent–teacher rating scales have parallel self-report forms. It is also common to assess internalizing constructs such as anxiety and depression with narrow-band scales (e.g., Children's Depression Inventory, Kovacs, 1991; Multidimensional Anxiety Scale for Children, March, 1997). The most common self-report "personality" measure for adolescents is the Minnesota Multiphasic Personality Inventory–Adolescent (MMPI-A; Butcher et al., 1992). Although this instrument is used extensively in clinical practice, its use in the field of school psychology is still relatively limited. The limited use of this measure in the schools is likely for several reasons—including a lack of emphasis on this measure in training programs, the focus of this tool on pathology, the length of time it takes for a child to complete the measure (about an hour and a half), and the relatively limited age range of children evaluated in the schools (it is generally recommended that this test not be given to children under the age of 14). In Shapiro and Heick's (2004) study, school psychologists reported commonly using self-report rating scales but uncommonly using measures of personality assessment such as the MMPI-A. In fact, 70% of school psychologists reported that they had not used such measures at all in their previous 10 evaluations.

Self-report measures are advantageous because they allow clinicians to assess children's perceptions of the problems. Self-report measures may be particularly helpful when evaluating internalizing symptoms, as these symptoms are ones that frequently cannot be observed by others. Children do have to have adequate reading abilities to complete self-report measures, and for this reason, most self-report measures cannot be administered to children under the age of 8. Although self-report measures are helpful in providing the child's perspective on issues, self-report ratings typically do not correlate highly with ratings from parent and teacher measures. Thus the clinician is left to make sense of these differences and attempt to determine the "true" presence of symptoms. As with informant-based rating scales, self-report measures are more useful in assessing the severity of a child's problem compared with his or her peers than in identifying specific behaviors of concern for the child that might be targeted in an intervention.

## Functional Behavioral Assessment

In much the same way that the use of CBA methods has been increasing for evaluating academic problems, FBA methods are increasingly being used to link assessment to intervention for emotional and behavioral problems. However, according to Shapiro and Heick's (2004) survey, such methods are by no means commonplace. One-quarter of school psychologists reported not using such methods at all in their previous 10 evaluations of children suspected of having emotional and behavioral problems, and only 14% reported using these methods in almost all of their last 10 evaluations.

Functional assessment procedures are a broad group of procedures that are based on the concept of identifying the behavioral function, or purpose, of a behavior. In functional assessment, the antecedents and consequences of the behavior are identified, with the goal being to understand the environmental conditions that maintain the behavior in question. Through a better understanding of the relationship between the behavior of the individual and the contextual factors that precipitate and reinforce the behavior, interventions can be implemented that attempt to change the behavior by addressing the function (Watson & Steege, 2003). For example, if a student is disruptive in class (e.g., talks to other students, is out of his seat) and consistently receives attention (in the form of teacher reprimands) for this behavior but receives no positive feedback for appropriate classroom behaviors, we might hypothesize that the function of the behavior is to obtain attention. Our intervention recommendations would follow from this hypothesis and include recommendations to cease providing attention for the disruptive behavior. Instead this behavior should be ignored and attention should be provided to more positive behaviors (e.g., raising his hand to speak).

Watson and Steege (2003) outlined three forms of FBA: *indirect, direct descriptive*, and *functional behavioral analysis*. With indirect FBA, interviews, as well as rating scales and records reviews, are used to identify and describe the behavior of concern and to generate hypotheses regarding the function of the behavior. As described by Gresham, Watson, and Skinner (2001, p. 161) functional assessment interviews have four main purposes: (1) to identify and define the behavior of concern; (2) to identify antecedents of the target behavior; (3) to obtain initial information on the possible function of the target behavior; and (4) to identify behaviors that can be substituted for the target behavior. These purposes are accomplished through asking questions about what the behavior looks like, as well as the context and setting in which the behavior occurs. Although indirect FBA can provide valuable information, direct descriptive FBA, in which observations are conducted, should be used to help better identify functional relationships between the behavior(s) of concern and environmental factors. Observations allow the school psychologist to directly observe the behavior and to see the antecedents and consequences associated with the behavior in the context in which the behavior occurs. However, even observations do not allow one to confirm that a certain function is maintaining the behavior. In order to confirm hypotheses regarding behavioral function, a functional analysis would need to be conducted. This involves miniexperiments in which the behavior of concern is observed under different conditions (e.g., providing attention to the behavior, allowing escape from a task following the behavior). Although true functional analysis procedures are relatively common in inpatient clinical settings in which functional methods are employed, these procedures are less common in school settings.

The FBA framework encompasses three functions of behavior. These include obtaining attention or access to desired activities or tangibles for engaging in a certain behavior, escaping or avoiding an aversive task, and self-stimulation (Watson & Steege, 2003). It is important to remember that attention can be both positive (e.g., getting peers to laugh at a joke) or negative (e.g., teacher reprimands) in content and still positively reinforce the behavior in question. As long as the consequence (in this case, attention) increases the likelihood that the behavior will occur again, the consequence is considered to be positively reinforcing.

The information obtained from the functional assessment is used to develop a plan for intervention that addresses the function of the behavior. For example, as noted, if it is hypothesized that a student's disruptive behavior during class is reinforced by attention from his or her teacher, we would provide attention to positive, on-task behaviors and remove attention from disruptive behaviors. Because functional assessment techniques lead directly to interventions, they have significantly more treatment utility than many other methods of assessment. Functional assessment methods are particularly useful with behaviors that are externalized (e.g., oppositional behaviors) but are less useful with internalized behaviors (e.g., depression) that are not clearly tied to environmental contingencies. Although functional assessment methods were initially developed with children with severe behavior problems who were institutionalized, they have been adequately adapted to the school setting, and we expect that their use will continue to increase as more training programs emphasize these methods and more clinicians experience the utility of such methods in tying assessment to intervention.

## DIAGNOSIS AND CLASSIFICATION IN THE SCHOOLS

As with all assessment issues discussed thus far in this chapter, a lack of agreement exists in the field of school psychology on the usefulness of providing diagnostic and/ or classification labels for children. By way of definition, "classification" is the term typically used in the schools when assigning special education labels (e.g., learning disability, emotional disturbance), whereas "diagnosis" is the term typically used in clinical practice when assigning DSM-IV labels (e.g., ADHD, separation anxiety disorder). However, these terms are often used interchangeably, and they have in common the assignment of a label to a child.

One concern regarding the use of diagnostic and classification systems is that they may lead to "self-fulfilling prophecies." For example, a child labeled as having a learning disability may cease to try as hard and his or her parents and teachers may cease to expect as much, leading to a decline in academic performance. Concerns have also been expressed that the process of diagnosing or classifying children artificially places them in categories that are not reliable. In addition, because diagnostic systems typically used require categorical decisions to be made (i.e., either the child has the problem or does not), individuals with the same label can display different behaviors and varying levels of behavior severity, and children with "subclinical" problems (who may benefit from treatment) may not receive a classification because a certain threshold of symptoms is not met. One of the most commonly leveled criticisms against diagnostic systems in the field of school psychology is that they are not directly linked to intervention (Kamphaus, Reynolds, & Imperato-McCammon, 1999; Merrell, 2003). Although we acknowledge that there are significant problems with classification systems, we do believe that they serve a purpose. In many systems, classifications are required for individuals to access and/or be reimbursed for services. For example, although states can provide noncategorical services under IDEA, most states use the categories provided in the federal guidelines. This situation means that, for a student to receive special education services, he or she *must* be assigned to a certain special education category. In the private practice sector, almost all insurance companies require a DSM-IV diagnosis for insurance reimbursement. Although these issues of access to services are very practical and many would argue that we should work toward changing these system requirements, it seems unlikely that significant change will occur any time in the near future.

Practical issues aside, there are other, more theoretically based arguments for the use of diagnostic systems. Such systems do allow for better communication between professionals (Merrell, 2003). For example, if as a school psychologist you are speaking with the physician of a child who has been diagnosed with ADHD, you can both use this term and know that you are referring to generally the same set of symptoms. Although there is variability in the specific behaviors exhibited by children with ADHD, the use of this term nevertheless provides some common understanding. Of course, this enhanced communication does assume that the diagnosis was correctly made. If the diagnosis was made in error, the communication ceases to be helpful and meaningful. In addition, although we acknowledge that classification systems do not directly lead to interventions, we believe they can help guide the selection of appropriate intervention techniques. Increasing emphasis is being placed on "evidence-based practice" and "empirically supported interventions" (i.e., those that have well-conducted research to support their use) in the psychology literature. The participants in the studies that support these interventions are typically labeled in some manner, either with specific DSM-IV labels (e.g., children with separation anxiety disorder) or with general categories (e.g., children with anxiety). Thus by classifying a child we can know in general what treatments might be effective for that child. Our job is then to implement the treatment in a manner that is compatible with the child's specific symptom presentation and the context in which these symptoms are being exhibited. This may involve conducting additional assessments to better understand the function of the child's behavior in the context in which the behavior is occurring. It is important to remember that just because most children within a certain diagnostic category respond to a certain treatment (e.g., the majority of children with anxiety respond positively to cognitive-behavioral interventions) does not mean that all children with a certain label will respond to a certain treatment. Thus it is still important to take into account individual differences and to continuously evaluate the effectiveness of an intervention on the individual child.

Although the purpose of an assessment is not always to provide a label for the difficulties a child is experiencing, frequently in schools at least part of the purpose of an evaluation is to determine whether a child meets criteria for a certain special education category. Because of this, school psychologists frequently are faced with making decisions (as a member of a multidisciplinary team) about the appropriate classification for a child. Thus, regardless of a school psychologist's philosophy on the use of labels, all school psychologists will need to be knowledgeable about classification systems. However, we do not believe that classification should be the primary goal of assessment. Assessment may lead to a determination of which, if any, diagnostic labels fit the child's symptom presentation, but assessment should also, and more important, lead to intervention recommendations. Although it may appear that this state of events would naturally follow (especially given our point that classifications can help lead to intervention selection), this is certainly not always the case. For example, if a child is diagnosed as having ADHD, we know from the research that behavioral interventions are likely to reduce ADHD-related behaviors in the classroom setting. However, we do not know what specific behaviors we should target. Does the child engage in significant out-of-seat behavior? Does the child have difficulty following instructions? Does the child have peer relationship problems because he or she is always acting impulsively? In addition, we do not know the function of these behaviors through the diagnostic process. Is the child engaging in out-of-seat behavior for attention, to escape an aversive task, or as a self-stimulatory behavior? These types of questions must also be answered as part of the assessment process so that, in addition to providing a diagnostic label for a child, we can provide parents and teachers with recommendations about what can be done to help reduce the child's problem behaviors and to increase the child's positive behaviors. As more research is conducted on formal classification systems, there is a hope that they may become more functional in nature (Scotti et al., 1996). Currently, we contend that school psychologists should view the assignment of a classification or diagnosis as one part of the assessment process in many cases, while at the same time realizing that a label by itself is likely to be of minimal benefit to the child and those who interact with the child.

## ASSESSMENT AS A PROBLEM-SOLVING PROCESS

Much has been written about assessment as a problem-solving process (e.g., Flanagan & Ortiz, 2002; Witt, Elliott, Daly, Gresham, & Kramer, 1997), and in Chapter 7 of this text we provide an in-depth discussion of the data-driven problem-solving approach to school psychology. Within this approach, assessment information is collected to guide decision making throughout each of the steps. We strongly believe this approach to school psychology is the most useful one for effectively addressing the academic and behavioral problems facing today's children and youth. As discussed in Chapter 7, when using the problem-solving model, one seeks to identify the discrepancy between a child's current academic and/or behavioral performance and the desired performance for the child. Given this model, the goal of an evaluation should not simply be to provide numerical values regarding the child's functioning and to choose a category that best fits the child. Rather, the goal is to identify conditions that will enable a child to most effectively learn (Tilly, 2002). Assessment as part of the problem-solving process is directly linked to intervention. This is in contrast to more traditional assessment activities in which assessment is not directly linked to intervention and the goal is typically to make a diagnostic decision. We stress that the traditional approach to assessment is not inherently bad; it just serves a different purpose than does the problem-solving approach. In addition, traditional assessment requires a higher degree of inference to generate intervention strategies than does assessment under the problem-solving method, which obtains a direct measure of a student's skills in the context in which they occur. Higher inference is a problem in that the greater the inference, the less confidence we can have that the intervention will be effective in remediating the student's problem (Tilly, 2002).

Next we outline the problem-solving process of assessment and use a hypothetical example to help illustrate this process. We also provide a graphic representation of this process in Figure 8.1.

### Identification of the Problem: The Referral and Clarification

An assessment begins with a referral. Typically, the referral is from a child's teacher or parent. The referral contains some information on the problem(s) of concern but typically does not provide detailed information. For example, the referral issue might be, "Tony is having difficulty learning and attending in class." After receiving the referral, the school psychologist should clarify the nature of the problem with the referring source via an interview. The goal of this interview is to obtain more information on the behaviors of concern, the context in which these behaviors occur, and the desired level of performance. Information should be obtained on the following: specific behaviors of concern, expectancies for the behavior, opportunities for the expected behaviors to occur, how long the problem behaviors have been occurring, situations in which the

Receive Referral Question

↓

Clarify / Obtain Additional Details

↓

Develop Hypotheses

↓

Choose Assessment Procedures/Methods

↓

Conduct Assessments

↓

Review All Data

↓

Develop Intervention Plan

↓

Implement Intervention

↓

Evaluate Intervention

↓

If No Improvement, Reassess Problem

**FIGURE 8.1.** Problem-solving process in assessment.

behaviors occur, situations in which the behaviors do not occur, any changes that have occurred in the child's life (including exposure to traumatic events), and positive aspects of the child's behaviors. This initial interview can also be used to help clarify the discrepancy between the actual performance of the child and the desired performance.

In addition to clarifying details regarding the referral problem, the school psychologist should obtain additional background information on the student to help put the behaviors in context and potentially rule out other contributing factors. For example: Does the child have any major health problems? Did the child meet developmental milestones on time? Is the child currently on any medications? This information is most likely obtained via an interview with the child's parents.

Observations of the child may also be conducted by the psychologist. These observations may help clarify the nature of the problem, as well as identify potential antecedents and consequences surrounding the problem.

### Analysis of the Problem: Development of Hypotheses and Collection of Assessment Data

Once the referral question has been clarified, the psychologist should develop hypotheses that will guide additional assessment. In our example referral problem, let's assume that there have been no significant changes in Tony's life, that he has no medical problems, and that he has reached major development milestones as expected. He is now in the third grade but has struggled with school since beginning kindergarten. He is currently behind his peers in reading, according to this classroom teacher. In addition, his parents report that he has always been a bit on the active side and that they have had difficulties getting him to attend to and follow their instructions. His teacher reports many of the same problems. His parents and his teacher agree that they would like to see Tony reading on grade level, being more attentive to academic work, and being more compliant with their requests.

At this point, we conclude that there is a discrepancy between Tony's actual current performance and his desired performance in reading. In a traditional approach to assessment, it is likely that Tony would be administered standardized measures of intellectual ability (e.g., WISC-IV) and achievement (e.g., WJ-III) to determine whether he meets criteria for a learning disability. However, in the problem-solving model, our primary goal is to identify interventions that may help improve Tony's reading skills and decrease his problematic behaviors in the context of his current classroom setting. As discussed earlier in this chapter, as well as in Chapter 7, there are a variety of reasons Tony may not be performing well, including that he does not want to complete his reading assignments, he has not spent enough time on his assignments, he has not had enough help to complete assignments, he has not had to do the tasks in that manner before, or the reading material is too difficult for him. Following the functional approach outlined by Daly et al. (1997), we administer Tony a variety of curriculum-based reading probes under different conditions (e.g., incentives for reading at a certain rate, repeated reading practices), alternating with a baseline probe with no modifications. We ascertain that Tony is reading at the frustrational level in third-grade material but is at the instructional level when reading first-grade material. In addition, Tony's performance improves when he is provided with a reinforcer for improving his performance.

Regarding assessment of Tony's behavioral and attention problems, if our goal was to decide whether Tony's behaviors were symptomatic of ADHD, we would likely have Tony's parents and teachers complete norm-based behavior rating scales. However, as noted earlier, in the problem-solving model, diagnosis is not the focus of our assessment. Thus, to help us learn more about conditions in which Tony exhibits inattentiveness and conditions in which he is on task, we conduct a more detailed classroom observation to obtain additional data on the times when Tony is inattentive and the antecedents and consequences of this behavior. We note that Tony is frequently off task and inattentive during reading and the that consequence for his behavior is typically to be sent away from the class group—either into the "quiet corner" in the classroom or to an isolated seat in the back of the classroom where the teacher cannot see what he is working on. In an interview with Tony's parents, they reported that they have difficulties getting Tony to do his homework—he often jumps up from the table, attempts to engage his parents in conversations, and doodles on his homework papers. They also noted that he was often noncompliant with their requests in general. They noted that they had tired of repeating commands and that once they asked him several times to do something, they dropped the request, even if he did not follow through.

## Review of Data

Once we have completed our assessments, we compile all the data (including our initial interview data) and attempt to draw some conclusions about the problems present, as well as what interventions may be effective in remediating these problems. As noted, Tony read more words per minute when provided with a reinforcer than with no reinforcer and is also finding grade-level reading to be too difficult. Thus it seems likely that Tony's difficulties with reading are a combination of the reading he is currently assigned being too difficult for him and of a lack of motivation to complete reading assignments.

Observations of Tony in class, as well as interview data from his parents, indicate that he is most likely to be inattentive and off task when engaged in tasks he finds aversive. Typically, the consequences of his behavior are removing him or allowing him to remove himself from the setting. Based on these data, it seems likely that the function of Tony's behavior is to escape from aversive tasks (e.g., reading time, homework time).

### Intervention Development

Once the data have been reviewed (and additional data collected if necessary to follow up on issues not initially presented as concerns), we are ready to make intervention recommendations. In Tony's case, based on our assessment of his reading skills and attention problems, we recommend that he be provided with frequent reinforcement for completing reading assignments. For example, Tony might earn points toward a larger reward or might be given the option to choose from a menu of reinforcers after completing a reading assignment at home or at school. In addition, we recommend that Tony be given reading assignments within his current instructional level. With regard to Tony's difficulties with inattentiveness and off-task behavior, we noted that Tony's teacher provides him little feedback in the classroom and that she allows him to escape from reading activities by separating him from the rest of the class. We recommend attending to Tony when he is on task and providing mild consequences for off-task behavior—but not allowing him to choose not to engage in reading. At home, we recommend that Tony's parents be consistent in their requirements and that they not allow Tony to escape an aversive situation by simply not complying with parental requests. We further recommend that Tony's homework time be broken into small chunks, with frequent reinforcement provided for completing assignments.

### Evaluation of the Intervention

To determine whether an intervention is successful, we must evaluate it in an ongoing manner. Observations can be repeated, CBM probes administered, and feedback obtained from parents and teachers. If an intervention is not having the desired effect, we must evaluate why it is not. Have we targeted the wrong problem? Did we target the right problem but not use an effective method? The evaluation process must be continuous so that we know when we must rethink our intervention plans to make them produce the desired results.

## FINAL THOUGHTS

We encourage school psychologists not to approach assessments with dread and not to think of assessment as a purely psychometric exercise. Let's face it: With some minimal training, almost anyone can administer the measures mentioned in this chapter. If all there were to assessment was administering and scoring a standardized measure or two, assessment would indeed be a tedious activity. However, we must learn to look beyond the numbers and beyond traditional assessment techniques. We must learn to *think* about the child who has been referred to us and the context in which the child interacts (school, home, community). We must remember that the goal of an evaluation is not simply to decide on an appropriate classification for a child but to improve the child's educational and/or social–emotional functioning. To do that, we must approach evaluations from a problem-solving model and must take our assessment duties seriously—not as something to endure until we can engage in a more interesting activity. Evaluations done right should be interesting—all children are unique, and our evaluations should reflect that.

## DISCUSSION QUESTIONS AND ACTIVITIES

1. Compare two of the recently revised measures of intellectual ability (e.g., WISC-IV, Stanford–Binet V, Woodcock–Johnson III). What theory of intelligence are the tests based on? What was the norming process for the tests? Are the test(s) psychometric properties adequate?

2. Interview school psychologists from different school districts regarding their opinions of the need for the achievement–ability discrepancy in identifying children with learning disabilities. Do they think their evaluation procedures will change with the changes to IDEA regarding the definition of a learning disability? If so, how?

3. Search for existing FBA interview and observation forms. Compare and contrast these and use them to create a form you can use when conducting functional assessments in the schools.

4. Interview parents and teachers for their opinions about requiring children to be classified as having a certain disability to receive special education services. Would they prefer a noncategorical system? Why or why not?

5. Talk with current school psychologists about their approach to conducting assessments. Are they using a problem-solving approach? If so, what makes their approach a problem-solving one? If not, how could they change their approach to more directly reflect the problem-solving approach?

# 9

# The School Psychologist's Role in Prevention and Intervention

## PART 1. ACADEMIC SKILLS

It has been our experience that one of the main reasons that individuals enter the field of school psychology is to "help" others—to assist children and youths who experience learning and/or behavioral difficulties. The development of knowledge and skills in prevention and intervention services is an integral part of school psychology training programs, deemed important by professional organizations and leaders in the field and valued by practitioners. Preference for this role is matched with evidence indicating the critical need for prevention and intervention services if we are to address pressing issues facing our children and youths (e.g., Carnine, 1999; Forness, 2003a, 2003b; Friedman, 2003; Hunter, 2003; Power, 2003; Shapiro, 2000; Ysseldyke, 2000). Despite the overwhelming consensus regarding the importance of this aspect of school psychology service provision and the evidence indicating its urgency, practicing school psychologists tend to spend a minimal portion of their time in this role (see Chapter 5). This apparent lack of attention to evidence-based prevention and intervention practices in school settings is not limited to the field of school psychology. For quite some time now, scholars have recognized gaps between our existing knowledge of effective prevention and intervention practices and actual adoption of those practices in educational settings (e.g., Abbott et al., 1999; Carnine, 1997; 1999; Forness, 2003a; Friedman, 2003; Gersten et al., 1997; Hunter, 2003). Recognition of this gap has led researchers to carefully consider issues essential to the promotion of evidence-based practices in school settings.

In this chapter and in Chapter 10, we discuss prevention and intervention issues in school psychology. We describe how a data-driven problem-solving approach is helpful in facilitating the provision of effective prevention and intervention services for addressing learning (this chapter), as well as social–emotional or mental health (Chapter 10) needs of children and youths. In addition, we summarize the key areas of knowledge and skills that school psychologists will need in order to embark on this endeavor. We include a discussion of the literature on resiliency, which provides a wealth of information regarding important risk and protective factors that influence development. Knowledge in this area is helpful as a starting point for prevention and intervention because it provides information regarding who should be the focus of intervention, what domains of functioning we should target, and when certain domains should be targeted. We also provide a brief overview of some of the effective prevention and intervention strategies that are supported in literature. Knowledge in this area is useful in guiding the problem-solving process toward intervention strategies that are likely to be effective. We end each chapter with a description of the process for using this information to inform treatment planning at each level of prevention (i.e., primary, secondary, and tertiary) in school settings. Throughout our discussion, emphasis is placed on the use of evidence (from the literature as well as from the immediate problem-solving context) to inform the decision-making process as it relates to intervention selection, implementation, and evaluation.

## PREVENTION AND INTERVENTION AS PART OF A DATA-DRIVEN PROBLEM-SOLVING PROCESS

When we view the entire process of schooling as an "intervention" that alters development (cognitive, affective, social, and physical) from its natural (i.e., unschooled) course (Deno, 2002), it is easy to see how prevention and intervention services are an essential part of education. As we discussed in Chapter 6, within domains of functioning important to schooling (e.g., reading), children learn and develop at different rates. Similarly, within individuals, developmental progress varies over time and across domains. We also know that individuals respond differently to various interventions. Taking these natural variations into account, it is clear that education and mental health professionals must monitor outcomes and be responsive by adapting intervention techniques to meet the individual needs of the students they serve.

Advancements in our knowledge regarding effective instructional strategies and intervention techniques can help build our capacity for improving educational services and creating school environments that promote positive outcomes and reduce the risk of learning and mental health problems. Despite these advances, we must still acknowledge that our ability to predict a priori how our knowledge from research studies will generalize beyond the research contexts and into real-world settings is limited. In light of this limitation, we advocate the use of an *experimenting society* approach to solving problems in school settings (e.g., Campbell, 1988; Cronbach, 1975). This approach relies on the scientific method to determine the efficacy of prevention and intervention strategies within the contexts in which they are used. Thus, as we discussed in Chapter 6, it is necessary to view prevention and intervention efforts as being embedded in a data-driven problem-solving process that focuses on the contexts in which problems occur.

Our current empirical knowledge base can inform and guide certain aspects of the decision-making process, but ongoing evaluation and feedback is necessary for ensuring effective outcomes. The problem-solving process does not provide us with a crystal ball so that we can predict in an *absolute* manner how successful various prevention and intervention efforts will be for different students, but it can help to facilitate the selection of strategies with a *higher probability* of being successful. Further, it incorporates measurement and evaluation methods so that we can at least answer the question, Did our prevention or intervention efforts work? As noted, we cannot assume that an intervention that has been effective in one setting with one individual or group of individuals will work with the same individual or group of individuals for a different problem or problem context or for a different individual within the same context. This uncertainty does not mean that group-level research is not useful in informing the decision-making process. We have neither the time nor the resources to haphazardly implement interventions on a trial-and-error basis. Thus we must find a balance between our current knowledge base (i.e., existing research on empirically sound prevention and intervention practices) and information we collect about the problem and its context. From this information, we can derive working hypotheses regarding what prevention and intervention strategies are *likely* to facilitate problem resolution. Then we need to test these hypotheses.

To illustrate the preceding points, consider the important domain of reading. Here it is easy to see how research can inform our decision-making process regarding prevention and intervention efforts. First, information from the research literature can help us determine *who to target* and *in what important domains of functioning*. Studies indicate that more than one in six children in the United States will have problems learning how to read in their first three years of school (National Reading Panel, 2000). These data are alarming when we consider the fact that reading is a pivotal and enabling skill that translates into meaningful personal, social, and economic outcomes for individuals (Simmons & Kame'enui, 1998). More specifically, children who develop poor reading skills are more likely to experience learning and behavioral difficulties in school and are at risk for later-life problems (e.g., dropout, unemployment, adjudication). Alternatively, those who develop strong reading skills are more likely to experience academic success and positive outcomes in later life. Further, children with special needs and those living in poverty are at an extremely high risk for the development of poor reading skills. Thus the research literature indicates that reading is an important skill and that some children are at higher risk for the development of reading problems, making them potential targets for prevention and intervention efforts.

Research literature can also inform the problem-solving process by indicating *when* we need to intervene (i.e., critical periods of development) and, sometimes, it helps inform *how* we should intervene (i.e., what intervention strategies are likely to work for particular problems, contexts, or populations). For example, some longitudinal research indicates that when children develop early reading difficulties, these problems tend to persist. According to Juel (1988), the probability of being a poor reader in fourth grade for those who were poor readers in first grade was 88%. Similarly, students with poor reading skills at the end of third grade failed to significantly improve their skills by the end of eighth grade (Felton & Pepper, 1995). Further, when we consider research examining the natural course of reading development for students with and without early reading problems, data indicate that a critical time exists in which we should focus on altering reading trajectories. Longitudinal research illustrates this point, demonstrating how the discrepancy in reading performance between groups of poor readers and strong readers becomes more pronounced as children progress through the early school grades (Good, Simmons, & Smith, 1998). Persistence of reading problems has been explained as emanating from early foundational skill deficits and being exacerbated by reduced exposure to print and eventual reductions in motivation and desire to read (Stanovich, 1986, 2000). By the time students with poor reading skills enter the third and fourth grades, they are performing well below their same-age peers, and, at this point in time, it is too late to simply modify initial reading instruction to facilitate the acquisition of beginning reading skills (Good et al., 2002).

As we noted in the previous paragraph, a critical and short period exists in which we can alter reading trajectories (Simmons & Kame'enui, 1998). Further, the evidence indicates that proficiency in foundational skills in beginning reading is causally linked to the development of reading competence (National Reading Panel, 2000; National Research Council, 1998). Development of these foundational skills differentiates successful from less successful readers (Kame'enui & Carnine, 2001; Simmons & Kame'enui, 1998). These foundational skills include: "(a) phonological awareness or the ability to hear and manipulate the sound structure of language, (b) alphabetic principle including alphabetic understanding or the mapping of print to speech and the phonological recoding of letter strings into corresponding sounds and blending stored sounds into words, and (c) accuracy and fluency with connected text or the facile and seemingly effortless recognition of words in connected text" (Good et al., 2002, p. 702). The good news is that, through instruction, these important skills are teachable. Furthermore, intervention research demonstrates that if low-achieving students can be brought up to grade level within the first 3 years of school, their reading performance tends to stay at grade level (Adams, 1990). Taking all of this into account, reading scholars have suggested that "what is needed for prevention of reading failure is to begin early and assess dynamically" (Good et al., 2002, p. 699).

From our rather brief review of the literature on the development of reading skills and reading intervention research, it is possible to surmise how knowledge in this area would be helpful in addressing the needs of students who are referred for reading problems. It tells us that reading is an important and pivotal skill that affects success in school and later-life outcomes. In addition, it tells us that many students experience reading problems and that some students (e.g., students who are economically disadvantaged or have special needs) are more at risk for the development of reading difficulties than others. It also indicates that we should intervene early and focus on teaching foundational reading skills as a means of primary prevention. Still, this wealth of empirical knowledge does not tell us the whole story regarding specifically how we should address Joey Smith's reading problems within the context of Sunshine Elementary School. In order to address Joey's reading concerns, we need to answer the questions in the problem-solving process as they relate to his particular situation (What is the problem? Why is it occurring? What can we do about it? Did it work?). It is our belief that effective problem solvers *integrate* knowledge of the factors that influence important developmental outcomes, knowledge of empirically supported treatments, and the information they collect about the problem and its context. Thus school psychologists who are involved in prevention and intervention of reading problems at an individual, small-group, or schoolwide level should be cognizant of the empirical literature on reading difficulties and should employ a data-oriented problem-solving approach to addressing such issues.

# FACTORS THAT INFLUENCE DEVELOPMENT

Research on child development, including risk and resiliency factors, has much to contribute to our understanding of effective prevention and intervention services in schools. Psychologists who study the natural course of development for typically and atypically (e.g., children with autism) developing children and youths have provided us with mapped trajectories of important developmental outcomes across various domains of functioning. This information helps inform the problem-solving process because it helps us to know when students typically meet various levels of performance across developmental domains. This information thus contributes to our definitions of "expected levels of functioning" as we try to determine discrepancies between current and desired levels of performance. In addition, knowing when we can expect students to obtain certain skills helps us to match our instructional techniques to a child's developmental level. For example, Friman and Blum (2002) argued that mismatches between parental expectations or assumptions about their child's knowledge and what children actually understand are central to problems of child compliance. One example is Jean Piaget's work on the development of a child's ability to understand abstractions and abstract relations. Piaget's work on *conservation* (i.e., the capacity to conserve and apply certain qualities of an object or event to another object or event) is helpful in understanding how children develop the concept of "sameness." Friman and Blum (2002) suggested that parents often assume that a child has the capacity to understand similarities across behavioral episodes even when that capacity may not be well developed. Parents may get frustrated when their child, who has just been disciplined in one situation, seemingly does the "same thing" again. Parents might comment, "That's the same thing I told you not to do yesterday" or "Didn't I warn you not to do that again?" When young children have underdeveloped capacities for understanding abstractions such as "sameness," it is very difficult for them to see how what they did yesterday in the living room at Aunt Michelle's house is in any way similar to what they did today at home in the kitchen. Similarly, mismatches between a child's capacity for understanding instructions and parental delivery of commands can lead to significant issues of noncompliance.

As Friman and Blum (2002) noted, when working with children to teach them new skills, it is helpful to know something about how children learn and develop the capacity for understanding language. Similarly, problems may occur in classroom settings when there is a mismatch between a student's level of understanding and a teacher's instructional cues. Psychologists who are interested in prevention and intervention services in the school or in other settings must have some understanding of the natural course of development, as their focus may be on detecting progress along a particular domain (e.g., reading, capacity to understand language and abstractions) and intervening to alter trajectories when they detect a gap between actual and expected rates of progress.

## Risk Factors

In addition to knowing the natural course of development, psychologists interested in prevention and intervention services should be familiar with research regarding the factors that tend to influence development and subsequent later-life outcomes. An extensive amount of research has demonstrated that children who are raised under certain conditions (e.g., poverty, abuse, family dysfunction) are at significantly higher risk for problems in their adult lives (e.g., marital discord, unemployment). This line of research has focused on the identification of *risk factors* that are predictive of later life dysfunction. Research consistently indicates that poverty is the most powerful risk factor that predicts adult dysfunction. Poverty, or a lack of resources, can result in certain adverse living situations, such as economic dependence, overcrowding, and disorganization within the family system (for a review, see Doll & Lyon, 1998). Another powerful predictor of negative adult outcomes is an ineffective or uncaring parenting environment. The importance of warm, caring, consistent parental environments to the development and general well-being of children has been well documented (see Masten & Coatsworth, 1998). The occurrence of physical or emotional maltreatment in childhood is a third predictor of negative adult outcomes, particularly the development of adult psychopathology. A fourth factor predicting adult problems is marital discord and/or family dysfunction. Children raised in conditions of chronic family conflict tend to end up in similarly dysfunctional family conditions in adulthood. All four factors (poverty, uncaring parental environments, abuse or maltreatment, and family conflict) have been linked to negative later-life outcomes. Further, evidence suggests that "factors tend to be chronic life conditions rather than acute hazards" and that "the rate and intensity of undesirable outcomes appears to increase geometrically with exposure to each successive risk factor" (Doll & Lyon, 1998, p. 356). This information tells us that children with prolonged exposure to multiple risk factors are at the greatest risk of developing problems and are, therefore, in great need of support services. They also, however, are likely to be the most difficult to treat (i.e., they fall at the "top of the prevention triangle").

## Protective Factors

In addition to risk factors, some research has examined factors associated with the development of competence in spite of adversity (i.e., *protective factors*). The concept of resilience refers to "manifested competence in the context of significant challenges to adaptation or development" (Masten & Coatsworth, 1998, p. 206). Researchers who study resilience are often interested in the questions Why do some children succeed amidst a sea of adversity? and Is there something special or unique about these children? In a recent review of this literature, Masten and Coatsworth (1998) reported that "converging evidence suggests that the same powerful adaptive systems protect development in both favorable and unfavorable environments" (p. 205). These include: (1) quality parent–child relationships (i.e., warm, caring, competent relationships with a parent or surrogate caregiver figure); (2) good cognitive development; and (3) self-regulation of attention, emotion, and behavior. Further, research indicates that early prevention and intervention to foster the development of competence and prevent problems is critical to successful later-life outcomes.

Our knowledge base of protective and risk factors is increasing. In this section we provided a very cursory overview of the risk and resiliency literature, the major findings of this work, and its implications. "Development is biased towards competence, but there is no such thing as an invulnerable child" (Masten & Coatsworth, 1998, p. 216). Thus it is important for prevention and intervention efforts to focus on ameliorating risk factors and enhancing protective factors for children in school settings. We encourage school psychologists to advance their knowledge of this literature and to keep abreast of new findings, as these will have important implications for our prevention and intervention work (e.g., Doll & Lyon, 1998; Egeland, Carlson, & Sroufe, 1993; Luthar & Cicchetti, 2000; Masten & Coatsworth, 1998; Miller, Brehm, & Whitehouse, 1998; Nettles, Mucherah, & Jones, 2000; Pianta & Walsh, 1998).

# EVIDENCE-BASED INSTRUCTION AND INTERVENTION STRATEGIES

Equally important to our understanding of the natural course of child development and of important risk and protective factors that influence this development is our knowledge of empirically supported instructional techniques and intervention strategies. This literature is enormous, and sifting through it can be overwhelming. Thus in this chapter we highlight some of the major findings in the effective-teaching and -intervention literature. As we do so, we caution readers to keep in mind that when selecting intervention practices, one should consider practices with demonstrated: (1) trustworthiness and effectiveness, (2) relevance to the current problem and its context, and (3) efficiency. One should also keep in mind the following limitations to evidence-based practices: (1) research findings may not generalize to the problem situation that you are working with; (2) when empirical findings indicate that the intervention was effective for a group of students, individual differences in response to the intervention are also likely to be noted; (3) intervention strategies found to be *efficacious* (i.e., to produce desired outcomes in controlled research) may not be *effective* (i.e., efficient, practical, acceptable, feasible in practice contexts); and (4) we cannot know whether a prevention or intervention strategy works with the problem we are addressing until we evaluate it.

## Literature on Effective Instruction

As Shapiro (1996) aptly notes, "a substantial literature has demonstrated that a child's academic failure may reside in the instructional environment rather than in the child's inadequate mastery of skills" (p. 27). Over the past few decades, researchers have examined how effective teachers structure their classrooms and utilize strategies to create instructional environments conducive to learning (e.g., Good & Brophy, 1994). The literature on effective teaching indicates that quality of instruction is influenced by what effective teachers *think* about teaching and learning as well as what they *do*. What teachers think about how children learn influences what the teachers do in the classroom. Research indicates that teacher expectations about learning characteristics of particular students can have a profound impact on the manner in which they interact with those students. Further, students are more likely to learn when teachers hold high expectations and less likely to learn when they hold low expectations.

With regard to classroom management, it is interesting to note that effective teachers generally use the same kinds of consequences for misbehavior that ineffective teachers do. How they tend to differ from ineffective teachers is in the manner in which they tend to manage problem situations before they arise (Kounin, 1970). Effective teachers prevent problems by establishing classroom environments in which students are engaged in functional, interesting, worthwhile materials and activities so that participation in classroom activities is meaningful, a focus is placed on group aspects of classroom management, and there are fewer incentives to misbehave (Gettinger, 1988; Wolery, Bailey, & Sugai, 1989).

When learning problems arise, effective teachers tend to be *active problem solvers* and to focus on *alterable variables* (i.e., what they can change) when deciding what to do to improve outcomes for students (Howell & Nolet, 2000). Moreover, "effective teachers know *when* and *how* to make changes to meet the needs of students who are not progressing" (Howell & Nolet, 2000, p. 10). Teaching requires knowledge of the *content* of instruction, as well as the *structure* or *format* of instructional delivery. Lesson preview, explanation, demonstration, guided practice, correction, and independent practice are a few examples of the structure or formats that effective teachers use in the classroom. What teachers do or the instructional practices that teachers employ is only one part of the equation for effective teaching. In order for learning to occur, there needs to be consideration of the interaction between and alignment of three important factors (Howell & Nolet, 2000): (1) *students* (i.e., who is being taught or what the learner brings to the instructional context), (2) *curriculum* (what is being taught or the set of learning outcomes and expectations), and (3) *instruction* (how things are taught or what the teacher does). "The interactive nature of learning points out the truism that evaluations designed to guide instruction must focus on the learning interaction, not on individual components of the interaction" (Howell & Nolet, 2000, p. 19). As we have noted in earlier chapters, one limitation of traditional approaches to assessment is the focus on child factors to the exclusion of the learning context. The effective-teaching literature suggests that decisions about interventions should be determined by consideration of the interaction of student, curriculum, and instructional factors. Further, the focus should be on *alterable* (i.e., those amenable to change) characteristics of these factors.

## The Student (*Who* Is Being Taught?)

What the learner brings to the instructional context is one aspect of the learning equation. For example, as Howell and Nolet (2000) note, one important alterable variable that a student brings to the learning context is his or her *prior knowledge* (i.e., skills, strategies, perceptions, expectations, and beliefs). When a student does not have adequate prior knowledge or skill in a particular area, tasks become difficult. Tasks that have missing information or ambiguous cues or that lack predictability are considered difficult. Of course, whether or not a task is difficult varies for individuals with different prior knowledge bases and skills (e.g., novices vs. experts). Thus task difficulty has more to do with the interaction of the task and the learner's prior knowledge than with the task itself. Unfortunately, "many people attribute difficulty in school to deficits in a student's fixed capacity to learn—not missing prior knowledge" (Howell & Nolet, 2000, p. 21). In addition to task-specific knowledge (i.e., content knowledge and skills in the subject matter being taught), students need to have sufficient task-related knowledge (i.e., skills required to learn). Task-related knowledge is learned and therefore alterable. It includes such things as attention, motivation, and problem-solving skills. Students who are effective learners, for example, are able to analyze task demands and, from this information, select strategies for task completion. They are good at *solving problems* (Carnine, 1989; Howell & Nolet, 2000; Pressley, 1996), and they are able to *self-regulate* and *self-monitor* their behavior and their learning with respect to awareness of their skills and the requirements of the task or situation at hand. Students who do not have strong problem-solving skills should be taught these skills within the context of existing instructional objectives rather than in isolation (e.g., Derry & Murphy, 1986). Similarly, students who are deficient in self-regulation or self-monitoring skills may need explicit instruction in these areas (Howell & Nolet, 2000).

*Selective attention* to task, ability to *recall* information, and *motivation* are three additional student variables that affect learning and that are alterable through instruction. For example, in order for learning to occur, students must selectively attend to important information and ignore irrelevant or unimportant information. Certain instructional techniques (e.g., the use of previewing, prereading questions, and discriminated practice) can help to facilitate selective attention to important aspects of the task (e.g., Kryzanowski & Carnine, 1980). Effective learners are also skilled at recalling important information. Recall of information is important for comprehension tasks, and success-ful students use strategies (e.g., looking back through text, story webs) to facilitate recall. These strategies can be explicitly taught and embedded within the instructional contexts in which they are useful (e.g., Pressley et al., 1995; Swanson & De La Paz, 1998). Another important student variable is motivation to learn. Students who perse-vere (work harder and longer at something despite difficulty or negative feedback) are said to be more motivated than students who tend to give up. Thus strategies designed to improve sustained engagement in task activities are useful. It is important to note that, although individual differences may exist with respect to the degree to which stu-dents have difficulties in each of these areas (i.e., attention to task, recall, and motiva-tion), these task-related skills are *alterable* via various instructional strategies. Thus emphasis should be placed on identifying these deficit areas with the intent to match them with instructional supports designed to improve such difficulties.

Another important student variable is the degree to which a student is proficient in a particular skill, or where the student falls with respect to *skill development* on the learn-ing hierarchy (Haring, Lovitt, Eaton, & Hansen, 1978). Daly, Lentz, and Boyer (1996) describe the learning hierarchy in the following way:

> As the learner is gaining a new skill, he or she will first *acquire* it. The learner then becomes *fluent* in skill use. Next, he or she learns to *generalize* its use to novel contexts. Finally, he or she *adapts* its use to modify the response as necessary according to novel demands. (p. 370)

Different instructional techniques are useful in helping students progress through each stage of the learning hierarchy (Daly et al., 1996; Haring et al., 1978; Howell & Nolet, 2000). For example, students who are just acquiring new skills (e.g., beginning reading skills) and who are developing accuracy are in need of modeling, demonstration, prompt-ing, cueing, and corrective feedback. In contrast, students who have mastered a certain level of accuracy with a skill must practice that skill to achieve proficiency and fluency. Strategies for improving fluency include increased opportunities for drill and practice, as well as reinforcement for such activities. Instructional strategies have also been developed to promote generalization and adaptation of skills (e.g., Alessi, 1987; Stokes & Baer, 1977). When considering a student's level of proficiency from a cognitive psychology per-spective, researchers have described this concept as the student's "automaticity" with that skill (e.g., LaBerge & Samuels, 1974). More specifically, "automatic skilled performance develops with extended practice after a level of high accuracy has been reached, and when one is automatic, the skill can be performed with minimum attention and effort" (Samuels & Flor, 1997, p. 109). Evidence indicates that knowledge and skills that are developed to automaticity are retained and that, when students are performing at an automatic level, they are able to devote attention to other tasks. For example, in the area of reading, when students are able to decode at an automatic level, fewer demands are placed on working memory, and they are better able to comprehend what they read (Samuels, LaBerge, & Bremer, 1978). Regardless of the theoretical background of the researcher, much atten-tion in the intervention literature has focused on strategies and instructional techniques that facilitate the development of fluency or the degree to which students are able to per-form tasks with some level of automaticity (e.g., Carnine, 1989; Fuchs, Fuchs, Hosp, & Jenkins, 2001; Mastropieri, Leinart, & Scruggs, 1999).

During the problem-solving process, information collected about a student's prior knowledge (i.e., task-specific knowledge, as well as task-related knowledge) can be use-ful in the development of hypotheses about the reasons problems are occurring and, subsequently, in selecting appropriate intervention strategies. We have highlighted some important alterable student variables that might be targets of assessment. Processes and procedures for assessing these student variables are available in the literature (e.g., Howell & Nolet, 2000; Shapiro, 1996, 2004; Witt, Daly, & Noell, 2000), and we encourage school psychologists to consult these resources and to become proficient in using a data-driven problem-solving approach to assess student variables and their alignment with curricular variables and instructional strategies.

## The Curriculum (*What* to Teach)

In addition to considering *who* is being taught, teachers need to consider *what* to teach. The *curriculum* is a set of learning outcomes and expectations—the "what" of teaching (Howell & Nolet, 2000). When thinking about curriculum, Howell and Nolet (2000) argue that it is important to distinguish between the *intended* curriculum (the formally recommended, sanctioned, or adopted curriculum), the *taught* curriculum (the one that is based on what teachers do and use—the actual curriculum), and the *learned* curriculum (what students actually learn). Problems occur when the intended curriculum does not match the learned curriculum. This is evident when discrepancies exist between actual and expected levels of student progress. If students are not making adequate progress in a specific domain, then it is important to ask whether the curriculum is aligned with student needs and instruction.

In a well-designed curriculum, we know when a student is not making adequate progress because student progress in meeting instructional objectives is monitored. A strong curriculum is organized with instructional goals and objectives. According to Howell and Nolet (2000), instructional objectives include the following specifications: (1) content (i.e., what the student is expected to learn), (2) behavior (i.e., what the student does that indicates that he or she has learned), (3) criterion (i.e., the expected level of performance), and (4) conditions (i.e., the context or situation in which the student will work). When objectives are established, it is easy to measure student progress and compare it with the criterion to determine whether a problem exists (i.e., a discrepancy between student progress and the criterion).

Part of curriculum development includes organizing and sequencing the content of what is to be taught in a given area. One way to organize content is to think in terms of the *big ideas* in a particular domain of functioning. "Big ideas" are empirically validated foundational skills and strategies that are prerequisite to later skill development and success in particular content areas or domains (Kame'enui & Carnine, 2001). As we noted earlier in this chapter, for example, certain foundational reading skills (e.g., phonological awareness, the alphabetic principle) are valid indicator skills predictive of later success. Thus these skills should be part of the "big ideas" found in a reading curriculum (Simmons & Kame'enui, 1998). Similarly, at the secondary level, "big ideas" have been used to organize a variety of curricula (e.g., earth sciences, history), and this approach has helped to integrate content (see Grossen et al., 2002). To accelerate learning and to proactively address the needs of students, curricula can be organized or engineered around "big ideas" and can incorporate six important principles of accommodation for diverse learners (see Kame'enui & Carnine, 2001; Stein, Carnine, & Dixon, 1998). These include:

- Identifying "big ideas" and organizing curricula around them
- Teaching explicit problem-solving strategies within the curriculum

- Preteaching background knowledge
- Scaffolding instruction (i.e., providing instructional support via coaching, feed-back, cooperative learning activities, etc.)
- Integrating new and old skills and concepts
- Including adequate review that is distributed over time, cumulative, and varied to promote generalization and transfer

If the curriculum is carefully organized so that it moves along a *sequential hierarchical structure* (i.e., organized so that later concepts and skills build on earlier concepts and skills in a sequential fashion), then assessment of the match between student skills and placement in the curriculum can be very useful (Howell & Nolet, 2000). Further, *what* is being taught (e.g., factual information, conceptual information, rule relationships, strategic knowledge) also dictates to some extent *how* instruction should occur (see Howell & Nolet, 2000). The structure or format of a lesson should vary as a function of the type of information that is taught (e.g., factual, concept, rule relationships, strategic information). For example, learning of factual information involves memorization and is best achieved via explicit instruction, repeated practice, and error correction. Learning of facts can be hindered when students have difficulties with selective attention and recall. Thus teachers need to consider how to control the amount of new information to be learned and how to facilitate attention to the task. One procedure for facilitating this process is "folding-in" or "drill-sandwich" procedures, wherein tasks are organized such that students are slowly introduced to unknown material that is embedded with known material (see Shapiro, 1996). Another important consideration in teaching factual information is facilitating discrimination between new and old facts, and this can be accomplished through the organization of materials such that contrast between new and old facts is at first very large. Conceptual knowledge (i.e., knowing that certain objects, events, actions, or situations share common attributes) requires abstraction and understanding of rules for defining all relevant features of a member of a category. For example, learning to distinguish the category of "dogs" is best accomplished through presentation of examples and nonexamples that illustrate the full range of attributes that are involved in the concept of "dogs." Discrimination is also important in concept learning. Thus instructional concepts that are easily confused should be taught separately (see Howell & Nolet, 2000). Practice in accurately identifying the concept should occur prior to training in discrimination with other concepts. The teaching of rule relationships and strategic information also requires different instructional strategies. As should be evident from our brief description, the curriculum is just one part of the teaching equation, but like student variables and instructional techniques, it plays a significant role in the facilitation or hindrance of academic success (Howell & Nolet, 2000; Kame'enui & Carnine, 2001; Stein et al., 1998).

## Effective Instructional Approaches (*How* and *When* to Teach)

With student issues, we are concerned with "who" is being taught, with curriculum issues, we are concerned with "what" should be taught; and with instruction, we are concerned with "how" and "when" it should be taught. "It is the responsibility of a skilled teacher to make an informed, reasoned decision about which instructional approach is appropriate for a particular student at a particular time" (Howell & Nolet, 2000, p. 71). Some general findings in the effective-teaching literature indicate that students who fall behind in the curriculum benefit from instruction that teaches missing prior knowledge in a direct fashion. Further, "students with the least skills, who are making the least progress, need the most instructional support" (Howell & Nolet, 2000, p. 71). Research on effective teaching focuses on defining the qualities associated with maximum instructional support. Teachers can manipulate their use of time, assignments, and actions to match the curriculum and learning needs of the student (Howell & Nolet, 2000). Learning is facilitated via explanation, demonstration, guided practice, timely correction, and task-specific feedback. Teacher actions (e.g., planning for instruction, delivery of information, asking questions, responding to efforts, conducting activities, and evaluating for instruction) should be aligned with objectives in the curriculum. In addition, and as noted in the preceding sections, teachers can align instructional strategies with student needs, with the type of information they teach (i.e., factual, conceptual, rule relationships, strategic information), and with the learning hierarchy (i.e., acquisition, fluency, generalization, adaptation).

## PREVENTION AND INTERVENTION LITERATURE ON EFFECTIVE TEACHING

An extensive literature exists on empirically supported prevention and intervention practices, and countless resources and books are devoted to this topic. Further, guidelines for selecting evidence-based practices are available within the school psychology literature (e.g., Kratochwill & Shernoff, 2004; Kratochwill & Stoiber, 2000a, 2000b, 2002). This wealth of information is both good and bad for school psychologists interested in facilitating the application of prevention and intervention services in school settings. The good news is that, when working with parents and teachers, we do not need to start from scratch in developing specific intervention strategies or selecting techniques that have empirical support. The bad news is that, even when we select interventions from a list of those determined to have empirical support, the list is still quite long, and we have neither the time nor the resources to take a trial-and-error approach to implementing empirically supported practices. Thus the data-driven problem-solving model is essential to guiding the intervention selection process by linking assessment, intervention, and evaluation services. We also believe that the problem-solving process can be enhanced by knowledge of the literature on how children learn and develop over time, as well as by a thorough understanding of how different factors (i.e., student, curricula, and instruction) must be aligned to facilitate learning. As Tilly (2002) notes, effective problem solving involves careful analysis of information on the problem and its context to generate hypotheses and solutions with the least amount of inference. In other words, our knowledge base can help guide our decision-making process so that we can shrink the universe of options to a manageable form. For example, assessment of alterable student and curricular variables can help to narrow the focus of intervention strategies likely to improve learning (see Howell & Nolet, 2000). Still, it is important that intervention strategies are monitored to determine their effectiveness, feasibility, and acceptability.

In this section we highlight some prevention and intervention strategies that have been found to have empirical support in addressing important variables related to learning. In a problem-solving approach, the theoretical or philosophical basis for the intervention is less important than the efficacy of the intervention. Thus strategies should be selected based on their intended outcome and relevance to the problem situation rather than on their theoretical basis. As you read this section, you will notice that a variety of different intervention strategies are available to address important targeted outcomes. Further, intervention strategies do not necessarily fall neatly within one specific intended outcome category. In other words, one intervention may address multiple problems. For example, an intervention such as peer tutoring may help improve student engagement in task activities by creating increased opportunities to respond and also may improve skill development by providing instructional supports and corrective feedback on a more frequent basis. Our discussion of intervention strategies is brief and intended to provide readers with a *sample* of the range of strategies that might be used to address important learning outcomes. Further, our review is by no means comprehensive. Entire volumes (e.g., Lane, Gresham, & O'Shaughnessy, 2002; Rathvon, 1999; Shinn et al., 2002; Stoner et al., 1991; Walker et al., 1995), chapters (e.g., Lloyd, Hallahan, Kauffman, & Keller, 1998), special issues of journals (e.g., Lloyd et al., 1988) and meta-analyses (e.g., Quinn & McDougal, 1998) have been devoted to discussion of prevention and intervention strategies.

## Strategies Designed to Improve Academic Engagement, Motivation, Self-Regulation, and Problem Solving

In 1963, Carroll proposed that learning was a function of time engaged in learning relative to time needed to learn. Since that time, an extensive line of research has shown that there is a direct relationship between the amount of time students are engaged in a task (i.e., paying attention, working on tasks, participating in discussion) and academic performance (for a review, see Gettinger & Seibert, 2002). Differences exist in task engagement rates across classrooms and across students within classrooms. Further, students from lower socioeconomic levels and students with learning problems have been found to have lower rates of task engagement than their peers. In other words, in order for students to learn, they must have both opportunities to do so and access to instruction. Thus prevention and intervention strategies designed to increase engagement in the learning environment by addressing issues that may hinder such access (e.g., selective attention to task, motivation, self-regulation, and problem-solving skills) can be viewed as a first step in ensuring that students have the opportunity to benefit from the learning environment. Improving attention to task and task engagement involves consideration of the student's skills (selective attention, motivation, self-regulation, problem solving), as well as curriculum and instructional variables. Next we highlight a few strategies that address this issue (for a more comprehensive review, see Gettinger & Seibert, 2002).

### Structuring of the Classroom Environment

One way to facilitate task engagement is to create learning environments that encourage active participation and discourage disruptive and off-task behavior. Six tasks are "critical to successful classroom management: (1) organizing a productive classroom environment, (2) establishing classroom rules and procedures, (3) managing transitions, (4) managing independent seatwork, (5) communicating competently with students, and (6) teaching prosocial behaviors" (Rathvon, 1999, p. 70). Research indicates that when teachers are proactive and devote more time to structuring the learning environment at the beginning of the year, students are more engaged in tasks throughout the remainder of the year. Similarly, when teachers spend less time structuring their classrooms to promote academic success, students are less likely to be engaged in tasks and more likely to be disruptive. When students are more disruptive, teachers end up allocating more time to intervening with misbehavior than to instruction, and student task engagement rates drop. Further, it is more difficult for teachers to regain instructional control after losing it than it is for them to maintain it by establishing it proactively and early in the year. Thus structuring the classroom environment to promote engagement and academic success should be viewed as a prevention strategy that involves several interrelated components best achieved at the beginning of the year. Detailed descriptions of these components are available in the literature (e.g., Colvin, 2002; Gettinger, 1988; Paine, Radicchi, Roselli, Deutchman, & Darch, 1983; Rathvon, 1999).

## Contingency-Management Interventions

Early on, investigations indicated that providing incentives and contingent feedback resulted in improvements in attention to task (e.g., Ferritor, Buckholt, Hamblin, & Smith, 1972; Hall, Lund, & Jackson, 1968). Hall and colleagues (1968), for example, found that contingent praise was an effective means of increasing study behavior. Ferritor and colleagues (1972) examined the effects of contingent reinforcement on attending behavior and on work completion. Results indicated that contingent reinforcement for completing work affected levels of attention to task, but contingent reinforcement of attending behavior did not consistently affect work completion. Thus, when using contingency-based interventions, it is sometimes necessary to target more specific outcomes of task engagement, such as work productivity (e.g., number of items completed within a time frame) or accuracy (e.g., percent correct). Reinforcement contingencies can be applied to individual students or to groups of students (for a review, see Skinner, Skinner, & Sterling-Turner, 2002).

In addition to reinforcement contingencies, researchers have examined the use of contingent punishment (e.g., teacher reprimands or removal of privileges) with individuals and with groups of students. When used properly, punishment procedures have been found to be effective in increasing task engagement (e.g., Abramowitz, O'Leary, & Rosen, 1987; Acker & O'Leary, 1987) and academic productivity (e.g., Abramowitz, O'Leary, & Futtersak, 1988). We have not focused on contingent punishment in this section, however, because of certain complications that may arise with its use (Abramowitz et al., 1988; Hall et al., 1968).

## Increasing Student Engagement through Teaching Strategies

Research indicates that certain teaching strategies are associated with higher levels of student engagement than others (see Gettinger & Seibert, 2002). For example, when teachers utilize interactive teaching strategies (e.g., discussion, review, reading aloud), students are more likely to be engaged in task activities. Instruction that occurs at a faster pace is also associated with higher levels of engagement. In addition, evidence suggests that increasing opportunities for students to actively respond results in increased active task engagement. This can be accomplished via peer tutoring and cooperative learning activities and also through high levels of teacher questioning.

## Self-Monitoring

As Gettinger and Seibert (2002) noted, even when teachers consistently employ strategies designed to maximize student engagement, some students will spend less time than needed on a task as a result of other factors (e.g., low motivation, poor self-monitoring, ineffective problem-solving or self-regulation skills). Students can be taught to self-monitor their attention to task and thus can improve task engagement. According to Shapiro and Cole (1994), self-monitoring involves observing one's own behavior and recording it. It is one component of a set of strategies referred to as self-management. Other components of self-management are self-evaluation (i.e., comparing information collected about one's own behavior with a criterion) and self-reinforcement (i.e., administering consequences for meeting the criterion). These procedures, together or sometimes in isolation of each other, have been found to improve a variety of target behaviors (e.g., academic accuracy, attention to task) across various target populations (e.g., students with multiple handicaps and developmental delays, preschoolers, students with learning difficulties, students with behavior problems).

## Self-Instruction and Strategy Instruction

Teaching students to use self-instructional strategies as a way to verbally mediate tasks and task situations can facilitate the development of self-control skills (e.g., Meichenbaum & Goodman, 1971). In addition, self-instructional training has been employed to teach social (e.g., Maag, 1990) and academic (e.g., Johnson, Whitman, & Johnson, 1980) skills. Some studies investigating the efficacy of self-instruction have focused on teaching strategies relevant to solving academic problems in the areas of math (e.g., Cullinan, Lloyd, & Epstein, 1981), reading (e.g., Miller, Giovenco, & Rentiers, 1987), and written expression (Graham, Harris, MacArthur, & Schwartz, 1991). Teaching students strategies for approaching various academic tasks is useful when the type of information being taught involves rule relationships (e.g., "i" before "e" except after "c" or when sounded as "ay" as in "neighbor" and "weigh") or strategic knowledge (e.g., steps in solving arithmetic problems). Thus this approach to instruction is useful when students have difficulties with problem solving as well as when the type of information being taught involves rules or strategies. In addition to strategy training that is embedded within the context of specific academic tasks, some researchers (e.g., Deshler & Schumaker, 1986; Pressley, 1996) have examined the utility of training students in more general learning strategies (e.g., how to study, strategies for memorization, note-taking strategies) rather than those specific to learning a particular academic skill (e.g., long division). For example, strategy instruction can be used to teach students study skills and improve engagement in studying across a variety of academic domains (for a review, see Harvey, 2002, or Lentz, 1992).

## Strategies Designed to Improve Skill Development, Fluency, and Retention of Information

Although engagement in instructional activities and tasks is essential to learning, it is not necessarily sufficient (Gettinger & Seibert, 2002). In order for learning to occur, there also needs to be alignment of instruction with student skill proficiency on the learning hierarchy and with the nature of the curriculum being taught. As we have noted in earlier sections of this chapter, certain strategies for organizing curricular materials and instruction are recommended in the effective-teaching literature. We begin this section with a brief review of this work. Next, we describe a few empirically supported intervention strategies for addressing skill development in important academic domains.

## Organization of Material and Instruction to Promote Learning

Teachers can arrange instructional materials (e.g., identify "big ideas" and organize material around them) and employ instructional strategies (e.g., provide feedback and review) to facilitate learning. Some aspects of instruction are dictated by the type of information being taught (factual, conceptual, rule relations, strategies). Similarly, some aspects of instruction should vary to fit the student's skill level with respect to the learning hierarchy. According to Daly and colleagues (1996), instruction during acquisition of a skill should focus on the development of accuracy via demonstration, modeling, cueing, and prompting. Once accuracy is achieved, fluency building can be accomplished through increased opportunities to respond and drill and practice, with reinforcement for high rates of responding in context. When students are accurate and fluent in a particular skill within the learning context in which it was taught, instruction can move toward the development of generalization. This can be accomplished by modeling the skill across contexts, drilling across contexts, and reinforcing skill use across contexts. According to Carnine (1989) and Engelman (1997) some of the most important general considerations during instructional planning include:

- Introducing information in a cumulative fashion to avoid memory overload
- Preteaching easier concepts first to reduce errors in training
- Providing supervised practice in learning to discriminate concepts when topics are introduced that are similar and likely to be confused
- Spacing discriminated practice trials to reduce interference effects (i.e., introduce one concept and, once it is learned, introduce the other concept with discriminated practice)
- Relating new concepts or skills to learned information to make it more meaningful
- Providing a delayed review of difficult items
- Requiring quicker response times to promote fluency and automaticity
- Teaching to mastery or criterion.

## Strategies for Improving Academic Performance

It is important to note that the same effective instructional design principles described previously are applicable across the academic domains (e.g., reading, writing, mathematics, social studies, and science). For each instructional domain, it is important to establish the "big ideas" that need to be taught. For example, in reading, it is important to provide explicit instruction in early foundational skills such as phonemic awareness. In mathematics, *number sense*, or "a child's fluidity and flexibility with numbers, the sense of what numbers mean, and an ability to perform mental mathematics and to look at the world and make comparisons" (Gersten & Chard, 1999, pp. 19–20), seems to be an important foundational skill. Foundational skills such as phonemic awareness in reading and number sense in mathematics are important, as they relate to later success in these important domains. For example, research has indicated an "intricate relationship between conceptual understanding and consistent use of efficient strategies for computation and problem solving" (Gersten & Chard, 1999, p. 26). When students lack proficiency in these important foundational skills, teaching should emphasize explicit instruction such that students acquire and become fluent in them. Numerous intervention strategies have been designed to address particular academic skill areas, and it is not possible to review each of these strategies within this chapter. Instead, we have focused on describing factors important to learning (i.e., student variables, curricular variables, instructional variables) so that readers can consider how these relate to the vast intervention literature. Thus we encourage readers to consult the literature on intervention strategies designed to address various academic problems (e.g., reading fluency or comprehension) and to see if they are able to identify the underlying features of the strategy that fit with our discussion of effective teaching. For example, one strategy for improving reading fluency is the use of repeated readings, wherein students are asked to read and reread short passages that contain generally recognizable words several times until a certain criterion is reached (see Mastropieri et al., 1999). This strategy is useful when students have achieved a certain level of accuracy with regard to reading and when the goal of instruction is to improve fluency. In contrast, reading interventions such as self-questioning or story mapping are designed to improve comprehension (i.e., recall of information or understanding of text), and they involve explicit instruction in strategies and/or rules that are useful to facilitating comprehension (for a review, see Swanson & De La Paz, 1998). Examining intervention strategies with an eye toward how they incorporate principles of effective instruction and/or how they fit with the problem context and student learning needs is helpful in narrowing the universe of intervention options during the problem- solving process.

## DATA-DRIVEN PROBLEM SOLVING ACROSS LEVELS OF PREVENTION

In Chapter 7, we described the critical features of the data-driven problem-solving model as "outcome focused, data-driven, integrally linked to intervention, and context specific." These critical features are so interwoven that it would be inappropriate to discuss prevention and intervention practices independent of a problem-solving process that includes context-specific assessment and outcome-focused measurement and evaluation. Thus we instead focus on how prevention and intervention are integrally linked to each phase of the problem-solving process across each level of prevention (i.e., primary, secondary, and tertiary).

As illustrated in the triangle (Figure 7.2), at the level of *primary prevention*, problem-solving efforts (i.e., assessment, analysis, intervention, and evaluation) are focused on *all* students in the school. Primary prevention and intervention efforts are sometimes referred to as *universal supports* because they are applicable to all students. At this level of intervention, it is still important to consider the interaction of population, curriculum, and instructional variables. In other words, the selection of universal supports should involve consideration of *who* will receive these interventions (i.e., the students at the school), *what* will be the structure and content of these services (i.e., curriculum issues), and *how* and *when* instruction and interventions will be implemented (i.e., teaching and intervention delivery and monitoring issues). Further, just as problem solving is data driven when working with individual students, decisions at this level of the problem-solving process should be guided by data.

At the primary prevention level, all students at the school are the targets of universal supports or interventions. Thus information about the student population is useful in determining intervention needs. In addition, information from the literature on child development and risk and resiliency can be useful in determining domains to target for intervention. Once important domains of functioning are selected as a focus for primary prevention, it is important to gather information about the current school context and general performance of students in the domains of interest. For example, if a school decides to focus on establishing strong prevention and universal supports in the areas of reading and behavior, then it is important to assess how students are currently functioning in these domains. In addition, with regard to questions about curriculum or "what" to teach, it is important to assess whether the intended curriculum (i.e., the curriculum adopted for all students) is designed to address the "big ideas" within various instructional domains and to accelerate learning and meet the diverse needs of students (Kame'enui & Carnine, 2001). This is true when planning the curriculum for young students and for secondary students (Grossen et al., 2002). Further, the same curriculum considerations are needed when planning for basic academic areas (e.g., reading, writing, mathematics) and content areas (e.g., science, social studies) as when planning for behavioral and social skills areas (see Howell & Kelley, 2002, Howell & Nolet, 2000).

Once information is collected about current student performance, curriculum, and instructional practices in the target domain (e.g., reading), this information can be analyzed to determine how students fit within the triangle of need for support and how well instructional practices and curricula are aligned with student needs. For example, information on student performance on foundational reading skills assessments such as the DIBELS (Good et al., 2002) can be used to determine which students are: (1) not experiencing problems (i.e., achieving at benchmark or expected levels), (2) at risk for problems (i.e., achieving below expected levels and in need of strategic interventions), and (3) currently experiencing significant problems (i.e., achieving well below expected levels and in need of intensive supports). At this point in the problem-solving process, the information collected helps to determine discrepancies between actual and expected performance, as well as gaps in curriculum or instruction. Collecting this information helps to answer the question What is the problem?

The next step in the problem-solving process is to analyze the information to determine why the problem is occurring and what can be done to improve the situation. At the primary prevention level, the focus is on what can be done to address student needs at a universal or schoolwide level. Interventions at this level consider the curriculum as well as instructional practices and staff development needs. Once universal targets for intervention are selected, it is important to set goals and to plan for monitoring the implementation of interventions, as well as for formative assessment of student outcomes. An excellent illustration of the application of these steps of the problem-solving process on a schoolwide or primary prevention level is described by Simmons et al. (2000).

The same problem-solving steps occur at the secondary and tertiary levels of prevention, but the focus of data collection and intervention is on groups of students in need of strategic intervention (i.e., secondary prevention) or individual students in need of intensive supports (i.e., tertiary intervention). Across levels of problem solving, the process of questioning remains the same, but the intensity of prevention and intervention efforts and the frequency of monitoring of student outcomes may increase.

Howell and Nolet (2000) argued that students with the fewest skills are often in need of the most support. This is also true of our monitoring efforts. When students are at increased risk for learning and/or behavior problems (i.e., at the top portions of the triangle), it is important to monitor their responsiveness to interventions on a more frequent basis (e.g., Deno, Espin, & Fuchs, 2002).

## CONCLUSIONS

We believe that school psychologists who have strong foundational knowledge in learning and development, risk and resiliency research, the effective-teaching literature, and a framework for data-driven problem solving are in a strong position to facilitate the provision of prevention and intervention services in school settings. As with any learning process, beginning school psychologists should start by acquiring basic foundational knowledge and competencies in the data-driven problem-solving process. They should master the "big ideas" within the empirical literature and build fluency with the problem-solving process prior to attempting to expand their knowledge of the vast prevention and intervention literature. In this chapter we have attempted to highlight some of the "big ideas" relevant to prevention and intervention issues in school psychology. We encourage school psychologists in training and in practice to continue to expand and refine their knowledge of intervention options once they have established proficiency and fluency in the most robust of these strategies.

## DISCUSSION QUESTIONS AND ACTIVITIES

1. Consult the literature on risk and resiliency issues. Imagine that you were asked to design a preschool classroom that promoted the development of academic competence and reduced the exacerbation of risk factors. What would this classroom look like?

2. Visit an elementary classroom and observe instruction for at least one class period. Write a summary of the observation and note as many characteristics of the learning environment as you can in terms of student, curriculum, and instructional variables.

3. Search the empirical literature on a specific intervention topic in this chapter (e.g., reading fluency, comprehension, reading acquisition, strategy instruction, number sense in mathematics, group contingencies). Review the articles and write a brief (i.e., 3–5 pages) summary of the intervention strategy. Include a description of the strategy (e.g., its purpose, target group or skill deficit, procedures, and special considerations) and a summary of the relevant research, with a list of references.

4. Visit a local school or library and obtain a copy of an elementary school reading curriculum. The learning hierarchy would suggest that the curriculum should be sequenced such that concepts and skills build upon earlier concepts and skills in a sequential fashion. Examine the curricular materials and identify aspects of the curriculum that seem to target acquisition of skills and fluency building.

5. Imagine that you are asked to consult with a teacher about a child who is experiencing behavior problems in the classroom. The teacher emphasizes that Joey, who is in

her fourth-grade classroom, has difficulty in reading and comprehending stories. She has referred Joey because during reading exercises he is often off task and disruptive in the classroom. What problem-solving strategies would you utilize to effectively assist the teacher and Joey? What questions would you want to ask and what additional information would you gather?

# 10

# The School Psychologist's Role in Prevention and Intervention

## PART 2. MENTAL HEALTH AND SOCIAL–EMOTIONAL BEHAVIOR

In Chapter 9 we focused our attention on the role of school psychologists in prevention of and intervention with *academic* problems. We now turn our attention to the school psychologist's role in addressing students' *mental health* and *social–emotional* needs. As we enter the 21st century, the social and mental health challenges facing our children and youths are growing in number, diversity, severity, complexity, and scope. Demands on schools to meet the mental health and social–emotional needs of students are growing, yet the provision of prevention and intervention services for youths with mental health issues has been described as underutilized (Strein, Hoagwood, & Cohn, 2003) and fragmented (Greenberg et al., 2003; Hoagwood & Johnson, 2003). More specifically, data indicate that only a small percentage (i.e., approximately 20%) of children in need of specialty mental health services receive them and that, when they do, the overwhelming majority (i.e., 70–80%) receive these services within school contexts (Hoagwood & Johnson, 2003). With increasing recognition that schools often serve in the role of de facto mental health providers, researchers and policy shapers have begun to develop frameworks for the provision of evidence-based practices (EBPs) and policies to address the mental health needs of students in school settings (e.g., Forness, 2003a; Hoagwood & Johnson, 2003; Hunter, 2003; Power, 2000, 2003).

In this chapter we describe the role of the school psychologist in prevention of and intervention with mental health and social–emotional problems. We begin with an overview of the mental health and social–emotional challenges facing today's students.

206

Next, we discuss the application of a data-driven problem-solving approach to the prevention of and intervention with mental health and social–emotional needs of students. In doing so we highlight the importance of a public health prevention framework, consideration of evidence-based treatments, linking of systems of care, and adherence to a data-oriented problem-solving approach to management activities. We end the chapter with a description of the problem-solving process across levels of prevention, with an emphasis on mental health issues.

# MENTAL HEALTH AND SOCIAL–EMOTIONAL NEEDS OF STUDENTS

As many scholars have noted, schools are faced with growing numbers of students with or at risk for learning and/or social–emotional problems (e.g., Greenberg et al., 2003; OSEP Center on Positive Behavioral Interventions and Supports, 2000). These problems present themselves in varying degrees of severity and complexity. In this section, we provide an overview of the scope of mental health and social–emotional problems among school-age populations, as well as the impact of these issues in school settings.

## Prevalence of Disorders and Range of Problems in School-Age Populations

Kazdin (2004) described the range of student mental health and/or social–emotional concerns as fitting within three major categories: (1) psychiatric disorders, (2) problem and at-risk behaviors, and (3) delinquency.

### Psychiatric Disorders

Population-based epidemiological studies have indicated that "16% to 22% of children and adolescents up to the age of 18 have a diagnosable disorder; five to nine percent of youth can be classified as seriously emotionally disturbed" and "approximately 4–8% of children, ages 9–17, had severe psychiatric disorders" (Hoagwood & Johnson, 2003, p. 4). What do these estimates mean, exactly? To answer this question, it is important to start with a basic understanding of what is meant by the term "disorder." In addition, it is important to grasp the degree to which these prevalence estimates reflect *actual* rates of disorders and whether they truly represent the range of dysfunction present in children and adolescents (Kazdin, 2004).

Various diagnostic systems have been developed that describe criteria for the range of psychological dysfunctions or patterns of behavior associated with impairments in general life functioning, which are referred to as psychiatric or mental disorders. The *Diagnostic and Statistical Manual of Mental Disorders* (DSM-IV; American Psychiatric Association, 1994) and the *International Classification of Diseases* (ICD-10; World Health Organization [WHO], 1992) are two prominent diagnostic systems that catalog the range of disorders that individuals might experience in childhood, adolescence, and/or adulthood. The DSM is the most commonly used system, and it includes 10 broad categories of disorders that are first evidenced in infancy, childhood, or adolescence. These include *mental retardation, learning disorders, motor skills disorder, communication disorders, pervasive developmental disorders, attention-deficit and disruptive behavior disorders, feeding and eating disorders of infancy or early childhood, tic disorders, elimination disorders,* and *other disorders of infancy, childhood,* or *adolescence.* The DSM also includes a range of broad categories of disorders that are not unique to childhood but that are also relevant, as they can arise throughout the lifespan (e.g., *anxiety, mood, substance-related,* and *eating disorders*). It is important to note that although diagnostic systems such as the DSM provide specific criteria for diagnosing disorders, these criteria differ across different diagnostic systems, and criteria have been revised and changed considerably in various editions of the same diagnostic system.

In addition to the taxonomies of disorders available in formal diagnostic systems such as the DSM, some general categories of dysfunction are widely recognized by researchers and practitioners, and these are often used to categorize disorders in treatment studies. Kazdin (2004) describes five general categories: *externalizing disorders, internalizing disorders, substance-related disorders, learning and mental disabilities,* and *severe and pervasive psychopathology. Externalizing disorders,* which are problems directed toward others or the environment (e.g., oppositional behavior, aggression, hyperactivity, and antisocial behavior), are the most common reason for clinical referrals in children and adolescents, followed by *Internalizing disorders,* or problems directed internally (e.g., anxiety, depression).

When looking at prevalence rates of various psychiatric concerns and when considering outcomes of treatment studies, Kazdin (2004) notes several important considerations. First, he argues that general categories of disorders (e.g., internalizing disorders and externalizing disorders) are often more useful than specific diagnostic categories, as some treatment studies do not adhere to strict criteria for inclusion. This way of looking at general categories is also referred to as the *broad-band* approach (Merrell, 2003), which has its roots in multivariate statistical studies for classification of children's behavioral and emotional problems. In addition, Kazdin notes that regardless of which classification system is used to determine diagnosis, different assessment methods can result in different prevalence rates. Also, prevalence rates for different disorders do not necessarily capture the scope and severity of problems. More specifically, prevalence rates of disorders may underestimate problems, because a number of children may exhibit symptoms that approach but do not fully meet criteria for disorders (i.e., subsyndromal), yet these children still show significant impairment in functioning. Similarly, some children may meet criteria for severity of symptoms but may not meet criteria for duration or age of onset of symptoms. Finally, prevalence estimates may not capture the severity and complexity of problems, as many children and youths who meet criteria for one psychiatric disorder also qualify for a second or comorbid disorder.

### Problem and At-Risk Behavior

Research indicates that approximately "30% of 14- to 17-year-olds engage in multiple high risk behaviors that jeopardize their potential for life success" (Greenberg et al., 2003, p. 467). During adolescence, students are more likely to engage in a range of behaviors (e.g., risky sexual behavior, violence, truancy, drinking and driving, substance use) that are likely to place them at risk for psychological, social, and health concerns. Although many children who engage in such activities also meet criteria for a disorder, many more students engage in such behaviors but are able to manage daily functioning and do not meet criteria for a disorder (Kazdin, 2004). Regardless of whether these behaviors co-occur with a diagnosable disorder, the risk associated with such acts is often sufficient to warrant intervention.

## Delinquency

The third category of problem behavior, delinquency, is "a legal designation that includes behaviors that violate the law" (Kazdin, 2004, p. 546). Within the category of delinquency, some behaviors are deemed illegal for adults and juveniles. These are called *index* offenses and include such things as robbery, drug use, aggravated assault, and homicide. Other acts, referred to as *status* offenses, are designated as illegal for certain age groups (e.g., juveniles). Some examples of status offenses include running away, underage drinking, and truancy. Prevalence estimates are more difficult with delinquent behavior, as many of these offenses go undetected or unreported. As Kazdin (2004) notes, studies have indicated that a fairly large percentage of adolescents (e.g., 70%) engage in some form of delinquent behavior. Most of these youths engage in status offenses such as underage drinking or substance use and do not continue to engage in such behaviors. A much smaller percentage (e.g., 20% to 30%) are involved in more serious offenses, and only about 5% are responsible for committing greater than 50% of officially documented offenses.

### Issues of Complexity and Comorbidity: Need for Early Detection and Intervention

Children and youths who meet criteria for one psychiatric disorder, problem, or at-risk behavior and/or delinquency often meet criteria for an additional disorder or problem category. The cooccurrence of psychiatric disorders among children and youths is termed *comorbidity* and has been well established in the empirical literature (Angold, Costello, & Erkanli, 1999). In community samples, for example, roughly 50% of youths who meet criteria for one psychiatric disorder also meet criteria for a second, and rates are much higher for clinically referred samples (Kazdin, 2004). As problems increase in severity, it seems that a concomitant increase in comorbidity occurs. For example, the overlap between delinquency and psychiatric disorders is reportedly high, with estimates indicating that between 50 and 80% of delinquent youths meet criteria for at least one diagnosable disorder, the most common of which are ADHD, conduct, and substance abuse disorders (Kazdin, 2004). Research also indicates that the prevalence of mental health disorders is higher for students who are receiving special education services (i.e., 70.2%) than for any other group, including students who are served in the mental health system or the drug and alcohol treatment systems (Hoagwood & Johnson, 2003). Thus it should not be surprising that large numbers of students with mental health concerns and/or deficiencies in their social–emotional competence also have difficulty learning and may disrupt the learning of others (Greenberg et al., 2003).

The issue of comorbidity among psychiatric disorders and other problems can be illustrated with an example. Attention-deficit/hyperactivity disorder (ADHD) is now recognized as the most *common* neurobehavioral disorder of childhood and among the most *chronic* health conditions affecting school-age children (American Academy of Pediatrics [AAP], 2001). Estimates of the prevalence of the disorder range from 4 to 12% in nonreferred, school-age community samples (AAP, 2001), with higher estimates in clinically referred children. According to Barkley (2006), children with ADHD account for a significant percentage (i.e., 30–40%) of referrals to mental health practitioners. Among children and adolescents with ADHD, there is a high prevalence of associated disorders, including anxiety, learning disabilities, depression, and disruptive behavior disorders (Brown et al., 2001; Jensen et al., 2001). With regard to the co-occurrence of other psychiatric disorders, estimates indicate that approximately 44% have one, 33% have two, and 10% have three other disorders in addition to ADHD (Root & Resnick, 2003). The most common comorbid diagnosis is oppositional defiant disorder, followed by conduct disorder, anxiety disorder, and depression (Barkley, 2006; Root & Resnick, 2003). Estimates indicate that approximately 80% of children with ADHD experience academic difficulties and that approximately 50% are eligible for and are receiving special education or related services (Reid, Maag, Vasa, & Wright, 1994; Root & Resnick, 2003). Thus it is safe to say that school psychologists will be involved with children and adolescents who meet criteria for ADHD, and likely for comorbid disorders or learning difficulties, on a fairly regular basis. This does not mean, however, that *all* students with diagnoses of ADHD will have learning problems or comorbid psychiatric disorders. Instead, this means that, at a group level, children and/or adolescents who meet criteria for ADHD are more likely to experience learning or comorbid disorders than those who do not meet criteria for ADHD.

When psychiatric disorders such as ADHD co-occur with other psychiatric disorders, with problem or at-risk behaviors, with delinquency, and/or with learning and behavior problems, failure to detect such comorbidity may affect response to treatment. For children with ADHD, for example, findings from a large-scale, 14-month, comparative study conducted by a national consortium of researchers (i.e., MTA Cooperative Group, 1999a, 1999b) suggested that the presence of some comorbid disorders (e.g., anxiety) moderated the effects of medication treatment (Jensen et al., 2001). According to Forness (2003b), "by not attending to emergence of a psychiatric diagnosis and of possible comorbid diagnoses, we may not only be potentially mismanaging treatment resources but also may be missing critical opportunities for determining the most effective course for treatment-resistant disorders" (p. 322). Despite widespread recognition of the common co-occurrence of academic, social–emotional, and mental health concerns within the empirical literature, underidentification and misidentification rates for mental health problems in school settings appear to be fairly common (for discussion, see Forness, 2003a, 2003b). Forness (2003b) cites primary prevention research that demonstrates how classwide interventions in preschool have been found to result in significant improvements in symptoms and functional behavior of at-risk children (e.g., Serna, Lambros, Nielsen, & Forness, 2002), as well as possibly forestalling the actual development of psychopathology for those at highest risk (e.g., Serna, Nielson, Mattern, Schau, & Forness, 2002). Forness (2003b) argues that we must attend to comorbidity issues and early signs of pathology. In addition, he comments that educators in general and school psychologists in particular are guilty of "back-loading" our efforts and providing only reactive or tertiary care for mental health concerns rather than working from a public health or primary prevention framework wherein services are "front-loaded" to address the earliest signs of problems. We agree with this criticism and believe that the field of school psychology has great potential to make inroads in mental health promotion by moving increasingly toward a prevention and early intervention mode of service delivery.

## ADDRESSING MENTAL HEALTH ISSUES FROM A PROBLEM-SOLVING STANCE

Stepping back for a minute from the gravity of the mental health and social–emotional issues we described in the previous section, let's revisit the problem-solving approach to school psychology service delivery that we outlined in Chapter 7. To start, we argued that the traditional refer–test–place model of school psychology practice wherein the school psychologist's role is that of diagnostician was inadequate. More specifically, we described how assumptions in the philosophically based system that dominated early practice (i.e., that diagnosis informs treatment) were questionable (e.g., Deno, 2002; Tilly, 2002) and how school psychologists had been faced with enough practice failures from this approach to begin to consider alternatives. Next, we argued that school psychologists might approach problems from a data-oriented problem-solving approach that focused on using the scientific method to determine what works in contrast to the traditional model, which was more likely to produce recommendations based on diagnosis. We highlighted the fact that a problem-solving approach is outcome-focused, data-driven, integrally linked to intervention, and context-specific. Further, it follows a specific line of questioning: (1) what is the problem?, (2) why is it occurring?, (3) what can we do about it?, (4) did it work? The decision-making process in this model is guided by data with an emphasis on formative assessment (see Chapter 7) to determine the effectiveness of our prevention and intervention efforts. Thus, in a problem-solving approach, "instead of measuring student performance to find disabilities our purpose is to diagnose the conditions under which students' learning is *enabled*" (Tilly, 2002, p. 29). Further, from this perspective, "failure to profit from general education is relatively common and results to some extent from idiosyncratic, inappropriately arranged environmental events" (Lentz & Shapiro, 1985, p. 199). In Chapter 8, we described how a problem-solving model was applicable to addressing academic concerns. In particular, we described how learning problems are best solved through consideration or *diagnosis* of the alignment and interaction of student, curriculum, and instructional variables rather than from consideration of any one of these factors in isolation (Howell & Nolet, 2000).

In the beginning of this chapter, we described the scope of mental health and social emotional issues facing our youths. In doing so, we used diagnostic terms (e.g., ADHD) and labels (e.g., delinquency) that are based on structural taxonomies. When reading our description of mental health concerns, one might ask, Why should we place an emphasis on structural, diagnostic taxonomies of behavior, when we argued in Chapter 7 that diagnosis does not necessarily inform treatment? This is an excellent question—one that we believe warrants further discussion prior to describing the application of a data-oriented problem-solving approach to addressing mental health and social–emotional problems. So, we ask ourselves, What is the utility of a structural, diagnostic classification system such as the DSM and how can it possibly fit within a functional, data-oriented problem-solving approach to school psychology?

According to Scotti et al. (1996), "a basic first step in any scientific endeavor is classification" (p. 1179). Theories are often developed through deductive methods that start with observations of typical and atypical behavior, with efforts to sort these observations into categories of similarity and dissimilarity. Taxonomies that result from this process are again observed, and over time theories can be developed about these observations. The application of inductively derived theories and classification schemes must then be deductively applied in order to determine their practical use. This process and its importance in applied sciences is described by Scotti et al. (1996):

> Once we have amassed a number of critical observations about the behavior of many individuals, we summarize them (i.e., construct and theory development) and then apply these generalizations to the specific case. Without such a process, we would need to rediscover the principles of behavior anew for each client who seeks our services. "In effect, syndromal cat-

egories . . . provid[e] fundamental guidance to the *beginning* of a functional analysis" (Hayes & Follette, 1992, p. 352); that is, we begin an analysis at the nomothetic level and proceed deductively from what we know about persons with similar patterns of behavior (e.g., etiology, response covariation, prognosis, treatment design) to a focus on the target person in question. (p. 1179, emphasis added)

Thus one way to look at diagnosis and how it might fit within a problem-solving model is to consider these terms as describing constellations of covarying behaviors that can help to inform the "what" of behavior (i.e., delineating specific clusters of covarying behaviors [syndromes] and setting criteria for the duration of their occurrence).

Scotti and colleagues (1996) argued that the DSM structural categories are open to two levels of analysis. First, they can be viewed descriptively, as they point to other symptoms and/or behaviors to investigate and, therefore, can be helpful in defining problems (i.e., discrepancies between expected levels of functioning and developmentally inappropriate levels that meet criteria for a diagnosis). Second, when a syndrome or set of covarying behaviors is present across individuals, it is possible to raise more causal questions of common etiology, mechanism, or function. This is to say that, with continued research on the developmental trajectories of certain syndromes (i.e., clusters of systematically covarying behaviors), we might be able to come to some general conclusions regarding common etiologies, response covariation, associated risk factors, prognosis, and potentially common treatment strategies to address the covarying set of behaviors or symptoms. Currently, however, the utility of the DSM classification system in meeting this second aim is questionable.

Scotti and colleagues (1996) argued that there is much to be done before we can attempt to move in the direction of linking intervention strategies to certain clusters of covarying behaviors but that with continued research this might become possible. For example, at a descriptive or structural level, the behaviors of children with panic disorder resemble the behaviors of children with social phobia, yet at a functional level differences can be noted. Children with panic disorders and children with social phobia often exhibit a cluster of behaviors that is referred to as a "panic attack" (i.e., physiological responses and thoughts of losing control or being embarrassed that are associated with behavioral avoidance that significantly interferes with daily functioning). On a purely structural level, these two disorders appear very similar. Yet, at a functional level, this pattern of behaviors tends to be situationally specific for children with social phobia and more closely triggered by internal and physiological cues for children with panic disorders. In other words, a similar pattern of behavior can be triggered by different antecedents for different syndromes, and these functional relations (i.e., between the syndrome and the antecedent cue) can be useful in directing treatment for the different groups. Still, this analysis leaves out other potentially relevant functional relationships that may contribute to or exacerbate patterns of behavior exhibited by individuals (e.g., consequences connected to avoidance of social situations, skill deficits that may have contributed to the initial development of the social avoidance pattern). These finer-grained analyses might be accomplished through functional assessment methods conducted at the level of the individual child. Scotti and colleagues (1996) argue that we consider a melding of structural and more problem-solving or functionally based approaches to treatment by "augmenting the DSM with a system of functional analysis, using the best of both methods by moving from broad and nomothetic classification of the person to fine-grained idiographic analysis of the case, which includes the person and relevant social systems" (Scotti et al., 1996, p. 1187).

We now return to the problem-solving model and its application to prevention and intervention for mental health and social–emotional issues. As we noted in Chapter 7, the purpose of schooling is to alter development (cognitive, affective, social, and physical) from its natural or unschooled course (Deno, 2002). For example, from an academic learning standpoint, we expect that students' reading, writing, and math performances will be altered through the course of schooling. In addition, we recognize that students will learn to read at different rates and that problem solving will be necessary to determine proper alignment of student, instructional, and curriculum variables to facilitate literacy development. Although we often think of schooling in terms of academic development, it is also true that most of us (e.g., educators, parents, students, teachers, and community members) expect schools to address broader issues for students. Greenberg and colleagues (2003) capture this broader educational agenda:

> In addition to producing students who are culturally literate, intellectually reflective, and committed to lifelong learning, high-quality education should teach young people to interact in socially skilled and respectful ways; to practice positive, safe, and healthy behaviors; to contribute ethically and responsibly to their peer group, family, school, and community; and to posses basic competencies, work habits, and values as a foundation for meaningful employment and engaged citizenship. (Greenberg et al., 2003, pp. 466–467)

In other words, schools are expected to alter student development from its unschooled course across a wide range of domains, including mental health and social–emotional competence. Just as individual differences exist in how students develop literacy skills, the development of social competence is not a uniform process across students. Problems arise when gaps exist between current and expected levels of mental health and social–emotional well-being. As we described earlier, taxonomies of mental health problems, such as the DSM, can help to organize our thinking about what constitutes a significant discrepancy between expected and actual performance in domains of mental health and social–emotional functioning. In other words, they help us determine whether or not a problem exists (i.e., whether the child's functioning is discrepant from developmentally normal levels of functioning), and, from a structural standpoint, they assist us in a description of *what* the problem looks like and can potentially help direct the nature of additional inquiries (Scotti et al., 1996). When we move on to problem analysis, however, and we ask "why" or "what for" questions about problem behaviors, the utility of diagnostic classification systems is reduced, and we need to consider assessment procedures that have been found to be more directly linked to intervention development (e.g., functional assessment, functional analysis). Thus departure from structural classification systems begins in the second step of the problem-solving process when we ask why the problem is occurring. When we begin to think about intervention strategies (i.e., what can we do about the problem?) we may return to consideration of syndrome and the evidence-based practices that have been found to be effective for groups of students with particular disorders (e.g., the use of psychostimulants for children with ADHD or the use of cognitive-behavioral therapy for children with anxiety problems). We do so with caution, however, knowing that we need to carefully consider issues of contextual fit and individual responsiveness to intervention. Thus, during the fourth step in the problem-solving process (i.e., did it work?), it is important to directly evaluate the effectiveness of the intervention.

As we enter the 21st century, school psychologists are faced with growing social-emotional and mental health concerns of students. These problems are often complex and rarely occur in isolation from other problems. In order to properly address these issues, we believe school psychologists need to be:

1. Aware of the nature, scope, complexity, and developmental trajectories of student mental health and social–emotional issues that point to the need for early detection, primary prevention, and intervention
2. Knowledgeable about evidence-based treatments for addressing these concerns
3. Prepared to interact with professionals from medicine, clinical psychology, and community care to ensure access to treatment
4. Experts in the application of a data-oriented problem-solving approach to management of primary, secondary, and tertiary intervention efforts

In the remaining sections of this chapter, we describe how the integration of a public health prevention model, emphasis on evidence-based prevention and intervention practices, coordination of systems of care, and adherence to a data-oriented problem-solving approach to school psychology practice provides a promising framework from which to address the mental health and social emotional needs of students.

## ADAPTATION OF A PUBLIC HEALTH PREVENTION FRAMEWORK TO SCHOOLS

The adaptation of public health models to developing systems of support for students within school settings will clearly play an integral role in the shaping of the future provision of prevention and intervention services for children and youths with or at risk for mental health concerns. Public health notions of *primary, secondary*, and *tertiary* prevention, which grew out of public concern over medical threats (e.g., communicable diseases), are currently being used across a variety of disciplines. For example, these approaches were adapted for use in the field of community psychology (e.g., Adams, Hampton, Gullotta, Wiessberg, & Ryan, 1997; Cowen et al., 1996; Edelstein & Mickelson, 1986) and have more recently been applied to educational settings and school psychology (e.g., Hoagwood & Johnson, 2003; Strein et al., 2003).

Returning to the river parable that we presented in Chapter 7, a public health prevention framework considers not only the needs of students who are already experiencing difficulties (i.e., children in the river) or at risk for experiencing difficulties (i.e., children close to the river) but also those who are not at risk or experiencing difficulties (i.e., children who are safely on dry land). Using a triangle of support (e.g., Figure 7.2), *primary* prevention services or *universal supports* are delivered to *all* students. *Secondary* prevention services are targeted toward students who are identified as at risk for the development of problems, and more intensive *tertiary* prevention efforts are directed at children who are already experiencing problems (i.e., children at the top of the triangle).

Arguably, the bulk of school psychology and special education practice has focused on the provision of tertiary services to children who are already experiencing difficulties (Forness, 2003a; Hoagwood & Johnson, 2003; Shapiro, 2000). As Shapiro (2000) aptly noted, "the difficulty with a child-by-child focus is that while we are solving little problems, we are missing the big problem" (p. 561). Shapiro argues for a shift in our approach to solving instructional problems from a reactive stance to a proactive and preventative position that considers the instructional needs of *all* students and emphasizes the prevention of academic problems through primary and secondary prevention efforts. The same argument can and has been made regarding the provision of mental health and social–emotional services to students in school settings (e.g., Hoagwood & Johnson, 2003; Strein et al., 2003; Walker et al., 1996). One potentially positive outcome of this shift in focus is the likelihood that through prevention and early intervention efforts we may reduce the number of students with or at risk for the development of more severe problems. This is indeed a meaningful goal when one considers the enormous amount of time and resources that are spent in reactive management of the most severe problems. For example, students with severe behavior problems account for a relatively small portion of the school population (1–5%), yet they are often the focus of greater than 50% of office/discipline referrals and may take up a significant amount of educator and administrator time (Sugai, Sprague, Horner, & Walker, 2000). Further, with early prevention and intervention efforts in place, it may be possible to alter developmental psychopathology trajectories in such a way that we reduce the incidence of psychopathology in our children and youths (Forness, 2003a, 2003b).

The public health framework also fits nicely with a data-oriented problem-solving approach for several reasons. First, "the framework for constructing levels of risk, causality, and health promotion depends upon data-based decision making" (Strein et al., 2003, p. 25). Second, in addition to being data-driven, emphasis is placed on the development of prevention and intervention strategies. The focus of "research" in this approach is to gather information to determine relationships among variables (e.g., biological, physiological, genetic, behavioral, social, economic) "with the explicit aim of ascertaining causality and developing interventions to promote health" (Strein et al., 2003, p. 25). Finally, research is conducted within the natural context to promote generality of findings to target settings and populations and, consistent with a data-driven problem-solving model, there is a strong reliance on the scientific method rather than expert judgment to determine what works.

## EVIDENCE-BASED PRACTICE MOVEMENT

Evidence-based practice (EBP) is another movement that has gained momentum and that is directly relevant to applying data-oriented problem solving to students' mental health and social–emotional needs. According to Hoagwood and Johnson (2003), "the term 'evidence-based practice' (EBP) refers to a body of scientific knowledge, defined usually by reference to research methods or designs, about a range of service practices (e.g., referral, assessment, case management, therapies, or support services)" (p. 5). Although different terms have been used (e.g., empirically supported treatments, evidence-based treatments, empirically validated treatments), much attention to EBPs has been generated by individuals and/or groups within the fields of medicine and, more recently, clinical psychology, school psychology, and education. Emphasis is placed on determining inclusion criteria for studies (e.g., random assignment of participants to conditions, specification of target population, use of treatment manuals, outcome measures), and reviews are conducted to evaluate the evidence for various treatment approaches. The overarching goal of EBP research is to evaluate the treatment literature according to the weight of the evidence (e.g., validity, quality, robustness).

In clinical psychology, for example, criteria have been developed and employed to evaluate the empirical literature on treatments for a range of common childhood syndromes. The result has produced two categories for referencing treatments. Findings from work in this area are described by Hoagwood and Johnson (2003):

> "Well-established" treatments were required to have two or more studies that demonstrated their superiority to medication, placebo, an alternative treatment, equivalence to an already established treatment, or a single-subject case study. "Well-established" treatments were consequently identified for Attention-deficit/Hyperactivity Disorder, or ADHD (e.g., behavioral parent training, classroom behavior modification; Pelham, Wheeler, & Chronis, 1998), conduct problems (e.g., parent training; Brestan & Eyberg, 1998), and phobias (e.g., participant modeling, reinforced practice; Ollendick & King, 1998). The second category, "Probably efficacious" interventions, were required to have two or more studies that demonstrated their superiority to wait-list control, one experiment meeting the criteria for a "well-established" treatment, or three single-case studies. "Probably efficacious" treatments were identified for the treatment of depression (e.g., cognitive behavioral therapy; Kaslow & Thompson, 1998), anxiety disorders (e.g., cognitive behavioral therapy; Ollendick & King, 1998), along with other treatments related to ADHD, conduct problems, and phobias. Studies of psychosocial interventions for autism, anorexia/bulimia, post-traumatic stress disorder, bipolar disorder, obsessive-compulsive disorder, panic disorder, and substance abuse had not yet met criteria for either of these categories. (p. 6)

The development and articulation of a methodology and framework for evaluating and selecting evidence-based interventions has also occurred in other fields (for an overview, see Hoagwood & Johnson, 2003). For example, within the field of school psychology, the Task Force on Evidence-Based Interventions in School Psychology has begun to identify evidence-based interventions to address behavioral, emotional, and academic needs of children in school settings (e.g., Kratochwill & Shernoff, 2004; Kratochwill & Stoiber, 2000a, 2000b, 2002). The task force in school psychology has aimed to "improve the quality of research training, extend knowledge of evaluation criteria for evidence-based interventions (EBIs), and report this information to the profession of school psychology" (Kratochwill & Shernoff, 2004, p. 34).

Although a complete synopsis of the literature on EBPs or EBIs is beyond the scope of this chapter, a few of the major issues and findings are worth noting. School psychologists who are new to the field should be aware of some of the criticisms that have been raised about the preceding approach to determining EBPs and the gaps that exist between our research and practice-based knowledge. For example, within the EBP literature an important distinction has been made between the concepts of *efficacy* and *effectiveness* whereby *efficacy* refers to standards for evaluating treatments in controlled research studies and *effectiveness* standards require demonstrated utility in the practice context (Kratochwill & Shernoff, 2004). According to the school psychology task force, "an intervention should carry the *evidence-based* designation when information about its contextual application in actual practice is specified and when it has demonstrated efficacy under the conditions of implementation and evaluation in practice" (Kratochwill & Shernoff, 2004, p. 35)—in other words, school psychologists should concern themselves with EBPs that have met standards for *effectiveness* (as well as *efficacy*).

In addition to the distinction between efficacy and effectiveness, a host of other issues are relevant to the integration of EBPs into school-based practice. Kratochwill and Shernoff (2004) highlight four of these. The first issue they raise is the difficulty in reviewing and summarizing the literature despite attempts to delineate clear criteria. The literature and the groups who are attempting to summarize the evidence are diverse, and this makes it difficult to organize a unified, consistent approach. Second, organizational and systems issues present in practice may not be considered in controlled research studies. This factor limits the generality of some research findings to school settings. Third, as we noted in Chapter 7, school psychology is a relatively immature profession, and as such practitioners may be more likely to rely on clinical judgment rather than the scientific method or the empirical literature to determine what works. Thus movement toward the adoption of EBPs will require a shift in this tradition. We find this shift a positive one, yet we recognize that any shift in tradition is often met with resistance. Finally, bridging the research-to-practice gaps in the implementation of EBPs (once they are identified) is likely to require additional training in these practices. Similar training issues are likely to arise for teachers and special educators.

We believe the movement toward identification of EBPs will continue to be important to practicing school psychologists and to school psychologists in training. Thus school psychologists should engage in continued professional development activities to keep abreast of the treatment research as new findings are integrated. In addition, the implementation of EBPs should be done with careful adherence to a problem-solving model that incorporates a formative assessment process to determine whether, in fact, the EBP was effective for the individual or group of individuals in the practice context. This approach is not unlike Cronbach's (1975) argument for the use of "short-run empiricism," as discussed in Chapter 7.

In the sections that follow, we highlight some EBPs that have been found to have empirical support in addressing the problems associated with the most common mental health and social–emotional needs of students. This is not an exhaustive list of EBPs. Instead, we have attempted to describe a range of EBPs that illustrate the diversity of this literature and capture some of the major issues that arise. First, we discuss parent management training as a well-established treatment for aggression and oppositional behavior. This treatment is also indicated as an EBP for children with ADHD (Kazdin, 2003, 2004) and incorporates the application of operant principles not unlike those found in another EBP for ADHD—classroom contingency management—which we discussed in Chapter 8. Next, we describe cognitive-behavioral therapy and its application and evidence in treating a variety of disorders (i.e., anxiety, depression). We end with a description of the evidence for the use of psychostimulant medication in the treatment of problems associated with ADHD. Forness (2003b) argues that educators have virtually ignored the psychopharmacology literature and that doing so places us "at risk of not choosing the most effective intervention for children in our care" (p. 322). Of course, school psychologists are not in a position to prescribe medication. The point Forness is making is that we need to be careful not to ignore or argue against potentially efficacious treatments such as the use of psychostimulants for children with ADHD. We include this example because it raises important questions regarding the current limitations of our practice and the need to link systems of care. Although additional examples are beyond the scope of this chapter, readers are encouraged to examine the literature for a wider range of EBP descriptions (e.g., Hunter, 2003; Kazdin, 2003, 2004). Finally, it is important to recognize that any list of EBPs is essentially a work in progress and will need to be altered to accommodate and integrate more recent findings.

## Parent Management Training for the Treatment of Aggression and Oppositional Behavior

Parent management training (PMT) is perhaps the most well-researched treatment for oppositional and aggressive behavior in children and adolescents (Brestan & Eyberg,

1998; Kazdin, 1997, 2003, 2004). Within the literature, one can find a number of empirically based PMT programs. Some of these programs are more generally targeted toward children with externalizing or disruptive behaviors (e.g., Forehand & McMahon, 2003; Webster Stratton, Reid, & Hammond, 2004), whereas others focus on children with specific diagnoses, such as ADHD (e.g., Barkley, 1997). Although specific procedures may vary across programs, the majority of PMT approaches emphasize teaching parents to use contingency management techniques to effectively manage their child's behavior in the home setting. Underlying this approach is a fundamental assumption that oppositional and aggressive behaviors are established and maintained by maladaptive parent–child interactions. Much of this emphasis is grounded in the work of Patterson and colleagues (e.g., Patterson, 1982; Patterson, Reid, & Dishion, 1992). PMT instructs parents in behavior management strategies (based on principles of operant conditioning) and teaches parents to be more positive, predictable, and consistent with their children. The goal is to shift interaction patterns so that prosocial, positive, and compliant behaviors are reinforced. Most PMT interventions follow a similar format wherein parents are taught techniques to increase positive behaviors (e.g., positive attention) before moving on to discipline strategies (e.g., time-out). According to Gimpel and Collett (2003), this format is based on a two-part model originally developed by Hanf (1969) and subsequently adapted by others (e.g., Barkley, 1997; Forehand & McMahon, 2003; Hembree-Kigin & McNeil, 1995). The process generally involves having parents meet with a therapist, who trains them in a variety of specific parenting behaviors (e.g., establishing rules, administering positive reinforcement for appropriate behavior). Program duration varies and may be dependent on the severity of presenting problems. For example, for young children with milder oppositional problems, PMT may last approximately 4–8 weeks, but for more complicated problems (e.g., clinically referred conduct disorders), PMT might last as long as 12–25 weeks (Kazdin, 2003).

The empirical literature on PMT is quite extensive (for reviews see Brestan & Eyberg, 1998; Kazdin, 1997). The treatment utility of PMT has been evaluated for children and adolescents, who range in age from 2 to 17 years and who exhibit varying degrees of oppositional and conduct problems. These studies have employed randomized control designs and have examined the maintenance of effects over time. Results indicate that PMT has resulted in significant improvements in targeted oppositional (e.g., defiance) and conduct problems (e.g., truancy, arrest rates) across multiple outcome assessment methods (e.g., parent and teacher reports, direct observation, record reviews). Improvements occur to normative levels and have been found to be maintained in follow-up studies extending as long as 10–14 years following treatment. PMT has been employed as an intervention approach for children already experiencing problems with oppositional or aggressive behaviors and has also been used as a prevention strategy for children at risk for such problems. Finally, PMT has been extended for use in group and community settings, attesting to its generality.

### Cognitive-Behavioral Therapy for the Treatment of Internalizing Problems

Cognitive-behavioral therapy (CBT) is currently recognized as an evidence-based practice and treatment of choice for internalizing problems such as child anxiety and depression (for a recent review, see Compton et al., 2004). This approach focuses on cognitive distortions or maladaptive cognitions and their role in problems of anxiety (Kendall, Panichelli-Mindel, Sugarman, & Callahan, 1997) and depression (Lewinsohn

& Clarke, 1999). In addition, there is a concomitant focus on modification of patterns of behavior and the development of more adaptive skills (Compton et al., 2004; Kazdin, 2003, 2004).

## CBT and Anxiety

In the treatment of anxiety, CBT employs cognitive restructuring and exposure-based interventions to promote the use of cognitions and behaviors resulting in habituation or extinction of inappropriate fears (Compton et al., 2004; Kazdin, 2003, 2004; Kendall, Aschenbrand, & Hudson, 2003). The exposure-based component of the intervention rests on the notion that "anxiety is a set of classically conditioned responses that can be unlearned or counterconditioned through associative pairing with anxiety-incompatible stimuli and responses" (Compton et al., 2004, p. 941). With systematic desensitization, for example, stimuli that are anxiety arousing are paired gradually and systematically with competing stimuli that produce relaxation (e.g., food, praise, cues for muscle relaxation). This can be accomplished through imagery or in vivo exposure. Treatment involves modeling and direct reinforcement of new skills and behaviors designed to mediate anxiety. For example, children are taught to recognize the physiological symptoms (e.g., muscle tension) and the internal dialogue (e.g., negative "what if" statements) associated with anxiety. Therapy focuses on the development of coping skills, including strategies for recognizing and reconceptualizing anxiety-provoking situations, as well as problem-solving alternatives for coping with the situation. Emphasis is placed on generating alternative explanations to correct maladaptive self-talk. In addition, children are taught to generate alternative actions or plans for how to cope with anxiety-provoking situations. Finally, children are taught to evaluate their alternative coping plans through self-evaluation and self-reinforcement procedures. CBT for anxiety problems typically involves 16–20 individually administered sessions. The first 8–10 sessions are devoted to learning new coping skills, and the second 8–10 sessions focus on application of these skills to varying levels of anxiety-producing situations.

A substantive research base supports the utility of CBT for the treatment of child anxiety (Compton et al., 2004; Kazdin, 2003, 2004; Kendall et al., 2003). This treatment has been evaluated in both single-case and randomized control trials with children ages 9–13 years. Multimethod and multi-informant outcome data indicate improvements in anxiety, as well as other areas (e.g., depression, aggression, social problems, hyperactivity). Further effects of treatment have been replicated by independent investigators, and effects have been maintained for periods of up to 6 years. As Kazdin (2003, 2004) notes, the treatment research on CBT for anxiety is exemplary because: (1) studies have included children who met diagnostic criteria for anxiety; (2) treatment findings have been consistent across studies; and (3) following treatment, many children fall within the normative range of functioning. Thus CBT is considered to be an "evidence-based" treatment for anxiety disorders.

## CBT and Depression

In the treatment of depression, CBT focuses on reinstating behavioral patterns associated with pleasant experiences and confrontation of maladaptive cognitions such as helplessness or hopelessness (Compton et al., 2004; Kazdin, 2004). CBT for depression is based on an assumption that "symptom change is most likely to occur through inter-

ventions that modify patterns of behavior through skills acquisition and patterns of cognition, with changes in depressed mood following in turn" (Compton et al., 2004, p.
952). Some aspects of CBT are standard (i.e., psychoeducation about depression and its
causes, goal setting, general problem-solving skills), whereas other aspects are tailored
to the specific skill deficits and needs of the individual (e.g., addressing negative
self-attributes, poor self-assertion skills, failure to attribute positive outcomes to internal, stable, or global causes). In addition, current CBT packages integrate parent and
family sessions with individual CBT (Compton et al., 2004).

Research also supports the use of CBT in the treatment of depression (Compton et
al., 2004; Kazdin, 2004). These studies adhere to the same methodological rigor as CBT
studies focused on anxiety disorders, but there are significantly fewer studies that focus
on youths with depression. Some limitations of the literature on CBT for depression are
important to note. For example, some studies had too few participants across conditions, resulting in insufficient power to determine between-group effects (Compton et
al., 2004). In addition, no studies to date have systematically evaluated components of
the treatment. Similarly, no studies have provided systematic replication by independent
investigators (Compton et al., 2004; Kazdin, 2004). With regard to long-term follow-up
data, studies indicate that there is a high risk of reoccurrence of depression for adolescents and a need for more research investigating the impact of treatment continuation
on long-term outcomes (Compton et al., 2004). Despite some of these limitations, there
is still a widespread consensus that CBT approaches are the best supported methods of
intervention for depression among older children and adolescents, including applications of this approach in school settings (Merrell, 2001).

## Psychostimulants for the Treatment of ADHD Symptoms

Psychostimulants are a well-established treatment for the symptoms of ADHD (Kazdin,
2003, 2004). When compared with nontreatment controls, psychostimulant medication
has proven effective in approximately 70–80% of children with ADHD (e.g., Barkley,
2006; Greenhill et al., 2001; Spencer et al., 1996). Further, in cases in which multiple
psychostimulants are employed (i.e., a second medication is tried when a child does not
respond to the first medication), response to medication has been shown to reach as
high as 90% (American Academy of Pediatrics, 2001). In a recent large-scale 14-month
comparative study conducted by a national consortium of researchers, "medication
management, alone or combined with intensive behavioral treatment, was superior to
behavioral treatment and community care in reducing ADHD symptoms; but only combined treatment showed consistently greater benefit than community care across other
outcome domains (disruptive and internalizing symptoms, achievement, parent–child
relations, and social skills)" (MTA Cooperative Group, 1999b, p. 1088).

Currently, literature documenting the short-term effectiveness of psychostimulant
medication on symptoms of ADHD represents the largest body of treatment literature
for any childhood psychiatric disorder (Spencer, Biederman, & Wilens, 2000). Psychostimulants are also associated with positive gains in academic, behavioral, social, emotional, and physical functioning (for reviews see Bennett, Brown, Craver, & Anderson,
1999; DuPaul, Barkley, & Connor, 1998; DuPaul & Stoner, 2003). To date, however,
long-term benefits on academic achievement have not been documented (e.g., Greenhill et al., 1999), yet some scholars have suggested that this may be partly due to the fact
that some academic outcome measures (e.g., standardized achievement tests) may not

be specific enough to capture differences in academic performance (DuPaul & Stoner, 2003).

Although the short-term effects of stimulant medication on ADHD are well established (Brown & Sammons, 2002), less information is available on the long-term effects of psychostimulants, with one exception. In the MTA study, parent and teacher ratings indicated that school-age children who received either medication alone (i.e., titrated to optimize stimulant dosage) or a combination of medication and psychosocial intervention displayed a marked reduction in core ADHD behaviors beyond participants in the community care sample and that these effects were maintained over a 14-month period (Greenhill et al., 1999; Jensen et al., 1999). Although these results are impressive, one might still argue that 14 months is not necessarily a "long" period of time and that much more research is needed in this area.

The issue of side effects of medication has also been studied extensively. Research has indicated that psychostimulants can have adverse side effects that may be short or long term and that the severity of adverse effects tends to increase linearly with dosage increases (Brown & Sammons, 2002). Approximately 4–10% of children experience adverse effects to stimulant medication (e.g., delayed onset of sleep, jitteriness, headaches, stomachaches, reduced appetite, irritability, anxiety, and social withdrawal), yet such adverse side effects are typically transient and dissipate after medication is discontinued (American Academy of Pediatrics, 2001; Barkley, McMurray, Edelbrock, & Robbins, 1990; Brown & Sammons, 2002; DuPaul et al., 1998). A smaller percentage of children (i.e., less than 1%) may be affected by tics as a result of psychostimulant use, particularly if the child has Tourette syndrome, another tic disorder, or a family history of such symptoms. To date, popular concerns with potential long-term adverse side effects such as drug use and abuse, growth suppression, or reduced cardiovascular functioning have not been empirically supported (American Academy of Pediatrics, 2001; Brown & Sammons, 2002). It should be noted, however, that the long-term adverse effects of stimulant medication have not been well studied; thus ongoing monitoring of psychotropic medication by a physician trained in their use is critical (Greenhill et al., 1999).

## Concluding Comments Regarding EBPs

In the preceding sections, we described three EBPs for the treatment of mental health or social–emotional concerns of children and youths. Our examples (i.e., PMT, CBT, and psychopharmacology) are intended to illustrate some of the commonly used strategies that have been found to be *efficacious* as well as *effective* for a variety of commonly occurring problems. They also illustrate the need to coordinate services across systems of care, a topic that we discuss in more detail in the next section. Other EBPs have been identified in the literature (e.g., multisystemic therapy, classroom contingency management, problem-solving skills training) for the treatment of various problem domains, and the list is constantly evolving with additional research. Thus school psychologists should keep abreast of the literature and frequently update their knowledge and skills. For information on the current state of our knowledge of EBPs and other issues relevant to mental health and social–emotional issues of children, readers should consult the recent literature (e.g., Kazdin & Weisz, 2004; Lambert, 2004; Lane et al., 2002; Merrell, 2003).

# LINKING SUPPORTS ACROSS SERVICE DELIVERY SYSTEMS AND PROVIDERS

Limitations associated with traditional approaches to training psychologists to work in specific settings and to restrict their work to addressing the needs of individuals who are experiencing difficulties have led scholars to argue for changes in the manner in which we deliver services (e.g., Power, Shapiro, & DuPaul, 2003), as well as the manner in which we train psychologists (Power, 2000; Power, DuPaul, Shapiro, & Parrish, 1995). Beyond important issues of the adoption of public health frameworks for prevention and the need to consider EBPs is the need to consider how we can link health, educational, community, and family systems to better meet the diverse needs of children and adolescents (e.g., Power et al., 2003). To build capacity for linking services across these systems, it is important that service providers (including school psychologists) build competencies in particular domains that will promote integration of services. For example, in an attempt to facilitate the linking of systems to address the prevention and management of chronic health conditions, Lehigh University and The Children's Hospital of Philadelphia (CHOP) have embarked on a joint endeavor to train doctoral-level pediatric school psychologists (see Power et al., 2003, for a description). Competency domains in training include: (1) interventions for chronic illnesses (e.g., knowledge and application of assessment and intervention methods), (2) prevention programming (e.g., knowledge of risk and protective factors related to chronic health problems and ability to apply core prevention programming components), (3) program evaluation (e.g., use of single-case and quasi-experimental research methods in program evaluation, use of participatory action research), and (4) intersystem collaboration (e.g., expertise in addressing health problems across settings, knowledge of methods for promoting interdisciplinary collaboration). Training is accomplished via course work, practicum experiences, and research training that mirror the notions behind linking systems by providing integrated training experiences (e.g., practicum experiences occur across school and health care settings). This movement toward explicit training in competencies relevant to linking systems of care is promising. It is likely that school psychologists will continue to work with other service providers (e.g., physicians, community agency personnel, clinical psychologists) and that efforts to facilitate coordination of services will enhance the delivery of mental health prevention and intervention services to children and youths. This work is still in its infancy, yet we believe it will play an integral role for school psychologists of the future.

# DATA-DRIVEN PROBLEM SOLVING ACROSS LEVELS OF PREVENTION

In Chapter 9, we discussed the application of a problem-solving model to various levels of prevention in addressing academic problems. The same process applies to the application of this model to address levels of prevention of mental health and social–emotional health. The work of Sugai, Horner, and colleagues provides an excellent example of prevention and intervention efforts aimed at addressing violence prevention through a positive behavioral support (PBS) process (e.g., Sugai, 2003; Sugai & Horner, 2002a, 2002b; Sugai et al., 2000). PBS is a process through which schools begin to improve services for *all* students by creating systems wherein intervention and management decisions are data-driven and guided by what has been demonstrated to be effective in the empirical literature.

As we noted earlier in this chapter, it is perhaps an understatement that student learning and social–behavioral needs are increasing. Longitudinal research points to the chronic nature of such problems and the critical need for *early* intervention if we are to offset negative long-term outcomes. The poor prognosis for students who experience early academic or behavior problems has been well documented. Irrespective of whether or not students receive special education or related services from schools, both academic and learning difficulties are associated with increased risk of negative outcomes, with a high cost to society (e.g. school dropout, substance abuse, unemployment, and incarceration). Moreover, when efforts toward intervention are provided in a crisis or reactive manner, the chronic nature of learning and behavior problems becomes more pronounced and is potentially more resistant to change (Forness, 2003a, 2003b).

With regard to social–behavioral difficulties, although students with severe behavioral problems account for a relatively small percentage of the student population, their needs tend to be chronic, as well as time and resource intensive (Sugai et al., 2000). Further, research reviews suggest that the rise in adoption of "zero tolerance" discipline policies, which rely heavily on suspension and expulsion practices, are not working and may in fact be exacerbating these problems (see Skiba & Peterson, 2000). Thus there is a need to shift our efforts from reactive and punitive methods to the development of more proactive, preventative, and educationally focused methods. PBS approaches are responsive to these issues. More specifically, PBS employs a public health prevention framework in providing a continuum of supports and prevention for: (1) students who currently are not experiencing learning and/or social–behavioral difficulties (*primary prevention*); (2) students determined to be at risk for the development of learning and/or social–behavioral difficulties (*secondary prevention*); and (3) students who currently are experiencing significant learning and/or social–behavioral difficulties (*tertiary prevention*).

*Primary prevention* efforts, or universal supports, are provided to all students through schoolwide reform that involves the consistent use of research-based effective teaching and behavior management practices, ongoing monitoring of these practices and student outcomes, staff training and professional development, and systems-level decision making. The goal of primary prevention is to create school and classroom environments that promote student learning and ultimately decrease the number of students at risk for learning and/or social–behavioral problems. The selection of universal supports should involve consideration of *who* will receive these interventions (i.e., the school population and risk and protective factors in the local community), *what* will be the structure and content of these services (i.e., EBPs for prevention of mental health and social emotional problems), and *how* and *when* instruction and interventions will be implemented. Further, just as problem solving is data-driven when we are working with academic concerns, decisions at this level of the problem-solving process should be guided by data.

Within PBS, *secondary* prevention and *tertiary* prevention efforts often involve the employment of a data-driven problem-solving process that includes the use of functional behavioral assessment (FBA) procedures. As we discussed in earlier chapters (i.e., Chapter 6 and Chapter 7) FBA has been defined as a structured problem-solving process through which a broad range of information is gathered through various methods (e.g., teacher interviews, rating scales, direct observations) to develop hypotheses regarding the "functional" or "causal" relationship between specific events (e.g., teacher attention) and the occurrence of problem behaviors (e.g., disruptive behavior).

The same problem-solving steps occur at all levels of prevention, but the focus of data collection and intervention is on varying numbers of students at each level (i.e., school, small group, individual). Like the application of this process to academic problems, problem solving to address students' mental health and social–emotional needs follows the same line of questioning at each level, yet the intensity of prevention and intervention efforts and the frequency of monitoring of student outcomes may increase with the intensity of student needs. When students are at increased risk for mental health or social–emotional problems (i.e., at the top portions of the triangle), it is important to monitor their responsiveness to interventions on a more frequent basis and to coordinate services across systems of care (Power et al., 2003).

# CONCLUSIONS

In this chapter, we have highlighted some of the important issues relevant to prevention of and intervention with mental health and social–emotional concerns in school settings. We believe school psychologists are in a unique position to make a significant contribution to prevention and intervention efforts. In order to do so, we believe there needs to be a shift in intervention focus from one that is predominately tertiary in nature to one that addresses primary and secondary prevention from a public health framework. Further, it is essential that practicing and preservice school psychologists are knowledgeable about (1) developmental trajectories relevant to various social–emotional and mental health problems, comorbidity issues, and risk and resiliency factors associated with such concerns; (2) EBPs for the treatment of such problems; and (3) strategies to link systems of care to support such endeavors. Finally, we consider a data-driven problem-solving model approach to be essential in comprehensively addressing the growing mental health and social–emotional needs of students in school.

# DISCUSSION QUESTIONS AND ACTIVITIES

1. Interview a teacher and ask him or her to describe some of the current mental health and social–emotional challenges that are affecting children and youth in school settings. Consider how the problems described fit within the categories discussed in the beginning of the chapter (i.e., psychiatric disorders, risky behaviors, delinquency).

2. What is comorbidity and why is it an important consideration when working with children with or at risk for mental health and social–emotional concerns?

3. Should school professionals be concerned with psychiatric diagnoses and diagnostic classification systems such as the DSM? Why or why not? Support your answer. If your answer is yes, how can diagnostic classification systems fit within a data-oriented problem-solving approach to school psychology?

4. What is an EBP? Describe the distinction that is made between *efficacy* and *effectiveness* in the EBP literature. Why is this distinction important to school psychologists?

5. Interview a practicing school psychologist about the role that he or she plays in addressing students' mental health and social–emotional issues. Ask about his or her involvement in primary, secondary, and tertiary levels of care. Does the role involve linking to other systems of care? If so, how does this occur? What interventions does he or she employ? Does he or she employ a data-driven problem-solving model in his or her approach to addressing these issues?

# 11

# The School Psychologist's Role in Facilitating Systems Change

In earlier chapters of this volume, we mapped our vision for the future of school psychology practice with a focus on the roles that we believe school psychologists should pursue. Thus far, we have provided an overview of a data-oriented problem-solving approach to defining problems, assessing problems, and linking these activities to the provision of evidence-based prevention and intervention services. We now turn to considering the *context* in which these practices occur and the *systems* issues important to their use. As we noted in Chapter 7, in order for any shifts in practices to be adopted and sustained, the question of how new practices will fit within existing organizational structures and systems must be addressed.

In this chapter, we provide an overview of the systems change literature and its relevance to schools and to school psychology. We describe how the current school context and the challenges facing educators highlight the need for systemic reform efforts. Next, we discuss systems change theory and its application to school systems. Emphasis is placed on viewing school organizations as systems and addressing levels of performance and performance needs within these systems. Drawing from lessons learned from previous attempts at systems change, as well as from best practices in the literature on this topic, we describe important stages of successful systems-level change in schools. We end this chapter with a discussion of the school psychologist's role in these endeavors.

## THE SCHOOL CONTEXT: CHALLENGES FACING SCHOOLS

Schools are faced with an array of interrelated challenges as they try to address the academic, social–emotional, and mental health needs of students. In this section, we highlight some of the most salient contextual issues facing schools today, including: (1) technological advances and changing dynamics of the workforce; (2) increased heterogeneity of the student population and increased number, severity, and complexity of student needs; and (3) the push for evidence-based practices and increased accountability despite diminishing resources. Consideration of the interplay of these challenges helps to illuminate the need for coordinated and systemic reform efforts.

## Technological Advances and Changing Dynamics of the Workforce

Greenberg and colleagues (2003) noted several societal changes that affect life circumstances of today's children and youths, including "increased economic and social pressures on families; weakening of community institutions that nurture children's social, emotional, and moral development; and easier access by children to media that encourage health-damaging behavior" (p. 467). These external, economic, and sociopolitical factors can alter the development of students who enter our school systems and play a role in shaping the heterogeneity of student needs. Just as the climate in schools is constantly changing as a function of an increasingly diverse student body, competencies required to enter the workforce have become a moving target in response to changing global dynamics and exploding informational and technological advances. Clearly, schools are struggling as they attempt to prepare an increasingly diverse student population for constantly changing demands in the workplace.

## Changes in the Student Demographics and Student Needs

As we enter the 21st century, schools are faced with rising numbers, diversity, and severity and complexity of student needs. In comparison to schools that were formed in the 1900s, today's schools serve significantly larger student bodies. Higher enrollments and class sizes can affect the general culture within a school setting and thus have an impact on how services are provided (Greenberg et al., 2003). In addition, student populations are increasingly heterogeneous (Greenberg et al., 2003; OSEP Center on Positive Behavioral Interventions and Supports, 2000). This is true with respect to social and economic disparities, ethnicity, race, range of abilities, and motivation (Greenberg et al., 2003). Not only are schools challenged with meeting the needs of an expanding and increasingly diverse student population, but, as we noted in earlier chapters, they are also faced with growing numbers of students with or at risk for learning and/or social–emotional problems (OSEP Center on Positive Behavioral Interventions and Supports, 2000). In sum, the rapidly changing nature of student characteristics creates new contextual demands on schools. As a result of these changes, educational systems must adapt and change if they are to be effective in meeting the needs of a complex and diverse student population.

## Increased Demands for EBPs and Accountability Despite Diminishing Resources

As Fullan (2000) aptly notes, "forces that were previously outside are now in teachers' faces every day" (p. 3). In an era of evidence-based practice and accountability, schools are increasingly expected to do more to address the needs of students (academic, social–emotional, and mental health) despite diminishing resources (Greenberg et al., 2003; OSEP Center on Positive Behavioral Interventions and Supports, 2000). In order to address the increasing numbers, diversity, and severity of student needs, schools must create systems of support that, on the one hand, work proactively to anticipate and prevent problems before they occur and that, on the other hand, provide a responsive continuum of secondary and tertiary supports for students with or at risk of developing more severe problems. The level of intensity of problem-solving and intervention efforts required to ameliorate concerns must vary as a function of the durability, complexity, and severity of the presenting problem. Thus increasingly more resources are necessary to match the growing issues in school settings. Given the finite nature of resources available for such efforts, schools must be proactive in anticipating needs, as well as flexible in making adjustments to new challenges and changing demands as they present themselves.

### Change as a Unifying Feature of the Challenges Facing School Systems

When one considers the top challenges facing school systems today (i.e., technological advances and changing dynamics of the workforce, increased heterogeneity of the student population and growing student needs, push for evidence-based practices and increased accountability), it is noteworthy that one unifying feature of these challenges is "change." Just as the pressures facing managers (e.g., global competition, increasingly demanding customers, and technological advances) are in a constant state of change— "relentless, multifaceted, unforgiving, blindingly rapid change" (Rummler & Brache, 1995, p. 1), the pressures and challenges facing school systems are a moving target. Schools, like businesses, are evolving systems. Thus they are affected by and reciprocally influence the contexts in which they exist. When contextual factors are changing at a rapid pace, pressures on the system to adapt are great. This situation exists because organizations respond to their external environments in an attempt to seek equilibrium. In the business world, "a processing system (organization) will either adapt to its environment, especially its receiving system (market), or cease to exist" (Rummler & Brache, 1995, p. 12). In a similar vein, "organizational change and strategic planning should be natural, necessary, and ongoing components of a healthy, evolving school" (Knoff, 2002, p. 237).

It is important to note that "adaptation is a process, not an event" (Rummler & Brache, 1995, p. 13). Systems that are healthy continually "demonstrate the capacity to analyze problems and to solve them in a manner that facilitates the attainment of their goals" (Curtis & Stollar, 2002, p. 225). Thus the concept of *lasting change* is an oxymoron. Problems occur when the focus of change is on an *innovation* (e.g., EBP, piecemeal solution) rather than on the *healthy evolution of the system* (e.g., Grimes & Tilly, 1996). This distinction is paramount to the development of school systems that are responsive to the changing contextual demands that we described earlier. School psychologists who are involved in systemic reform efforts will need to keep abreast of the demands and challenges that affect school systems. They also need to have knowledge and skills in a problem-solving approach to systems change.

## PROBLEM SOLVING, SYSTEMS CHANGE, AND SCHOOL PSYCHOLOGY

As the river parable described in Chapter 7 illustrates, we must consider primary and secondary prevention if we are to adequately address the continuum of students' needs. In the past, school psychology practice has almost exclusively focused on tertiary care (e.g., Forness & Kavale, 2001; Reschly, 2000; Shapiro, 2000; Ysseldyke, 2000). Thus it should not be surprising that systems-level change has not been a focus of service provision within our profession.

Despite the limited focus on systems change within our field, some scholars in school psychology have long been proponents of systems change as an integral part of practice (e.g., Curtis & Stollar, 2002; Knoff, 2002). They have argued that school psychologists are well suited to a systems-change role, as they are likely to "understand human behavior within the ecology of the school as part of a larger system" (Curtis & Stollar, 2002, p. 224). When discussing the competencies necessary for school psychologists to effectively engage in this process, the following descriptions have been offered:

> In order to engage effectively in system-level consultation, school psychologists need to call upon three areas of expertise: (a) understanding human behavior from a social systems perspective, (b) ability to use collaborative planning and problem-solving procedures, and (c) familiarity with principles for organizational change. (Curtis & Stollar, 2004, p. 224)

> To coordinate and facilitate a school-based organizational change and strategic planning process, school psychologists must understand and have expertise in three primary areas: (a) the problem-solving and planning cycles of a school from an organizational perspective, (b) the characteristics of an operating school district from a systemic perspective, and (c) the steps in a strategic planning process. (Knoff, 2002, p. 238)

Drawing from these two descriptions, one can identify several key competencies for school psychologists interested in the systems-change process. These competencies include knowledge of systems theory and the principles of organizational change, a basic understanding of schools as systems (e.g., their social ecology, structural aspects, and component parts), and skills in collaborative planning and problem solving. We believe that school psychologists of the future will play an increasingly integral role in the systems-change process and, therefore, should build competencies in these areas. Further, preparation and practice in systems-level influence and change are included in the most recent *Standards for Training and Field Placement Programs in School Psychology* (NASP, 2000d) and *Guidelines for the Provision of School Psychological Services* (NASP, 2000a). In the sections that follow, we discuss the systems-change literature and its application to school settings.

## SYSTEMS-CHANGE THEORY

One important prerequisite for serving in the role of a systems-change agent is a basic understanding of systems and systems theory. According to Curtis and Stollar (2002), general systems theory provides the theoretical foundation for systems-level intervention and organizational development. Early applications of general systems theory focused primarily on military and industrial settings, and extensions were made to behavioral sciences in the 1950s and to schools in the early 1960s (Curtis & Stollar, 2002).

A *system* can be defined as "an orderly combination of parts that interact to produce a desired outcome or product" (Curtis & Stollar, 2002, p. 224). For example, at a very small level, a human system might be defined as "the orderly combination of two or more individuals whose interaction is intended to produce a desired outcome" (Curtis & Stollar, 2002, p. 224). Further, and in contrast to mechanical systems, which are inorganic and more static or fixed, schools are organic or "living" systems. One manner in which living systems differ from inert systems is the way in which these systems are influenced by and in turn influence the environment and other systems. This *reciprocal influence* is captured in the manner in which some scholars have described child development. Bandura (1978) and Bijou (1993), for example, have suggested that from a systems or ecological perspective the child is influenced by and in turn influences the environment or system of which he or she is a part.

All living systems also are considered "open systems" wherein each part is interconnected with and reciprocally influences all other parts of the system, as well as the system as a whole (Curtis & Stollar, 2002). For example, school building systems are part of larger systems (e.g., a school district) and contain inner systems or "subsystems" (e.g., classrooms, intervention assistance teams, school improvement teams). When change occurs in one aspect of the system (e.g., change in personnel, change in student needs), the system is affected. In a similar fashion, changes in the surrounding contexts or larger systems affect the system as well as its subsystems. For example, policy changes (e.g., mandated testing for *all* students) or catastrophic events (e.g., a student suicide) can affect the system at all levels (e.g., policy, staff, administrator, and student levels).

The broad nature of the interlocking contingencies that govern living systems is captured within the following often cited statement attributed to the pioneering environmentalist John Muir: "When we try to pick out anything by itself, we find it hitched to everything else in the universe." Learning how various aspects of the system are interconnected and how they work together is one challenge that presents itself in systemic reform efforts. According to Curtis and Stollar (2002), *organizational development* is "the planned and sustained effort to bring about system-level improvement through self-analytic and problem-solving methods" (p. 227). For this process to be effective it must be planned and systematic.

As we noted in the preceding section, the early application of systems theory to real-world settings focused primarily on industrial and military settings. Thus the literature on improving performance within business settings is quite extensive. This section draws from this literature to describe the important distinction between viewing an organization from a vertical and functional standpoint and viewing it from a horizontal or systems perspective (Rummler & Brache, 1995).

Rummler and Brache (1995) argued that most business managers view their organizations from a fundamentally flawed perspective. More specifically, the typical view of an organization is *vertical* and *functional*, in which separate units within the organization (e.g., research and development, manufacturing, marketing and sales) are depicted as operating independently from one another and vertically via reporting relationships to other entities such as managers (see Figure 11.1). Within this vertical and functional view of an organization, the structures built around units are referred to by Rummler and Brache (1995) as " 'Silos' (tall, thick, windowless structures)" (p. 6). A similar picture could be drawn of a school organization, wherein grade-level units are depicted as separate entities that report vertically to the principal (see Figure 11.2). In high school settings, the units might be organized according to content areas (e.g., science, mathematics, social studies, language arts, music) or grade-level instructional teams. Regardless of how the units are organized, this vertical and functional approach to viewing organizations is limiting, as it fails to depict how work flows. Further, it does not illustrate what happens, for whom, or how. When managers and/or school leaders have this view of an organization, they tend to manage each unit separately (e.g., meeting sepa-

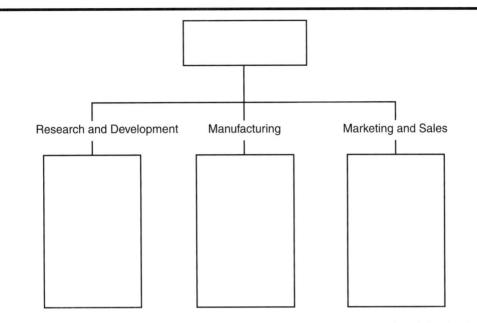

**FIGURE 11.1.** Traditional (vertical) view of an organization. From Rummler and Brache (1995). Reprinted with permission of John Wiley & Sons, Inc.

rately with grade level teams, or area units). This approach can result in a perpetuation of the vertical and functional view and can create competition across units. Conflict can arise when decisions are made that have implications across units. In school settings, for example, decisions such as scheduling or additional resource allocation can result in conflict. When units function independent of each other, it is difficult to

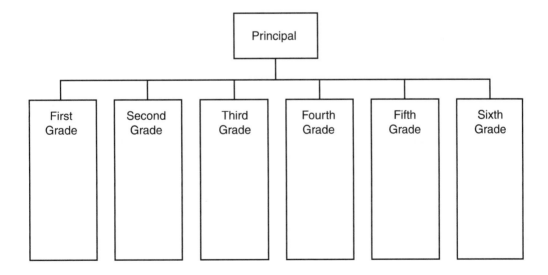

**FIGURE 11.2.** Vertical view of a school organization.

address these broader, schoolwide issues in a comprehensive manner. For example, a principal who is given additional funding and personnel to address reading at an elementary school must decide how best to utilize those resources. If the units within the school are viewed vertically and functionally independent from one another, then each grade-level unit might make a separate case for the use of these resources with little integration of information across grades. The result is that the principal must make some hard decisions, and some grade-level units will no doubt be unhappy with the outcome.

An alternative to viewing organizations vertically and functionally is to view them *horizontally* and from a *systems perspective* (Rummler & Brache, 1995). Figure 11.3 is an example of a systems or horizontal view of a business organization. This view helps to illustrate the flow of work and includes a description of what the organization does and for whom. Further, it allows one to see how the work is done by illustrating the connections between components of the system. Viewing systems in this manner allows one to examine where potential problems might arise in the flow. It also allows managers to proactively adapt to change by anticipating its impact on the flow of work within the system. Systems charts can be drawn to illustrate the flow of work for organizational sys-

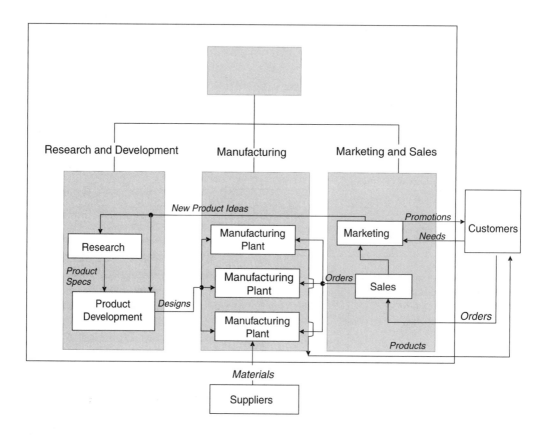

**FIGURE 11.3.** Systems (horizontal) view of an organization. From Rummler and Brache (1995). Reprinted with permission of John Wiley & Sons, Inc.

tems, as well as for the subsystems that operate within organizations. As we described in an earlier section, healthy organizations adapt to changing demands. "If an organization survives, it has adapted," yet "its health is a function of *how well* it has adapted" (Rummler & Brache, 1995, p. 12). From a systems perspective, managers can contribute to the health of an organization by using the systems framework to anticipate and adapt to change in a proactive manner.

Beyond this level of analysis, systems approaches to solving organizational performance problems also examine the connections between an organization's internal and external ecosystems and how these connections can be understood by examining how three *levels of performance* (i.e., organizational, process, and job/performer) interact with three *performance needs* (i.e., goals, design, and management). According to Rummler and Brache (1995), "the overall performance of an organization (how well it meets the expectations of its customers) is the result of goals, structures, and management actions at all Three Levels of Performance" (p. 17). A discussion of these interactions is beyond the scope of this chapter, but readers interested in systems-change issues are encouraged to explore this literature further (see Rummler & Brache, 1995).

## LESSONS LEARNED FROM PAST SYSTEMIC REFORM EFFORTS

Some of what we know of the systems-change process is a result of lessons learned from past attempts at implementing and sustaining innovations in school settings (e.g., Fullan, 2000; Fullan, Bertani, & Quinn, 2004; Gersten, Chard, & Baker, 2000). In an effort to address gaps between research and practice in school settings, attempts have been made to import "research-based" models into school settings (e.g., Fuchs et al., 1996). Unfortunately, and despite initially positive results, follow-up data indicated that projects often fail to sustain innovations when external supports were removed (Fuchs et al., 1996; McDougal et al., 2000). For example, one study conducted by Fuchs and colleagues (1996) trained schools to employ mainstream assistance teams (MATs) to support students experiencing learning problems. Despite providing training and ongoing support to 120 general educators and 30 special educators, school psychologists, and guidance counselors over several years and despite evidence that the MATs were successful in improving outcomes for children and that they could be run independently by school staff, MATs were not sustained at follow-up.

Failures to produce sustained adoption of evidenced-based practices, such as the study by Fuchs and colleagues, point to a critical need to understand systems and organizational issues (Curtis & Stollar, 2002; Fuchs et al., 1996; Knoff, 2002; McDougal et al., 2000). In recent years, there has been a shift in the focus of some educational reform efforts from simply advocating for the use of evidence-based practices toward *building the capacity* for school systems to adopt such practices. This has been facilitated by working directly with systems, policy makers, and important stakeholders to facilitate lasting change (Grimes & Tilly, 1996). According to Grimes and Tilly (1996), "school improvement becomes institutionalized when: (a) improvement is established as the school's direction; (b) agency personnel contribute to new policies that will guide services; (c) leadership provides ongoing support for innovative practices; (d) staff develop essential skills, knowledge, and attitudes; and, (e) agency procedures, goals, roles, and assignments are aligned with the change" (p. 466).

## PHASES OF THE SYSTEMS-CHANGE PROCESS

Adelman and Taylor (1997) analyzed the psychological and organizational literature to delineate a working framework for *scaling up* reform efforts in school settings. In a scale-up model, the framework that guides the systems-change process includes four overlapping phases: (1) *creating readiness* by enhancing the climate or culture for change; (2) *initial implementation*, whereby well-designed guidance and support structures are utilized to carry out replication in stages; (3) *institutionalization*, wherein there is a focus on ensuring that an infrastructure exists to sustain and enhance productive changes over time; and (4) *ongoing evolution*, which involves the development of mechanisms to improve quality and to provide continuing support in the face of new challenges and changing contexts.

We work from this framework and integrate additional concepts from the literature as we describe the phases of systems change in school settings. Before we start this discussion, however, we acknowledge an additional step that may be necessary prior to embarking on any systems-change initiative. According to Carnine (1999), important changes in professional practice are usually triggered by some *catalyst*. For example, potential catalysts for change in school systems include increasing global economic competitiveness, growing diversity in student demographics, and the fact that educational performance determines economic well-being for individuals and society. Carnine argues that it may be necessary to *campaign* for systemic reform efforts in education prior to initiating these changes. He defines a campaign as "any course of systematic aggressive action toward a specific purpose [that is] concrete, comprehensible, and to some degree urgent" (Carnine, 1999, p. 3).

A campaign involves six important steps. First, the campaign should *target visible problems* that are important and of broad interest to stakeholders. For example, issues such as literacy, school violence, and math or science performance are known to the general public and affect schools and the community broadly. Thus it is more likely that stakeholders will support systems-level initiatives that target these issues. The second step in a campaign is *establishing a coalition of groups* (e.g., private and public sector groups, advocacy groups) dedicated to the issue. Third, this coalition should be headed by a prominent credible leader to help ensure that a critical mass is built. *Staffing the campaign* is the fourth step in the process. The staff is responsible for lobbying, for translating research findings into practical summaries, and for disseminating information to relevant groups (e.g., researchers, policy makers, practitioners, community members). The fifth step is to *assemble the right information*. Information should be organized on the basis of its importance, trustworthiness, practicality, and accessibility. The sixth and final step in the campaign process is to *launch the campaign*. Like the problem-solving process we described in Chapter 7, this final step is outcome- or solution-focused.

Where Carnine (1999) leaves off in the final step in a campaign initiative (i.e., launching the campaign) is where the phases in systems-change process begin in the scale-up model described by Adelman and Taylor (1997). A scale-up project includes "a necessary organizational base and skilled personnel for disseminating a prototype, negotiating decisions about replication, and dispensing the expertise to facilitate scale up" (Taylor, Nelson, & Adelman, 1999, p. 306). Thus the process will typically be facilitated by a core team (i.e., 2–4 individuals), with additional members added when necessary to assist with new curricula, advanced technology, restructuring of education support programs, and other processes. Further, the scale-up process will likely require the addition of temporary infrastructure mechanisms to facilitate changes. The first phase of the process begins by laying the groundwork for change—creating an "official and psychological climate for change" (Taylor et al., 1999, p. 306). We believe that school psychologists should be involved in core teams focused on systems change. Following our discussion of the phases of change in a scale-up model of reform, we highlight the potential role that school psychologists might play in this process.

## Phase 1: Creating Readiness

As a first step in initiating the systems-change process, it is important to create a culture or context of readiness. According to Elias, Zins, Graczyk, and Weissberg (2003), "genuine collaboration is a form of collective ownership and it takes time to develop. . . . Thus, when an initiative begins it may signal not the beginning of change, but, at best, the beginning of readiness for change" (p. 312). Taylor and colleagues (1999) describe the tasks associated with creating readiness as the following: (1) disseminating the desired prototype and pursuing activities to build interest and consensus for change, (2) negotiating a policy framework and agreements for engagement, and (3) modifying institutional infrastructure. These tasks should be undertaken in a manner that reflects an understanding of the nature of the organization and its stakeholders. Stakeholders should play an integral role throughout the process. In particular, they should be involved in the decision-making process and in the redesign of mechanisms of the systems infrastructure. Further, in developing a sense of community and commitment, it is important that efforts be made to clarify potential benefits of the change efforts, with an emphasis on their personal relevance to stakeholders. Taylor and colleagues (1999) describe the steps in this process, as well as the potential barriers or pitfalls.

When creating readiness for change, the first consideration is the development of *vision* and *leadership*. It is important to have a vision of what the new approach would look like, as well as an understanding of how to facilitate necessary changes to move in that direction. Major objectives in this part of the process include the careful delineation of desired outcomes of the intended change, anticipated costs, and potential incentives and establishing which aspects of the prototype are nonnegotiable to change and which aspects can be adapted. A variety of assessment tools can be useful in this process (e.g., Smith & Freeman, 2002). For example, diagnostic evaluation methods that attempt to identify the needs of the system through multiple sources (e.g., surveys, questionnaires, interviews and observations, and input evaluations) can be useful in identifying potential goals (e.g., Curtis & Stollar, 2002). Input evaluations that focus on the assessment of skills and available resources for addressing needs identified in diagnostic evaluations are also helpful in this regard. Knoff (2002) describes additional tools (e.g., external environmental scan and analysis, internal organizational scan and analysis, stakeholder perception analysis) that are useful in this stage of the process.

An important part of this process is involving a critical mass of stakeholders (e.g., policy makers, staff, and parents) in the development of a vision. In fact, "*all* stakeholders should be meaningfully involved in every aspect of system-level change efforts, beginning with initial discussions regarding *potential* change and continuing through implementation" (Curtis & Stollar, 2002, p. 228). Some stakeholders function as "gatekeepers" in the system. They hold decision-making power and authority within the system, so their participation and sanction of the change is essential. It also is important to involve other stakeholders and, in particular, members of the system who will be affected by the change (e.g., teachers, parents). One strategy for gaining support from practitioners is to demonstrate innovations (Curtis & Stollar, 2002) and encourage staff to experiment with new practices that may eventually become policies (Grimes & Tilly, 1996).

Leadership and policy commitment are important, as they help to ensure the availability of appropriate resources to support the change initiative (e.g., time, space, funding, and administrative support), and they also provide safeguards for risk taking (Taylor et al., 1999). Administrators and policy statements should identify reform efforts as a high priority. Taylor and colleagues (1999) recommend the negotiation of formal agreements among the various stakeholders at each jurisdictional level. They suggest that this process be accomplished through three essential steps. First, to establish a basis for consensus, the scale-up team should provide in-depth information by building on introductory presentations. The goal should be to ensure informed and voluntary consent for participation. Second, a policy framework and set of rules for engagement should be negotiated. This should include a realistic budget. Third, representatives of all major stakeholders should ratify the agreements and policies in an informed and voluntary manner. The aspects of the systems-change process (e.g., principles, components, standards) that fall into the category of *nonnegotiable* considerations should be stated up front (e.g., need for the establishment of temporary infrastructures to facilitate change).

Another essential consideration in a scale-up model is *infrastructure redesign* to ensure ownership, support, and participation. Five fundamental components to redesigning infrastructure are: (1) governance, (2) planning and implementation of specific organizational and program objectives, (3) coordination and integration, (4) daily leadership, and (5) communication and information management (Taylor et al., 1999). Each of these endeavors involves a time commitment. In fact, time is one of the most common barriers to the change process.

Problems may occur if enough time is not set aside to create readiness and lay the groundwork needed for substantive change (Taylor et al., 1999). For example, considerable time and resources are needed to develop policy agreements, yet these are essential to sustained change. In addition, consensus and capacity building among key stakeholders is also time-consuming, yet critical, as is establishing time for planning. Thus restructuring of time is one of the most difficult problems associated with any scale-up method.

## Phase 2: Initial Implementation

The next phase in the scaling-up process is initial implementation of the prototype (Taylor et al., 1999). Temporary mechanisms are added in the redesign of the organizational infrastructure to provide guidance and support as the prototype is adapted and phased into the system. The first of these mechanisms is the addition of a site-based steering team that works with the scale-up team (from Phase 1) to guide program development and to provide support for implementation and replication. This team works directly with the school's administration, specific planning groups, and other stakeholders and is responsible for determining the sequence for change, as well as the strategies to facilitate implementation. The second mechanism involves having a change agent from the scale-up team work together with stakeholders on a change team. Curtis and Stollar (2002) identify this person as the on-site facilitator, whose purpose is to monitor implementation and refocus the group when necessary. Finally, mentors and coaches are trained to model and to subsequently teach elements of the prototype.

During this initial implementation phase, emphasis is placed on capacity building, which is accomplished through intensive coaching or mentorship, as well as follow-up consultation and technical assistance. Another critical feature of the implementation phase is the use of formative evaluation procedures to provide ongoing feedback for program development. Formative assessment information is collected on the implementation of the prototype (i.e., implementation integrity, acceptability), as well as on changes in processes (e.g., planning processes, governance structures, policies and resources) and initial outcomes (e.g., student outcomes). Summative assessments are less useful here, as sufficient implementation time is required to fully implement and adapt the prototype to fit within the existing context.

Some common problems during initial implementation result from a failure to create readiness in Phase 1. If there is a failure to establish consensus and commitment from stakeholders directly involved in the implementation process, for example, the result may be implementation of form rather than substance of the change. Top-down or administratively mandated policies that are established without active and meaningful involvement of staff members can lead to resistance to change, lack of understanding, and fault-finding behaviors on the part of staff members (Grimes & Tilly, 1996). Thus a failure to establish readiness in Phase 1 can have serious deleterious effects on initial implementation. Other potential difficulties in this phase might be those associated with the establishment of temporary infrastructures. If these mechanisms are not sufficiently in place, it may be difficult to facilitate productive working relationships and to anticipate and address problems promptly.

## Phase 3: Institutionalization

According to Taylor and colleagues (1999), "institutionalizing a prototype entails ensuring that the organization assumes long-term ownership and that there is a blueprint for countering forces that can erode the changes" (p. 317). Thus, in addition to maintaining implementation over time, emphasis is placed on creating mechanisms to address the evolution or enhancement of the system in the face of changing contextual demands. In order for this to occur, it is important that the organization assumes ownership and program advocacy (e.g., taking over the temporary steering group's functions, addressing ongoing policy and long-range planning concerns, and maintaining financial support). Institutionalization, however, is not ensured through ownership alone. "Over time, mechanisms for planning, implementation, and coordination are maintained by ensuring the activity is an official part of the infrastructure, has appropriate leadership, and is effectively supported" (Taylor et al., 1999, p. 318). Accomplishing these goals requires a critical mass of team members so that there is a broad base of involvement and so that the workload is manageable. Adequate resources (e.g., time, technical support, recognition and incentives for participation, continued professional development) are needed to support the institutionalization process. When approaches are newly institutionalized, it is also important to provide mechanisms for ongoing capacity building, particularly with regard to addressing staff turnover.

## Phase 4: Ongoing Evolution

"Ongoing evolution of organizations and programs is the product of efforts to account for accomplishments, deal with changing times and conditions, incorporate new knowledge, and create a sense of renewal as the excitement of newness wears off and the demands of change sap energy" (Taylor et al., 1999, p. 319). The key to fostering this process is the use of formative and summative evaluation—that is, data. These data are used to document accomplishments and to provide information to guide decision making. Beyond data on the efficacy of outcomes for students, formative data to facilitate program development and organizational change must be gathered. For schools to sustain this process without support, it is essential that mechanisms be in place for collecting, analyzing, and interpreting evaluation data. Thus the scale-up team should help to establish an evaluation team and should build capacity for this team to conduct evaluations. Although this aspect of the systems-change process may appear straightforward, this evaluation process may be financially costly, and it has the potential to have a "negative psychological impact on those evaluated, and the ways it can inappropriately reshape new approaches" (Taylor et al., 1999, p. 321). In particular, overemphasis on *accountability* tends to result in negative reactions, regardless of the type of organization or its focus. With this potentially problematic issue in mind, it is important to emphasize the use of formative evaluation methods to guide problem-solving efforts.

## THE ROLE OF THE SCHOOL PSYCHOLOGIST

As we have described in this chapter, the work of school psychologists does not occur in a vacuum or in isolation. School psychologists play a role in school systems. Thus their work influences and is influenced by the systems in which they work. In Chapter 1, we introduced our vision for school psychology practice in the 21st century. The roles we described included data-oriented problem solving, assessment, prevention and intervention, systems-level change, and being involved as a consumer and producer of research. These roles are interrelated, and the context in which they occur is a living, open, constantly evolving school system.

As we described in this chapter, school systems also exist as part of larger systems (e.g., districts, communities) and contain smaller subsystems (e.g., classrooms). These systems are complex and integrally interconnected. They provide the context for our work. School psychologists who are data-oriented problem solvers cannot and should not attempt to disconnect the problems they solve from the contexts in which they occur. We believe that school psychologists who possess knowledge and skills in systems change are in a position to play a role in problem-solving efforts designed to facilitate the development of healthy, evolving school systems. In this chapter, we provided a brief introduction to some of the important concepts that are relevant to systems-change theory and its application to school settings. In addition, we described some of the phases of the systems-change process.

Practicing school psychologists and those who are new to the profession should seek opportunities to develop their knowledge and skills in systems change, as we believe that competencies in this area can only enhance our effectiveness in other roles. We also believe that some of the skills and competencies that are already well developed in school psychologists (e.g., consultation, problem solving, assessment, research, and intervention skills) make school psychologists ideal participants in the systems-change process. In fact, we might argue that one potentially promising shift in our professional roles is from that of diagnosticians who primarily work in a tertiary care role to a data-oriented problem solvers who address prevention and intervention across all systems of care (i.e., primary, secondary, and tertiary) and work to facilitate the development of healthy, evolving school systems.

An example of this shift in role was illustrated in Chapter 1 in our description of the work of Margaret McGlinchey, who has been a practicing school psychologist for over two decades. Margaret's role has expanded over the years to include program development and leadership responsibilities. In particular, she has established part of her role to focus on developing systems capacity in the areas of data-driven problem solving, curriculum-based measurement, and systems change to address early literacy. Much of her shift in role grew out of frustration with problems associated with the traditional approaches. Of course, and as Margaret noted in Chapter 1, any shift in role will have its struggles, yet she also claimed that this is "definitely the most exciting time in my career and in school psychology" and that she was "thrilled to see the positive changes in the field—the increasing emphasis on prevention, intervention, function-based assessment, building-wide systems of service delivery, and the move to a problem-solving role." Our sentiments mirror Margaret's as we look toward the future of school psychology and its potential to emphasize a systems approach to solving problems facing schools. We are convinced that knowledge of systems and possession of systems-level change skills are becoming increasingly important for the effective practice of school psychology.

## DISCUSSION QUESTIONS AND ACTIVITIES

1. What are some of the major challenges facing schools today?

2. What is a system? What kind of systems are schools? Describe the subsystems that make up the school system, as well as the larger systems of which this system is a part.

3. Interview a principal and ask for a description of the organization of the school. Does the description given provide a vertical or horizontal view of the school organization?

4. The school principal you are working for would like to implement a research-based program to promote social competence. She attended a conference and learned of a packaged program that helped a school in another district. She wants you to take the lead on the project. Given your awareness of the systems-change literature, how would you go about this process? Who would you involve in the process? Where would you start? What questions would you have?

5. Find an article in the school-based literature that describes attempts made to produce lasting change or adoption of a process or EBP in a school setting. Was the approach successful or unsuccessful? Critique the article and identify components that were consistent with a systems-change approach to facilitating lasting change. What would you recommend to improve the process?

# 12

# The School Psychologist's Role in Research and Evaluation

As indicated in Chapter 5, most school psychology practitioners do not spend a significant amount of time engaged in research activities. Although research may not be a key role for the majority of practitioners, it is nevertheless important for all school psychologists to have a basic understanding of research methods. Even school psychologists who do not formally conduct research must be good consumers of research in order to stay up-to-date on effective practices and to answer questions from parents and teachers regarding best practices in educational and psychological issues. For school psychologists to respond knowledgeably to such questions, they must read and be able to critically evaluate research-based articles, including methodology and research design. All school psychologists, in addition to being consumers of research, should utilize some aspects of research design methodology to engage in data-based decision making in their everyday practice. It is essential that data-based decision making occur to ensure that students are actually benefiting from the services they receive. Of course, some school psychologists will also conduct formal research studies. For those who wish to engage in research, the schools are a prime place to conduct research studies, including applied research and program evaluation. Although program evaluation has traditionally received little emphasis in school psychology training programs, we believe that well-trained school psychologists have the potential to play an important role in evaluating the impact of educational and mental health programs in schools and related settings. In this era of increasing accountability, it is essential for those in educational systems to be able to conduct evaluations of their programs to provide evidence for their continued use to various stakeholders, such as school board members, administrators, and community members. School psychologists who have basic training in program evaluation can provide an important service in this regard. In this chapter, we provide an overview of the different aspects of research and evaluation in the schools. We encourage all school psychologists to use these skills to help improve outcomes for the students, families, and teachers they serve.

# SCHOOL PSYCHOLOGISTS AS CONSUMERS OF RESEARCH

School psychologists must be able to understand and critically evaluate journal articles so that they can stay abreast of changes in the fields of education and psychology and share this information with parents and teachers as appropriate. School psychologists should be familiar with the four primary school psychology journals: *School Psychology Review* (the official NASP journal), *School Psychology Quarterly* (the official journal of Division 16 of APA), *Psychology in the Schools*, and the *Journal of School Psychology*. In addition to these journals, numerous other journals are available on topics of interest to school psychologists. These include assessment-focused journals (e.g., *Journal of Psycho-educational Assessment*), consultation-focused journals (e.g., *Journal of Educational and Psychological Consultation*), journals focused on early intervention (e.g., *Journal of Early Intervention*), journals focused on single-subject design studies (e.g., *Journal of Applied Behavior Analysis*), and journals devoted to a multitude of applied topics related to mental health issues in children and adolescents (e.g., *Journal of Clinical Child and Adolescent Psychology; Journal of the American Academy of Child and Adolescent Psychiatry*). Obviously it is impossible for school psychologists to subscribe to all journals that may be relevant to the field. However, we encourage school psychologists to subscribe to at least a couple of journals. School psychologists who are members of NASP will automatically receive *School Psychology Review*, and those who are members of Division 16 of APA will automatically receive *School Psychology Quarterly*.

Of course, subscribing to a journal is only the first step in keeping up-to-date with developments in the field. Plenty of journals sit on bookshelves and desks without ever being opened. Sometimes this is due to a lack of time to read; often, though, it is due to being intimidated by reading research-based articles. We admit that these articles are not always the most scintillating pieces of literature and that evaluating the merits of a research article can be difficult—especially if it has been a long time since one has had a research methods or statistics course. However, this skill is important, as not all published articles are of high quality. Although all of the journals mentioned here are peer-reviewed journals (meaning that the research is evaluated by members of the journals' editorial boards who offer opinions regarding the quality of the manuscript), this does not mean that the research that appears in these journals is without flaw. In fact, no research is perfect. Later in this section, we provide some guidelines to assist in evaluating research articles, but first we turn to the general types of journal articles school psychologists are likely to read.

## Types of Journal Articles

You will encounter three general types of articles when perusing a journal. These are original research studies, meta-analyses, and narrative reviews.

### Original Research Studies

Original research studies provide data in an attempt to answer specific research questions. There are numerous types of research studies that vary in their complexity and the stringency of their research methods and designs.

Some less complex original research studies involve survey research in which data are analyzed mainly via descriptive statistics (e.g., frequencies, means, and standard deviations). Such studies typically attempt to describe a general population. For example, many of the studies on the roles and functions of school psychologists that were cited in Chapter 5 were survey studies in which the researchers mailed survey questionnaires to school psychologists. These surveys contained questions regarding basic demographic information about school psychologists, as well as questions regarding how much of their time is spent engaged in various professional activities (e.g., assessment, consultation, intervention). Survey research can provide useful information regarding trends and practices in the field of school psychology, but it is less useful in guiding practice, because the purpose of such research is to describe what is currently being done or to evaluate perceptions of what should be done rather than to evaluate what assessment methods or intervention procedures might be the most valid for a certain population.

Correlational studies, which look at the relationships between different variables, are another common type of research. Much of the research on assessment instruments is correlational in nature. For example, when creating a new measure of anxiety, the developers would correlate the new measure with existing measures of anxiety—the higher the correlation between these measures, the stronger the relationship, and the more confident we can be that the new measure is assessing the same construct as the existing measures. Correlational studies can also be used to obtain information related to possible contributing factors to problems. For example, many studies examine how parent-related factors (e.g., parenting style, psychopathology, stress) relate to child behavior problems. When high correlations are found between parent factors and child behavior problems, we can say that these two constructs are related (e.g., the more behavior problems the child exhibits, the more stress parents report). However, as everyone who has taken a basic statistics course should remember, we *cannot* infer *causation* from correlational data. For example, even given a high correlation between parent stress and child behavior problems, we cannot conclude that high levels of child behavior problems *cause* parents to experience greater stress. It may be that this is the case. However, it also may be that parental stress leads to child behavior problems or that a third variable contributes to both stress and behavior problems—for example, a difficult child temperament may be related to the expression of both behavior problems in children and increased stress in parents. Only from a true experimental study can one draw conclusions regarding causation. However, true experimental studies are often difficult or impossible to conduct on many of the topics of interest in school psychology. For example, because of legal and ethical constraints, we can almost never randomly assign children to differing educational intervention groups—such as self-contained and mainstreamed special education instruction—as would be required in a true experimental design. Because of this design problem, we depend a great deal on correlational methods to draw inferences regarding possible correlates of childhood problems.

Experimental studies can be either group-design studies or single-subject design studies. Due to the prominence of single-subject design methodology in the practice of school psychology, we cover the use of these designs in a later, separate section of this chapter. Group-design experimental studies involve random selection of participants (in which potential participants within the population of interest have an equal chance of being selected to participate) and random assignment of the participants to the different experimental groups (in which participants have an equal chance of being assigned to any of the groups in the study). These designs can be either between-group studies (in which different groups of participants are compared) and/or within-group studies (in which participants are compared with themselves, as in pretest and posttest design studies). In addition to true experimental designs, there are quasi-experimental designs in which the researchers cannot truly randomize participants (e.g., a researcher plans to examine the effects of different bilingual education programs but children are placed in the different programs based on the schools they attend). Within the field of psychology, intervention or treatment studies are some of the most common types of studies that involve an experimental design. For example, if we were conducting a study designed to evaluate the effectiveness of an intervention for anxiety, children with anxiety would be selected from the general population (ideally this selection is random, but rarely is this truly the case) and randomly assigned to either an active treatment group (e.g., cognitive-behavioral therapy) or a control group in which children do not receive a treatment thought to affect anxiety (e.g., an attention-only group). Children in the study would be assessed at pre- and posttreatment. If children in the active-treatment group improved and children in the control group did not improve, we could tentatively conclude that the treatment led to the improvements. However, various threats to the design of studies (outlined in more detail later in this section) may hinder our conclusions and need to be considered when evaluating our data.

## Meta-Analyses

In addition to original research studies, meta-analyses, which are quantitative reviews of the literature, have gained in popularity over the years, and a well-done meta-analysis can be extremely valuable in integrating a variety of previous findings. When conducting a meta-analysis, the researcher examines original research studies on a certain topic. Results from individual studies are quantified using a common metric so that results from these individual studies can be combined and compared (Kazdin, 2000). For example, if one were conducting a meta-analysis on the effectiveness of medications versus cognitive-behavioral therapy (CBT) for anxiety, studies using each of these treatment modalities would be collected and coded so that all studies using medications could be compared with all studies using CBT. It should be noted that this is a simplistic explanation of meta-analyses, as there are many issues to consider when conducting this type of research. For example, how studies are selected for inclusion is an issue; typically, studies are excluded if their methodology is deemed to be inadequate. In addition, different researchers may define constructs differently (e.g., CBT may be defined as including different components in different studies), and results obtained via different assessment measures are combined. Different methods for quantifying outcomes of studies can also influence the outcomes of the meta-analysis and the conclusions reached (Kazdin, 2000). Even given these issues and the difficulties inherent in combining multiple studies in a common, quantifiable manner, the meta-analysis is the best method we currently have for summarizing information across studies in a meaningful way.

The use of effect sizes is the most common way of quantifying and comparing outcomes across studies in meta-analytic reviews. An effect size reflects the magnitude of a finding. Although there are different methods of calculating effect sizes, the most common method involves subtracting one mean from another mean (e.g., the CBT-group mean from the medication-group mean) and dividing by the pooled standard deviation. The result is a number expressed in standard deviation units that has a mean of 0 and a standard deviation of 1 (Kazdin, 2000). Higher effect sizes indicate a greater difference between groups. Cohen (1988) offered guidelines for interpreting these mean difference effect sizes. He suggested that effect sizes of 0.80 and greater are large; those from 0.50 to 0.80 are medium, and those from 0.20 to 0.50 are small.

## Narrative Reviews

Although meta-analyses offer a way to quantify findings from different studies, narrative reviews of the literature are also commonly conducted. In such a review, the researcher gathers original research articles on a certain topic area and simply summarizes the results in a qualitative fashion without attempting to create a common metric to combine results across studies. Narrative reviews are not as useful as meta-analyses because they provide no way to easily summarize and compare results across studies. In narrative reviews, it is more likely that studies of varying quality will be included and less likely that the authors will have specific criteria for the inclusion and exclusion of studies.

# Evaluating Research

As noted earlier, good consumers of research must be able to critically evaluate the research they read. In the following sections, we address some of the specific issues that should be considered (i.e., validity and clinical significance) when evaluating research articles, as well as general steps one can take when reading research to help evaluate the quality and contribution of the research.

## Internal Validity

Internal validity refers to the extent to which the results of a study can be attributed to differences in the independent variable in the study (e.g., the type of treatment) rather than to factors unrelated to the study. For example, if, following an intervention intended to decrease depression, children's depression decreases, then the stronger the internal validity of the study is, the more confident we can be that it was the intervention that led to the decrease in depression rather than some other factor (e.g., simple passage of time). In their classic text, Cook and Campbell (1979) outlined a number of threats to internal validity. Some of the more common threats are listed here, with brief definitions and examples related to an intervention study for children with depression. These threats are also summarized in Table 12.1.

- *History*: an event unrelated to the study occurs and influences the results of the study (e.g., a popular student commits suicide right before the postassessment period, and all children report increased symptoms of depression; obviously, this influences scores in the opposite direction than we would want to see)
- *Maturation*: events that occur with the normal passage of time (e.g., children report improvement on measures of depression due simply to the passage of time)
- *Testing*: repeated testing may influence results (e.g., children complete depression inventories every week, become bored with them, and begin answering all questions the same way)
- *Instrumentation*: changes in methods or measures used (e.g., children are rating how "down" they feel on a weekly basis; however, over time some children begin to interpret this term differently than they did originally)
- *Statistical regression*: the tendency of scores to get closer to the statistical mean on repeated testing (e.g., one would expect that a child who scored very high on a

**TABLE 12.1. Threats to Validity**

Threats to internal validity
- History: an event unrelated to the study occurs during the study
- Maturation: events that occur with the normal passage of time
- Testing: repeated testing at different time intervals during the study
- Instrumentation: changes in methods or measures used
- Statistical regression: tendency of extreme scores to regress to the statistical mean on repeated testing
- Selection: participants in one group differ from those in another group
- Mortality: participants withdraw from the research study
- Selection interactions: methods of selecting participants or assigning participants to conditions interact with other threats

Threats to external validity
- Sample characteristics: lack of similarity of participants to general population of interest
- Setting characteristics: lack of similarity of research setting to settings of interest
- Context characteristics: lack of similarity of participant behavior in research setting to behavior in natural setting

measure of depressive symptoms would not score as high at a second testing due simply to the fact that scores tend to regress to the mean)
- *Selection*: participants in one group may differ on some variables from participants in another group (e.g., children in the intervention group are primarily from high-socioeconomic status (SES) backgrounds, whereas those in the control group are primarily from low-SES backgrounds)
- *Mortality*: participants may withdraw from the research study (e.g., more children in the intervention group drop out than in the control group, leaving only the children most motivated to change in the intervention group)
- *Selection interactions*: methods of selecting participants or assigning participants to conditions may interact with any of the previously listed threats (e.g., children in the control group are all from the same classroom and children in the intervention group are from a different classroom; a child in the control classroom passed away during the intervention—possibly contributing to increased emotional distress in this group).

Given these threats to internal validity, what can be done to increase internal validity of research, and what should consumers of research look for when attempting to evaluate the internal validity of a study? In studies using different groups of participants, random assignment to groups is important. Random assignment helps to equalize the effects of these potential threats across the groups. Of course, this does not always occur. Participants in one group may drop out at a higher rate than those in another group, even though random assignment was used. Historical events may also differentially affect the groups. An additional difficulty in applied studies, as noted, is that true random assignment is often difficult—and sometimes impossible—to achieve. For example, when conducting research in the schools, often classrooms rather than students are randomly assigned to conditions. This situation leaves open the possibility that differences between classrooms, rather than the intervention, are contributing to the results. When random assignment is not possible (or even in cases in which it is), participants in the different groups may be "matched" on certain characteristics to ensure that the groups are equivalent (e.g., students in the intervention and control groups may be matched based on gender, SES, and grade point average [GPA]).

## External Validity

Even if a study has strong internal validity, the results may not be useful if they do not generalize beyond the experimental setting of the research study. External validity refers to the extent to which results from one study will generalize to other populations, settings, and so forth. Evaluating the external validity of a study is important because it helps consumers of research know to what extent the findings of the study may apply to the settings in which they work. Various factors have been noted to affect the external validity of research studies (Cook & Campbell, 1979; Kazdin, 1998; Scotti, Morris, & Cohen, 2003), and these are summarized in Table 12.1. One group of factors to consider are the characteristics of the sample used in the study. The more similar the participants in the research are to the individuals in the general population one wishes to know about, the more likely the results will generalize. For example, if a researcher were interested in crisis intervention practices of school psychologists in the United States, it would be best to obtain a sample of school psychologists from all areas of the United States rather than a sample of school psychologists from the specific state in which the researcher works. Alternatively, if one were interested in crisis intervention practices of school psychologists in rural areas, only school psychologists who work in rural school districts should be selected for participation.

The extent to which results will generalize also has to do with how the study was conducted. For example, if a study on the treatment of depression in children was conducted in a clinical setting with trained graduate student therapists following specific manuals, the results may not generalize to a school setting in which the school psychologist would be implementing the intervention without specific manuals and reliability checks.

How participants react to being in a research study can also limit the ability to generalize findings. For example, if a study on child compliance is conducted in a clinical setting, it is likely that children will be more compliant than in they are their home settings. Findings from this study may indicate that children are compliant with the majority of parental commands. However, because of the difference between the laboratory (clinic) setting and the home setting, this number is not likely to be reflective of the true rate of compliance in children across different settings. Thus the results would not generalize to other settings and would be specific to parent–child interactions in a clinic setting.

In order to attempt to produce results that will generalize, researchers should strive to randomly select participants from the population to which they are interested in generalizing and ensure that the methods of the study are similar to settings to which they wish to generalize. However, this is easier said than done—it is difficult to truly select participants randomly. For example, in selecting potential participants to be in the study on crisis intervention practices, a researcher might obtain a list of 500 school psychologists across the United States, randomly selected from NASP's and APA Division 16's membership lists (this being the simplest way to obtain a random sample of school psychologists across the country). Although this sample of potential participants may be a random sample of NASP and APA members, it is not truly a random sample of school psychologists, as only NASP or APA members could be selected. It may be that there is something different about school psychologists who are NASP or APA members from those who are not members (e.g., NASP and APA members may be more likely to seek continuing education opportunities and therefore be more knowledgeable about crisis intervention). Thus the results may generalize only to school psychologists who are members of NASP or APA. In addition, obtaining a random sample of individuals to whom the researcher will mail the survey does not guarantee that a random sample will be returned. Perhaps those school psychologists who are more involved in crisis intervention will be more likely to respond to the survey. Thus, although the target sample was randomly selected, those who responded are different from those who did not respond. Typically, there is no way to evaluate how those in the obtained sample may have answered differently from those who did not respond. However, in some situations it may be possible to compare those who responded with those who did not respond on certain characteristics (e.g., years of experience as school psychologists). Because true random selection can be difficult to achieve, when evaluating research studies one should attend to the extent to which random selection was attempted to help better understand the population to which the results will most clearly generalize.

## Construct Validity

The construct validity of a study has to do with the intervention (or experimental manipulation) in the study and its definition. If threats to internal validity have been ruled out, one can assume that the experimental intervention was responsible for the effect. Questions of construct validity relate to the extent to which factors considered not to be part of the intervention interfere with the interpretation of the intervention (Finger & Rand, 2003; Kazdin, 1998). For example, did children who received a cognitive-behavioral treatment for depression improve more than those children in a wait-list control group because of the cognitive-behavioral intervention specifically (as we might assume) or because they were receiving extra attention from a supportive adult? Threats to construct validity include experimenter contact with participants, demand characteristics, and experimenter expectancies. As in the preceding example, experimenter contact with participants may threaten the construct validity of a study if the experimenter has more contact with one group than with the other group. Demand characteristics can influence study outcomes when participants in research studies respond differently than they would naturally simply because they are in a research study. Participants may attempt to respond in a manner consistent with what they think the researcher wants or expects. For example, parents whose children are in a treatment study for depression may report that their children's symptoms are better because they know that the goal of treatment is to decrease symptoms of depression. Expectancies of the researcher can also limit the construct validity of a study. For example, a researcher may expect the children in the treatment group to improve and those in the control group not to improve. Because of this expectancy, the researcher may unknowingly and subtly treat the children in the two groups differently (e.g., being more positive with the children in the treatment group), and this difference may influence the outcomes of the study (Kazdin, 1998; Scotti et al., 2003).

To help reduce threats to construct validity, as well as internal validity, the "gold standard" when conducting intervention studies is to use double-blind placebo-control designs. In such studies, participants are randomly assigned to either a treatment group or a no-treatment placebo group, but neither the researchers nor the participants know who is in which group. This type of design is frequently used when evaluating the efficacy of medications. For example, if a new medicine for social phobia is being evaluated via a double-blind placebo-control study, half of the children in the study would be assigned to take the new medication and half to receive a placebo pill (a sugar pill), but neither the researcher nor the participants would know who was receiving the placebo pill and who was receiving the "real" medication. (Obviously, someone knows, via coded links, who has received what medication; however, this person is not involved in running the study nor interacting with the participants.) By using this design, the researcher can control for expectancy effects on the part of the participants and the researcher. Participants in both the placebo group and the medication group may expect that they will improve, but expectancy will not differentially affect the groups. In addition, the researcher will not treat those on medication differently from those taking a placebo because medication status is also unknown to the researcher.

Although double-blind placebo-control studies are relatively easy to implement when evaluating the efficacy of medications, such studies are much harder to implement when evaluating psychological or educational interventions. As of yet, no one has developed an adequate psychological placebo. Some researchers use an attention-control group as a placebo treatment. In this situation, a study therapist meets with the participants but does not engage in the active therapy being evaluated (e.g., CBT). Instead, he or she engages in nontherapeutic activities (e.g., play activities, academic tutoring if the treatment focus is not on academics). However, given that the relationship between the therapist and client seems to be an important factor in predicting who will improve in therapy, it is questionable as to whether this method truly represents a placebo treatment. In addition, it is very hard to double-blind psychological or educational intervention studies. Although participants may not be aware of whether they are receiving the active treatment, researchers most likely will be aware because the difference between an active treatment and a placebo treatment can be observed (whereas a placebo pill can be make to look just like the real medication).

## Statistical Conclusion Validity

This type of validity relates to errors in the use of measurement and statistical analysis techniques. Threats to statistical conclusion validity include: unreliability of measures, low statistical power, subject heterogeneity, and increasing the study error rate by making multiple statistical comparisons (and, therefore, likely getting a result that is statistically significant simply because of chance; Finger & Rand, 2003; Kazdin, 1998). The use of appropriate assessment methods and statistical procedures can help reduce threats to statistical conclusion validity.

## Clinical Significance versus Statistical Significance

In addition to evaluating the validity of a study, consumers of research should evaluate the clinical significance of the findings. Kazdin (2000) defines clinical significance as "the practical value or importance of the effect of an intervention, that is, whether it makes a real difference in everyday life" (p. 117). This issue of clinical significance and how it differs from statistical significance is one that has been receiving an increasing amount of attention in recent years. Statistical significance refers to conclusions reached about significance based on statistical hypothesis testing. This is the classic "$p$

value" with which one becomes familiar in introductory statistics courses. A $p$ value refers to the probability that the finding was obtained by chance. In order to be considered statistically significant, $p$ values have traditionally needed to be less than .05 (i.e., $p$ < .05). This statement asserts that there is only a 5% probability that the obtained result was due to chance. However, statistical significance testing does have drawbacks. One drawback is that it is heavily influenced by sample size. If a study has a large sample size, statistical significance is relatively easy to achieve. Conversely, if a study has a small sample size (and, therefore, low power—the ability to detect a meaningful effect when the effect is present), statistical significance is very difficult to achieve. In addition, statistical significance tells the reader nothing about whether the obtained result is meaningful in the real world. For example, if a researcher utilizes statistical significance testing to compare a CBT treatment with an attention-control "treatment" for children with anxiety and if those in the CBT group have a significantly greater reduction in anxiety symptoms at the posttest than children in the control group, we only know that, as a group, children in the CBT group improved more than children in the control group. We do not know whether children in the CBT group showed a meaningful decline in symptoms. It is possible that children in both groups were still experiencing high levels of anxiety at posttreatment.

Effect sizes (as discussed in the meta-analysis section of this chapter) have been used frequently as measures of clinical significance. However, although effect sizes are not influenced by sample size and do provide information about the magnitude of change, they still have limitations when evaluating the meaningfulness of a certain outcome. This issue is particularly relevant in treatment studies in which the question is whether a certain treatment is effective. In order to truly evaluate the effectiveness of a treatment, some measure of whether participants are functioning at a normative level is generally needed, given that the goal in treatment is typically (although not always, as discussed later) to return symptoms to a "normal" level. In addition to examining the effect size from pre- to postintervention for a given change, researchers can also determine whether scores at posttreatment fall in the normal range (as defined by normative information for that measure) and determine whether diagnostic criteria for the disorder for which the child was receiving treatment are still met (Kazdin, 2000). Jacobson and Truax (1991) proposed the idea of utilizing a *reliable change index* (RCI) in combination with statistically derived cutoff scores to help evaluate the clinical significance of results. The RCI involves determining whether reliable change took place from pre- to posttest and takes into account the standard error of measurement of the instrument used to assess change. A cutoff score denoting whether an individual is in the functional or dysfunctional range (obtained via various formulas presented by Jacobson and Truax) is used in combination with the RCI to determine whether an individual has achieved meaningful change.

Although methods of assessing clinical significance are increasingly being applied in studies (particularly therapy outcome studies), Kazdin (1999) argues that we should not assume that a person must be in the normal range on an outcome measure to conclude that change is clinically significant. He argues that, in some cases, change can be clinically significant when an individual shows some changes even though symptoms are not normalized (e.g., a child with severe separation anxiety, which led to school refusal, can now attend school even though he or she still has significant anxiety) or when the person is better able to deal with his or her symptoms even though no change has occurred (this would be especially true in the case of chronic problems such as tic disorders).

The topic of clinical significance and how to evaluate it is likely to continue to evoke much discussion. Consumers of research should be aware of this issue and, when reading research articles, attend to whether the authors have reported measures of clinical significance. This will help in the evaluation of whether the article provides meaningful information that can be applied to everyday practice.

### What to Look for When Reading Research Articles

In the preceding sections we have mentioned some aspects of research that the consumer should attend to when evaluating research studies. We now provide more details on how to evaluate the entirety of a research study. Pyrczak (1999) provides detailed information on evaluating research articles, and we have drawn extensively from his discussions.

Consumers of research should begin their critical evaluation of an article with the review of literature. The literature review should include recent research on the topic area, and the research should be discussed in an evaluative fashion. Contradictory findings from studies should be explained and an attempt made to integrate previous findings. In addition, within the literature review the authors should distinguish between theory-based literature and empirical literature. Literature reviews should be neither too broad nor too narrow but should provide sufficient background information to understand the importance of the study currently being conducted. The literature review should make it clear how the present study builds on previous studies and should lead directly to the research questions or objectives for the current study. After reading the literature review, the reader should understand how the current study will help advance knowledge and understanding of the particular topic area.

The method section follows the literature review. This section typically includes three subsections that provide detailed information on the participants involved in the study, the measures used, and the procedures followed. A close examination of the method section is key in assessing both the internal and external validity of a study. Participants should be adequately described, and the general population these participants were selected to reflect should be specified. Information on the number of participants and the demographic characteristics of participants should be included. Readers should evaluate whether the sample size is appropriate given the expectations of the study and the methods used to evaluate the results. In general, the more comparisons being made, the larger the sample size needed. For example, if a researcher is evaluating the outcome of a treatment program for depression and wants to look at outcomes for males versus females and children from two-parent homes versus one-parent homes, a larger sample size would be needed than if the researcher just wanted to examine overall outcomes. Measures used should be described and their psychometric properties mentioned. If the measures used were not psychometrically sound, the results may be questionable (e.g., findings may have been due simply to the unreliability of the measures used rather than the intervention). The procedures section should provide adequate details so that the reader is able to understand how the sample was chosen, how many eligible individuals participated, and what the dropout rate was. The uses of both random selection of participants and random assignment of participants should be clear from the method section.

Within the results section, the reader must attempt to determine whether appropriate methods of analysis were used and appropriate conclusions reached based on the results of these procedures. The analyses should be tied to the research questions proposed by the study authors, and it should be clear how each research question was addressed. Researchers should also include general descriptive statistics that describe the sample prior to presenting their main data analyses. For example, means and standard deviations for all measures used should be presented. If there are different groups in the study, this information should be presented for each group and compared in some manner. If the groups are not equivalent on these variables prior to the implementaion of an intervention the researchers should attempt to account for this in their data analysis. Statistical procedures used should be clearly described and limitations noted. In addition to evaluating the statistical significance of the results, the researchers should also discuss the practical or clinical significance of the findings and make clear when results may not be clinically significant even if they are statistically significant.

The discussion is the last section in an empirical research-based journal article. In the discussion, the authors summarize the findings and tie them back to the literature previously reviewed. Readers should attend to whether the discussion accurately reflects what is presented in the results. Researchers will sometimes overstate findings or play up significant findings while downplaying nonsignificant findings. In addition, the limitations of the study, including issues related to whether the results are likely to generalize, should be noted in the discussion. Conclusions that are based on data should be clearly differentiated from authors' hypotheses regarding what the results may mean. Because discussion sections do not always fully and accurately depict the actual results of a study, consumers of research should avoid skipping the results section and reading just the discussion section, although we realize it may be tempting to do this (especially in an analysis-heavy article).

The more one reads journal articles, the more familiar one will become with the different components of articles, and the easier it will become to evaluate research studies. We encourage school psychologists to take their journals off their shelves and read at least one article of interest each month.

## CONDUCTING APPLIED RESEARCH IN THE SCHOOLS

Thus far in this chapter we have focused on the school psychologist as a consumer of research. As important as it is to be a savvy consumer, we also believe there are great opportunities for school psychologists to become involved in conducting research. School psychologists have access to large populations of children, and children with a variety of problems are referred to them. This situation provides school psychologists with great opportunities to conduct research related to children. These opportunities may include intervention studies (e.g., does social problem solving increase children's use of prosocial skills?), as well as studies on assessment methods (e.g., is a new measure of depression psychometrically sound?) and studies that attempt to more fully describe a population (e.g., how do the social skills of children with depression differ from the social skills of children with anxiety?).

Although most school psychologists receive some training in research methods in graduate school, those in specialist-level programs and PsyD doctoral programs typically are not exposed to research as a primary focus of their training. If school psychologists wish to become involved in conducting research but are unsure how to proceed, it may be beneficial to contact faculty members in school psychology training programs to collaborate on projects.

If a school psychologist wishes to conduct research in the schools, he or she must take several steps before beginning the research. All research conducted in schools must be approved by the school district. Districts have different procedures for approving research, but most have an individual or a committee that reviews proposals to conduct research in the schools. In addition to obtaining district-level approval, it is also important to obtain building approval through the school principal. If a school practitioner is conducting research in collaboration with a graduate student or faculty member at a university, approval from the university's Institutional Review Board for the Protection of Human Participants will also need to be obtained. In addition to following required district procedures for conducting research, the school psychologist must adhere to ethical guidelines for conducting research. Ethically, participants must take part in the research voluntarily and must be allowed to cease participation in the study at any time without consequence. For example, a student's grade cannot be dependent on the student participating in a research study. Informed consent must be provided by a child's parent or guardian prior to the child's participation in the study. For parents to provide *informed* consent they must be fully informed of the procedures involved in the research, as well as the risks and benefits to them and their children from participating in the research. Child assent should also be obtained directly from the child prior to study participation. Above all, school psychologists should ensure that the welfare of the children they serve takes priority over their research agendas.

When developing a research study, school psychologists should review the literature in the area in which they are interested and develop specific, testable research questions they wish to answer (Keith, 2002). Broad questions should be clarified and broken into smaller, targeted questions. For example, the question How can the social skills of children with ADHD be improved? is a large and vague question with no specific testable research questions. Specific questions related to this global question might be: (1) Does a classwide social problem-solving skills intervention lead to increases in prosocial behavior in children with ADHD? (2) Does a pullout group program for children with ADHD that focuses on social problem-solving skills increase prosocial behavior in children with ADHD? (3) Does individual social problem-solving instruction result in an increase in prosocial behaviors in children with ADHD? A research project might focus on just one of these questions or might attempt to answer all of them and to make comparisons between the three methods of intervention. In addition to developing research questions, the researcher needs to define what is being measured and how the measurement will occur. For example, the researcher interested in social skills programs for children with ADHD would need to decide how to measure prosocial behaviors (e.g., observations of the students, teacher report, student self-report) and what specifically is defined as prosocial behavior. Obviously, in this case, the intervention program(s) would also need to be identified.

## Single-Subject Research

Although the previous example is likely to lend itself to a group-design study, as noted earlier in this chapter, single-subject design research is particularly applicable in the school setting. There are a variety of single-subject designs (as discussed later in this section), but all such designs have some commonalities. Freeman (2003) outlines four characteristics of single-subject designs. Single-subject designs involve *using participants as their own controls*, with the performance of participants being compared across several conditions, which at a minimum include a baseline and an intervention phase. In addition, single-subject designs involve the *repeated measurement* of the participants in the different conditions. Often observations are conducted in single-subject research, but this is not a necessary aspect of such research. Dependent variables can also be measured via other means that lend themselves to repeated use (e.g., words read correctly on a curriculum-based measure). Single-subject designs also involve *replication*. Instead of simply conducting a pre–postassessment, there is some replication of the intervention condition. This strategy allows the researcher to be more confident that it is the intervention that is leading to any observed changes. Within single-subject designs, only *one variable is manipulated at a time*. This practice allows the researcher to make stronger conclusions regarding the effects of an intervention. For example, in an intervention to increase reading fluency, participants might initially be offered a tangible reinforcer for a certain rate of fluency. This would be the only change made, so that the researcher can determine if this intervention leads to changes in fluency.

Because single-subject designs—unlike typical group designs—use participants as their own controls and do not require large sample sizes, they are well suited to research in the schools. School psychologists can obtain data on interventions they are implementing across just a couple of students and be able to draw strong conclusions. In addition, one of the appealing aspects of single-subject designs is the ease with which one can determine whether the intervention was effective. By simply graphing the pattern of responses under the different experimental conditions, one can *see* whether the intervention had an effect. There are no concerns with complicated statistical analyses, as there can be with group designs. School psychologists can use single-subject designs to do research without having to access large populations of certain children, which may be difficult given the low prevalence rates of many disorders. For example, it would be unusual for a school psychologist to have more than a handful of children with school refusal at any one time. Thus utilizing a group-design study to evaluate an intervention for school refusal would be difficult. However, using single-subject methodology, the school psychologist can research effective interventions for these children. The basic single-subject research designs are outlined subsequently. These designs are discussed in much more detail in a variety of sources (e.g., Cooper, Heron, & Heward, 1987; Freeman, 2003; Kazdin, 1998, 2001).

As noted previously, almost all single-subject designs begin with a baseline phase (typically referred to as A). Prior to beginning the intervention phase, it is important to ensure that the baseline data are stable. Baseline data should continue to be collected until such stability is achieved. Stability is typically reflected by a relatively flat line (indicating little change in the occurrence of the behavior) when data are graphed.

The simplest single-subject design is a baseline phase followed by a treatment phase (an *AB design*). However, this design lacks internal validity, as it does not allow the researcher to see whether the intervention accounted for the change or whether another factor did. Therefore, this design is not typically used in research published in the more prestigious journals, but variations on this design that have stronger internal validity are commonly utilized. In an *ABAB design*, baseline data are collected and the intervention implemented; then a return to baseline occurs and, after achieving a stable baseline a second time, the intervention is reimplemented. To conclude that the intervention is effective, the behavior should improve during the first treatment phase, reverse to close to initial baseline levels in the second baseline phase, and improve following the implementation of the second treatment phase. Figure 12.1 provides a hypothetical example of an ABAB design in which an intervention was implemented to decrease a young child's aggressive acts (e.g., hitting, kicking, biting). As can be seen in this graph, aggressive acts decreased in the B (intervention) phases compared with their frequency during the A (baseline) phases. Based on a graph such as this, we could conclude that our intervention had the desired effect. Variations to the ABAB design are numerous and include adding additional treatment components to study the effects of more than one intervention (e.g., ABACABAC, with B and C being different interventions).

*Multiple-baseline designs* are also commonly used in single-subject research. In this type of design, instead of withdrawing a treatment, the treatment is implemented across multiple behaviors, settings, or individuals at different points in time. If the treatment has an effect, the behavior should remain stable until the treatment is implemented for that behavior, setting, or individual. Figure 12.2 presents a hypothetical example of a multiple-baseline design across individuals. In this example, second-grade students

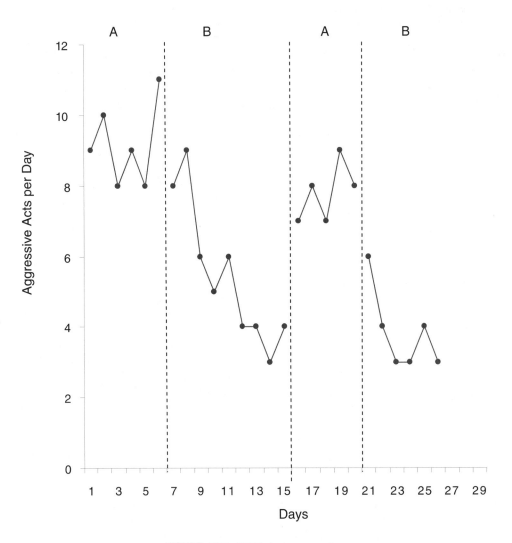

**FIGURE 12.1.** ABAB design example.

struggling with reading were initially provided with no intervention (baseline phase). A reading intervention was then implemented for one child, and this child's reading performance improved whereas the reading performance of the other two children remained stable at baseline levels. The intervention was then implemented for the second child, whereas the baseline condition remained in effect for the third child. Again, once the intervention was implemented, this child's reading performance improved. Finally, the intervention was implemented for the third child and, as with the other two children, reading performance improved from baseline levels. Because for each child reading performance improved only after the intervention was implemented, we can conclude that it was likely the intervention that led to this change.

If a researcher wishes to compare the effectiveness of two or more treatments, an *alternating-treatment design* may be appropriate. In such a design, two or more treatments (both intended to address the same target behavior) are presented in a random fashion (so that B does not always follow A) across observation periods. This procedure allows the researcher to determine whether one intervention produces more of an effect than another intervention. Although baseline phases are not required in alternating-treatment designs, they are frequently included prior to the presentation of the alternating treatments. Another variation on the alternating-treatment design is to include a final phase in which only the "best" treatment from the alternating-treatment phase is included.

*Changing-criterion designs* are used to evaluate the effectiveness of an intervention through making the criterion for success (and the associated reinforcement for this success) increasingly more stringent. In this design, the individual must reach a certain criterion to earn a reinforcer during the treatment phase. Once this initial criterion is met on a consistent basis, it is altered to require an increased level of performance. Once the second criterion level is met, the criterion is increased again, and so on. If the behavior changes only after the criterion is adjusted, the researcher can conclude that it was likely the intervention that resulted in the behavior change. For example, a child who is completing no math problems may initially have to complete 5 math problems to earn a reinforcer. Once he is consistently completing 5 math problems, the criterion may be changed to 10, and then 15, and so on until the child is regularly completing an entire math sheet of 25 problems.

Once a researcher has collected the data in a single-subject design, an evaluation of the data must take place. Unlike with group-design methods, there are no statistical significance testing methods appropriate for single-subject data. Data from these studies are typically graphed, and a visual analysis of these graphs is used to interpret the data and determine whether a meaningful change in behavior occurred and whether this change can be attributed to the intervention (Cooper et al., 1987; Kazdin, 2001). This visual inspection typically involves assessing the overall pattern of change in the data via examination of variability in the data, changes in the level or mean rate of responding, and trends (or directional paths) in the data. In some cases, it is quite easy to see that there was an effect. For example, if data are stable within each condition and no data points overlap between the baseline and treatment conditions, the researcher can conclude that the intervention had an effect. This is the case in the multiple-baseline example provided in Figure 12.2; for each child, there is no overlap between data points in the baseline and intervention phases. However, often there will be significant variability within phases and overlap in data points between phases (as there is in our ABAB design example shown in Figure 12.1). The more variability there is in the data

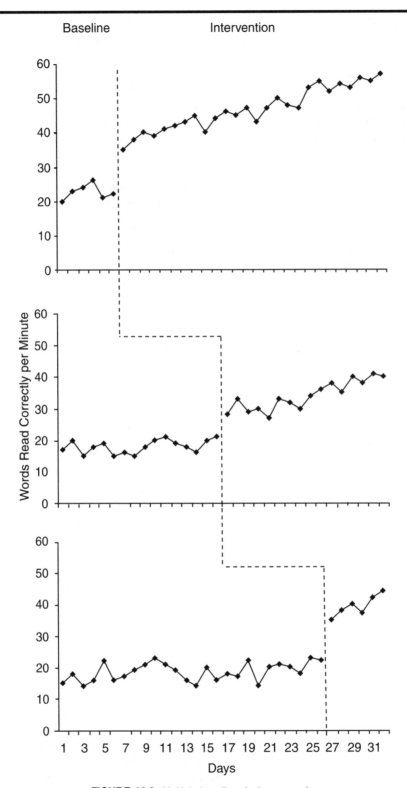

**FIGURE 12.2.** Multiple-baseline design example.

within a certain condition, the more the need for additional data to help spot a pattern of responding. Without a stable pattern of responding within each phase, drawing conclusions becomes more difficult—especially if there is a large overlap between data points in the different phases. The level of responding during each phase can also be examined to determine whether there is a difference in the behavior across conditions. For example, when switching from baseline to treatment, there may initially be a very dramatic change in level of the behavior. In an ABAB design, the same dramatic shift may also occur when returning to the baseline phase. The mean rate of behaviors in each condition is one method used to evaluate the level of responding. However, this method has drawbacks, particularly when there is significant variability in the data within conditions and a mean level line would not accurately reflect what was happening in each condition. When one examines the trend in data, an evaluation of the overall pattern of responses is conducted. This may be accomplished via examination of a trend line for each phase. For example, in our ABAB design in Figure 12.1, although there is some variability in responses in each of the phases, in general there is little change in the trend of the data in the baseline phases but a clear decreasing trend in the data following implementation of the intervention. In this example, there is both a change in the level of behavior and a change in the trend of the behavior between the baseline and treatment conditions.

As is discussed in more detail in the final section of this chapter, single-subject designs can be utilized not only when conducting formal research but also when evaluating the effects of interventions for individual students. As such, all school psychologists should be familiar with the basic single-subject designs and how to evaluate change when using these designs.

## PROGRAM EVALUATION

An additional type of applied research in which school psychologists may become involved is program evaluation. Program evaluation is a type of research that involves evaluation of social intervention programs (Rossi & Freeman, 1993). Worthen, Sanders, and Fitzpatrick (1997) define evaluation as "determining the worth or merit" of what is being evaluated (p. 5). Because a variety of ongoing programs are implemented in schools (e.g., drug-abuse prevention programs, English as a Second Language programs, bully prevention education), this type of research is sorely needed in the schools. Unfortunately, it seems that programs are often implemented with little research to support them, and then little research is conducted to evaluate these programs once they are in place. In some cases programs may become exceeding popular without any data to indicate that the programs are making the impact they are intended to make. One notable expert in special education and school psychology research has stated that "educators are notorious for embracing programs that look good but do no actual good" (Walker, 2001, p. 2). An example of this phenomenon of popular programs that are thin in supporting evidence is the Drug Abuse Resistance Education (DARE) program, a popular and well-intentioned program geared toward preventing substance abuse. Although DARE programs have been implemented in numerous schools across the country, outcome data on these programs have not been impressive. However, schools, families, and communities look favorably on this program and have expressed great distress in areas in which this program has been replaced with different drug-abuse prevention programs, including programs that have more supportive evidence behind them (e.g., Lynam et al., 1999).

Program evaluation is a broad and complex area. There are different types of evaluations, as well as numerous evaluation activities that may occur. One distinction that is often made is between formative and summative evaluations. Formative evaluation is ongoing and intended to provide feedback on how a program is working so that changes can be made, if needed. Summative evaluation is conducted after the program has been in place for some time or at the end of a program to determine how effective the program has been (Worthen et al., 1997). Often an evaluation incorporates both formative and summative activities. A distinction between internal and external evaluations is also often made. Internal evaluations are those completed by staff members from the agency running the program (e.g., a school psychologist employed by the school district evaluates the effectiveness of the school's drug education program). External evaluations are those completed by a group or individual outside of the agency (e.g., a group of researchers from the state department of health evaluates the school's drug education program). There are advantages and disadvantages to both internal and external evaluations. External evaluators are likely to be more objective about the program they are evaluating, whereas internal evaluators are more likely to be familiar with the program and the context in which it operates (Worthen et al., 1997). The activities within any type of evaluation are numerous. Rossi and Freeman (1993) group these activities into three categories: (1) program conceptualization and design, (2) monitoring and accountability of program implementation, and (3) assessment of program utility. Each of these activities is discussed here in more detail.

## Program Conceptualization and Design

At the program conceptualization and design stage, needs assessment activities are conducted (Greene, 2003; Rossi & Freeman, 1993). The main question to be addressed at this phase is whether there is a problem. Assuming that a problem is present (e.g., children are being bullied at school), the evaluator must clearly define the problem. This definition includes who is affected by the problem (e.g., children in middle school and high school), as well as the severity of the problem (e.g., about one-quarter of middle and high school children are victims of bullying). The identification of the problem can be achieved through a review of previous literature (including government reports), as well as by obtaining information directly from those involved in the organization. For example, in defining the bullying problem, we might look at previous research (which suggests that many middle school and high school students are bullied) and also obtain information directly from those in the schools in which we are considering implementing a program. We might conduct interviews with teachers, school staff, and students and review disciplinary records. In defining the problem, we should also ensure that the identified problem is an important issue for those involved. For example, if students indicate that bullying is a problem but rank alcohol use and school crime as greater problems, it may be better to address one of the more salient issues instead of bullying. It is also important to assess the demand for a program. For example, we may wish to implement a bully-prevention program that includes both a schoolwide component and a parent-education component about recognizing the signs of bullying and/or bully victimization and how parents can respond. However, it may be that parents (even those who perceive bullying as a problem) are not interested in actively participating in such an education program.

## Monitoring and Accountability

In the monitoring phase, the program has been implemented, and data are collected regarding its implementation. The data collected at this phase help determine whether the program is being implemented as intended. For example, is the program reaching those in need? Is the intervention being carried out as intended? Are the needed resources available (Rossi & Freeman, 1993)? Returning to our bullying program, let's assume that based on our needs assessment, we have chosen to implement a schoolwide intervention. It is likely that this program is reaching those in need because we did not select specific students to participate in the program. We have chosen to include more people than just those directly affected by the problem given the high prevalence of bullying, as well as for ease of program implementation (the program will be implemented in every homeroom class). However, in many situations the inclusion of those who do not need the intervention will be a waste of resources (Rossi & Freeman, 1993). For example, a universal program to target children with clinically elevated levels of depression would not likely be a good idea due to the relatively limited number of children who experience depression at any given time. In terms of evaluating whether the program is being carried out as intended and whether needed resources are available, we might observe in homeroom classes to make sure the lesson topics are being covered. In addition, we could interview teachers who are implementing the intervention and ask about coverage of certain issues, as well as their perceptions of whether they have the resources necessary to conduct the intervention (e.g., Are they receiving needed training in the intervention? Do they receive release time for preparing the intervention materials?).

## Assessing Program Utility

When assessing program utility, both the impact of the program (whether the program resulted in changes in the desired direction) and the efficiency of the program (the costs related to the benefits) are evaluated (Rossi & Freeman, 1993). These activities can be quite complicated, as there are numerous ways in which a program can be evaluated. The key idea behind assessing the impact of a program is determining whether the program produced the desired effect (e.g., a decrease in bullying) and whether this effect was greater than what would have occurred without the program or what would have occurred with an alternative program (Rossi & Freeman, 1993). Outcome measures must be identified (e.g., school discipline records, rating scales, observations), as well as who will provide outcome data (e.g., students, parents, teachers). It should also be recognized that the program may have an impact on more people than just the program participants. The families of participants, as well as staff members at the school where the program is implemented, may be affected. In addition, the immediate impact of the program may differ from its long-term impact (Greene, 2003). Thus the evaluator must decide who will be the focus of the impact assessment, as well as the time intervals that will be used to evaluate the impact. In addition, the evaluator must ensure that the design of the evaluation study allows the evaluator to draw conclusions regarding the effects of the evaluation (i.e., that there is internal validity). Rossi and Freeman (1993) outline a number of evaluation research designs that may be utilized in program evaluation. These include randomized experimental designs, as well as quasi-experimental designs.

The efficiency of a program may be evaluated through cost-effectiveness or cost–benefit analyses (Greene, 2003; Rossi & Freeman, 1993). In cost-effectiveness analysis, the cost of a program is evaluated relative to the results of the program. This allows comparison across programs (e.g., one bullying program, which cost $10 per student to implement, reduced bullying rates by 50%; another program, costing $50 per student, reduced bullying rates by 75%; thus the cheaper program is more cost effective). In cost–benefit analyses, the cost of the program is compared with the monetary value of the result. In this method, the outcome is expressed purely in monetary terms (e.g., difference in dollars expended on the antibullying program versus dollars saved from reduced negative consequences associated with bullying). The actual calculations of the efficiency of a program can, obviously, get quite complicated—especially when attempting to assign a monetary value to outcomes that are not easily quantifiable.

As should be evident from this brief discussion, program evaluation is an important yet complex activity. Rossi and Freeman (1993) stressed this point when they stated, "Doing evaluations only infrequently is a cut-and-dried activity. It is rarely like either putting up a prefabricated house or checking a document in a word processor's spelling program" (p. 27). Programs often have many more components, individuals involved, and desired outcomes than experimental research studies. In addition, programs tend to be ongoing rather than time limited, as traditional research studies are. Because program evaluations are complex, they are rarely carried out by a single person. School psychologists who wish to become involved in program evaluations should seek information on what is already being done in their districts and attempt to collaborate with individuals currently involved in such activities. In addition, school psychologists could collaborate with university faculty in developing and evaluating programs designed to address school-based issues.

## DATA-BASED DECISION MAKING

Although not all school psychologists will be engaged in formal research activities, all school psychologists should be engaged in data-based decision making. As discussed in detail in Chapter 7, the data-driven problem-solving model requires school psychologists to examine discrepancies between how a child is currently performing (what is) and how the child should be performing (what should be). Under this model, discrepancies are domain-specific (e.g., a child may have a discrepancy in social skills but not in reading skills), context-dependent (e.g., the problem may be present during independent seatwork but not small-group activities) and the assessment of the discrepancy is specific to the situation (e.g., using CBM probes to assess reading fluency). Interventions are then developed that target the discrepancy within the context in which the problem is occurring. Interventions should target the specific reason that the problem is occurring, as outlined in the overview of problem analysis in Chapter 7 (e.g., Is the work too difficult for the student? Does the student "get" something out of not doing the work?). Once the intervention is in place, it should be monitored via continuous collection of objective data (e.g., CBM probes, behavioral observations) to determine whether the intervention is having the intended effect and is, in fact, decreasing the discrepancy between "what is" and "what should be" for the student. At each of the steps in the problem-solving model, the school psychologist is required to use data to inform his or her decision-making process.

Data-based decision making as used within the problem-solving model closely parallels research activities, but also has some differences. Research activities are geared toward drawing conclusions that may generalize to other settings, individuals, and so forth. Research activities typically begin with specific research questions and hypotheses. Participants who meet certain criteria are then obtained to answer these questions. Data-based decision making is more focused on the individual student or client. The "question" to be answered is whether an intervention is having the intended effect for a specific individual in a specific situation. For example, Ella, a child with reading difficulties, is referred to the school psychologist for an evaluation. The evaluation is conducted, and recommendations are made for improving Ella's reading performance (e.g., conducting reading drills with overcorrection procedures). The question of interest in this case is, Do reading drills increase Ella's reading fluency? In data-based decision-making, our focus is on addressing the problem (i.e., discrepancy), and the question is whether or not the discrepancy was reduced by our intervention. When the presenting problem involves an individual child, the methods of evaluation are much the same as they are in single-subject research designs—we want to be able to draw an informed conclusion regarding whether the intervention is having the desired impact on the student.

To obtain a baseline level of Ella's reading fluency prior to implementing the reading drills, the school psychologist could administer CBM probes. Following the baseline phase, the reading intervention is implemented, and the school psychologist continues to evaluate Ella's reading fluency through regular CBM probes. Assuming Ella's reading performance improves, the school psychologist may be satisfied and conclude that this intervention is having the desired effect. If Ella's reading fluency does not improve, the school psychologist would likely conclude that the intervention is not having the desired effect and would implement another intervention. If Ella's performance is evaluated in this manner, the basic AB design described earlier is followed. However, as noted, with this design the school psychologist would be unable to attribute improved performance to the intervention specifically, as there might be something else influencing the outcomes. For example, in this case, perhaps it was noted that Ella's vision seemed to be poor, that she recently obtained glasses, and that it is really her improved vision that led to her improvement in reading. To be confident that it was truly the intervention that led to the improvement, the school psychologist would need to implement one of the other single-subject designs (e.g., an ABAB design) discussed earlier.

In addition to making data-based decisions regarding the effectiveness of specific interventions for children, school psychologists should also assist in making data-based decisions regarding students' educational programs. As discussed in Chapter 6, all students who are receiving special education services must have IEPs that outline specific goals they are to achieve. However, all too often there is little done to evaluate whether children are meeting their IEP goals. If it is unclear whether goals are being met, it is also unclear whether the special education program is having a positive impact on the child. Thus it is imperative that IEP goals be evaluated. For this to occur, IEP goals must be stated in measurable terms, and the child's performance on these goals must be evaluated on an ongoing basis. IEPs need to be reviewed only once a year. However, progress toward goals should be monitored much more frequently than this to determine whether the child is making adequate progress. Baseline levels of performance, as well as expected levels of performance, must be clear, and a system to measure change over time must be in place. If the child is not progressing, modifications may need to be made to that child's educational plan.

In addition to using data-based decision making to evaluate the outcomes for individual students, school psychologists who are involved in secondary or primary prevention efforts with groups of students (as discussed in Chapter 7) should also engage in data-based decision making. This data-based decision making may encompass both evaluation of the prevention program as a whole (which would parallel program evaluation methods discussed earlier in this chapter), as well as evaluation of individual student progress. As noted in Chapter 7, not all children respond in the same manner to prevention efforts. Thus for some children more intensive services may need to be implemented, whereas for other children, the services provided through a prevention program may be adequate to prevent learning or behavioral problems. Without monitoring of student progress, it becomes impossible to know which students involved in a primary prevention program may benefit from secondary or tertiary prevention and intervention efforts. In addition, if data are collected in a proactive manner (i.e., data are obtained on all students) on important domains of functioning (e.g., reading), then this information can help inform decisions regarding in which areas schools should focus their prevention efforts and which students should be the targets of secondary and tertiary level prevention and intervention.

Implementing interventions without evaluating their effectiveness is poor practice and is much less likely to lead to positive change for students than interventions that are evaluated in an ongoing fashion and are modified to as needed. As noted in Chapter 7, there is significant concern that traditional special education services are not effective in reducing the performance gap between children with disabilities and children without disabilities. If this is the case, clearly we are doing many students a disservice by not providing them with the skills they need to succeed within our school systems. We believe that by following the data-based problem-solving model in their daily practices, school psychologists can make a difference and can help students close that gap between where they are performing and where they should be performing. We strongly encourage all school psychologists to engage in this data-based decision-making process so that children are receiving the services most likely to meet their needs.

## DISCUSSION QUESTIONS AND ACTIVITIES

1. Obtain a copy of a recent issue of one of the four main school psychology journals. Examine the articles published in this issue and identify whether each is an original research article, a meta-analysis, or a narrative review. What differences do you see in the structure of these different articles?

2. Using a group-design experimental study from one of the main school psychology journals (or another journal focused on children), identify the possible threats to internal validity in the study. Also note whether the authors mention these in the discussion section of the article.

3. Locate a group-based intervention study focused on children (the *Journal of Clinical Child and Adolescent Psychology* is one good source of intervention studies). Do the authors evaluate the clinical significance of their results? If so, what method(s) do

they use? Do you agree with their conclusions regarding the meaningfulness of their findings?

4. Locate a single-subject design study (the *Journal of Applied Behavior Analysis* is one good source of such studies). What type of design do the researchers use? How do they evaluate the meaningfulness of the effects of their intervention?

5. Ask around in your school district about the types of programs that are run and the types of evaluation activities that occur. Are all programs evaluated? What room do you see for improvement in the way programs are evaluated?

6. Interview several school psychologists regarding their data-based decision-making practices. Do they regularly engage in this practice? If not, why not? If they do, obtain some examples of how they apply the methods and principles discussed in this chapter.

# 13

# Moving the Field Forward

MAPPING THE FUTURE
OF SCHOOL PSYCHOLOGY

One of us (KWM) recently visited with a prospective school psychologist—a woman who, having completed her undergraduate education several years ago and having worked in the fields of early childhood education and mental health for 10 years, was considering a career change into the field of school psychology. As the conversation progressed past the usual questions regarding application deadlines, selection procedures, financial support, training opportunities, and so forth, she asked some very pointed and intriguing questions regarding the future of school psychology. Understandably, she was concerned about the employment outlook in school psychology, considering that she would need to invest 3 or more years and change professions in order to gain entry into the field. On this issue, she was assured that the employment outlook for school psychologists was projected to be quite favorable for the next several years. Then she asked some more complicated questions: "Where is school psychology heading?" "What will the field look like in 10 years?" "What will happen to school psychology if public education undergoes major changes?" These questions led to an interesting discussion but also to some equivocation in providing answers to her questions. It is relatively easy to project certain aspects of the future of the field (employment trends, demographics, etc.) but much more complicated to predict with great confidence what the future will hold. In fact, what we can predict with the most confidence is that significant changes are ahead of us. From our present standpoint in time and experience, we can quite confidently describe *what we would like to see* as the future of school psychology, and in this volume we have attempted to provide a road map or model for the field. In fact, the title of this book, *School Psychology for the 21st Century: Foundations and Practices*, was developed from our very specific objective of writing a book on school psychology that went beyond merely describing the history and present status of school

264

psychology and actively advocated for what we consider to be models of good practice now and in the future. However, describing *what will be* is a more complicated matter, and we realize that prognosticating regarding the future is certainly risky business. Despite the necessary caveats that must be considered in writing a chapter on moving the field of school psychology forward, we believe that such a focus is a fitting way to conclude this volume. Although we recognize that there is some risk that our emphases and predictions might appear naive or off the mark 20 or 30 years from now, we don't think that will be the case. Rather, we are confident that our views are well considered and based on a solid foundation. That said, we recognize the challenge in promoting a view about the future of school psychology. Fortune-telling and soothsaying may be among the oldest of professions, but they are probably not held in as much esteem as even the purported oldest profession. Yogi Berra is credited with saying "Prediction is very hard, especially when it's about the future."

Near the turn of the last century—from about 1997 through about 2002—the future of school psychology was a major focus within the field. Several important publications and conferences were developed to address issues related to school psychology in the 21st century. Foremost among these sources include NASP's *School Psychology: A Blueprint for Training and Practice–II* (Ysseldyke et al., 1997); the proceedings of the Future of School Psychology Conference, which was held November 14–16, 2002, at several sites and "webcast" from Indianapolis, Indiana (see www.indiana.edu/~futures/ for more details and presentation summaries, some of which are included as articles in special issues of *School Psychology Quarterly*, vol. 18, no. 4, 2003, and *School Psychology Review*, vol. 33, no. 1, 2004); a special issue of *School Psychology Review* (vol. 29, no. 4, 2000) titled "School Psychology in the 21st Century"; and a chapter by Reschly and Ysseldyke (2002) titled "Paradigm Shift: The Past Is Not the Future" in *Best Practices in School Psychology: IV*. These sources are all important efforts to make an early-21st-century statement and vision regarding the future of school psychology. We have collectively been influenced by these efforts and have borrowed liberally from these sources in the preparation of this chapter.

This chapter includes a review of some issues related to the history of school psychology and how our past has shaped the present and future of the field in both positive and negative ways. Some prior efforts to predict the future of school psychology are reviewed. We should note that we owe a special debt to Fagan and Wise (2000) in developing our discussion of prior prognostication efforts, because their analysis of past attempts to predict the future of school psychology is simply the most comprehensive collection of information we have seen on this topic. Following this brief discussion, this chapter proceeds with our own carefully considered predictions regarding the future of the field. Perhaps most important, this chapter ends with our own analysis of a vision of where school psychology "should be" in the future, a summary of our own attempt in this volume to move the field forward and see it make the impact we know it is capable of making.

## FROM WHERE WE WERE TO WHERE WE ARE: THE EVOLUTION OF SCHOOL PSYCHOLOGY

Previous chapters in this volume, especially Chapters 2, 5, and 6, have provided an important historical context from which to understand the evolution of the field of school psychology. From its obscure and relatively recent beginnings within the larger fields of psychology and education, school psychology has struggled, grown, and finally arrived as a viable, strong, and mature profession and scientific discipline. There is no question regarding the arrival and maturation of the field, which has evolved into a large and potent force. Although school psychology is still small in comparison with its larger parent fields, there is no denying that it has made significant inroads in influence and that school psychologists are shaping practice, policy, and science at all levels—from the local school to the highest decision-making bodies.

One of the constants in this professional evolution has been the process of struggle and challenge. It is apparent that school psychology has grown and matured despite—or perhaps because of—both external and internal conflicts. Like a small tree that takes root in the rocky outcrops, the processes of opposition and constantly changing conditions have led to the growth of a stubborn, tough, and resilient organism whose roots have sunk in deep, having weathered a few storms. As the field of school psychology has arrived in the early part of the 21st century, it is interesting to consider what the future evolution of the field will bring and where it will be at the close of this century. In this regard, we can begin to think about the future by considering the forces that have brought us to the present, because it is quite likely that these same forces will continue to shape the field well beyond our own participation in it.

In this regard, we propose that two forces—changing social conditions or challenges and evolving legal aspects of education and psychology—will continue to have a major impact on the evolution of school psychology, just as they have had in its short history. We also expect that the two forces will continue to be integrally connected, with changing social conditions and attitudes spawning new legal conditions, and with both forces having an impact on the practice of school psychology. At the midpoint of the 20th century, who could have predicted that changing social attitudes and conditions regarding people with disabilities would have led to the enactment of the Education for All Handicapped Children Act of 1975 in the United States (now known as IDEA)? Who could have predicted that this federal law would serve as a major impetus for the field of school psychology, tripling in size in the United States in only two or three decades? Likewise, when the law was originated, who could have predicted that certain minor modifications to it, such as extending services to a younger age range (1987, 1990), or mandating the use of functional behavior assessment (1997) and no longer mandating the ability–achievement discrepancy model as the way in which learning disabilities are to be documented (2004) would have such a strong impact in professional practice, training, and research in the field?

In a similar vein, it is notable that changing economic and family conditions and social attitudes in the United States and Canada have had a dramatic impact on the demographics, status, and plight of children and that these conditions would result in major initiatives within the field of school psychology. For example, consider the major efforts within the field in recent years regarding providing services to "at risk" children and youths, predicting and reducing school violence, and providing appropriate conditions and support for gay and lesbian youths in school settings. Although important aspects of each of these concerns were evident in the 1960s and 1970s, they were certainly not considered to be central issues within school psychology at that time, a statement that can be supported by a quick perusal of the focus and titles of journal articles and books from that era. Thus we propose that the major changes or evolutions in the field of school psychology during the 21st century will not occur in isolation or in a social vacuum. Rather, we believe that the major changes in the field over the next several decades will develop in response to the ever-changing social, demographic, and legal conditions that affect the lives of children and their families and the delivery of school psychology services. It is also important to consider that change in professional practice often precedes changes in educational policy (Grimes & Tilly, 1996). In other words, although the field of school psychology must sometimes adapt practice to fit new policies, the reverse is also true. If practitioners, trainers, and researchers promote best practice in a reflective and proactive manner, it is quite possible that such practices will become codified into policy.

## THE CHALLENGES OF PROGNOSTICATION: PREVIOUS ATTEMPTS TO PREDICT THE FUTURE OF THE FIELD

Before we discuss our own views on the possible future of the field of school psychology, it is important to recognize the challenges and limits of such efforts at prognostication. Ever since school psychology emerged as a distinct field, there have been attempts to look forward and predict what the future might hold for the field. It is worth reviewing some of these earlier predictions in order to put the present state of the field within some context and to develop a lens through which our own views regarding the future of the field might be viewed.

Without question, the most detailed and comprehensive single compendium of prior efforts to provide viewpoints on the future of school psychology is "Perspectives on the Future of School Psychology," a chapter by Fagan and Wise (2000) in which they reviewed in depth the views of some of the most prominent writers in school psychology regarding the future of the field. This analysis considers prior predictions that proved to be accurate, as well as those predictions that did not come to pass, and discusses them within the context of ever-changing conditions the field has faced, which have made such prognostication difficult. A very brief review of a few of the more interesting viewpoints and predictions from this source is a useful addition to the current chapter.

The first well-known viewpoint or prediction regarding the future of school psychology was published in the 1930s, at a point at which the field really did not even have a clear identity. Leta Hollingworth (1933), one of the pioneers of school psychology, promoted her predictions regarding the future of psychological services in public schools in an article in a professional journal. Her predictions were more specifically aimed at the upcoming 25 years, or the period of time from 1933 to 1958. Hollingworth saw a future in which educational practice and the delivery of psychological services in schools would be informed by science and rational thinking, in which psychological services in schools would become commonplace, and in which the combination of these variables would eliminate many of the problems of the time. In her own words: "The school will be fitted to the child. Suicide of pupils, in despair at failure, will be unknown. Truancy will become a thing of the past. . . . Special talents and defects will be considered in school placements" (Hollingworth, 1933, p. 379). Her predictions proved to be both accurate and inaccurate, given that school psychology ultimately did emerge as a major player in public education but also that its influence obviously did not eliminate most of the major ills faced by children and youths in school settings.

With the advent of APA's Division of School Psychology (Division 16) in 1945, and with the convening of the historic Thayer Conference on the future of school psychology in 1954, the period surrounding the midpoint of the 20th century provided new opportunities for those engaged in leadership within the burgeoning field to reflect on its progress to date and to consider what the future might bring. The general view regarding the development of the field during that time period was that school psychologists should be firmly grounded in clinical psychology and group testing but that they would rely more heavily in the future on specialized, individualized assessment and intervention techniques (Luckey, 1951). Certainly, the role of school psychologists as skilled individual assessment specialists came to pass, although the specialized interventionist role has been accomplished with mixed success. At the Thayer conference, new initiatives for the young Division 16 included establishing credentialing guidelines for school psychologists in the various U.S. states and differentiating doctoral from master's- (or specialist-) level training in credentialing (Fagan & Wise, 2000). Division 16 was successful in promoting important developments in state department of education credentialing patterns, although the differentiating of doctoral and nondoctoral school psychologists never gained significant or widespread influence. In addition, prominent participants at this conference correctly anticipated the future growth opportunities in the field, although it is doubtful that they could have possibly predicted the explosive growth that occurred in response to the changing educational landscape in the United States after the original IDEA law was enacted.

As the field of school psychology began to come into its own in the 1960s and 1970s, the volume of professional literature increased substantially, and some of these writings addressed viewpoints regarding the future of the field. In our view, one of the most insightful efforts in this regard was Susan Gray's (1963) book, *The Psychologist in the Schools*. This volume was developed to provide a broad overview of the nascent field of school psychology and to provide a template for best practice. Perhaps the single greatest contribution of this work was the inclusion of two comprehensive chapters on the school psychologist as a *data-oriented problem solver*. Gray's work predated the current movement in data-based decision making and problem solving by two decades and established an important foundation for what in our view is one of the most significant roles that school psychologists can play. She foresaw a field in which school psychologists, armed with solid training in effective assessment, diagnosis, intervention, and scientific inquiry methods, would continually use these skills within a scientist-practitioner framework to propose testable hypotheses regarding learning and behavioral problems and would evaluate these hypotheses through carefully selecting and continually monitoring intervention efforts. Some other important future views during this era included Hirst's (1963) almost prescient prediction that there would be a strong increase in the professional workforce over the next two decades; Magary's (1967) discussion of the future emergence of the primary importance of the consultation role for school psychologists and the need for increased collaboration and cooperation on school teams and within professional organizations; Bardon and Bennet's (1974) call for more sophisticated and extensive training of school psychologists; and Tindall's (1979) comments regarding the emergence of increasing conflict between NASP and APA and the emerging problems of professional role constriction.

In sum, as we look retrospectively at the best known previous attempts to predict the future of school psychology, it is obvious that their accuracy and impact has been mixed. Some of these prior attempts ended up being far off the mark, whereas others were right on target. With the trepidation that comes from treading these well-traveled waters of prognostication, we now move our focus of this chapter to our own predictions regarding the future of school psychology.

# SCHOOL PSYCHOLOGY IN THE 21ST CENTURY: OUR PREDICTIONS

The predictions offered in this section have not simply been pulled out of the prover-bial hat. Rather, our views regarding the future of school psychology are implicit within the previous chapters of this volume and, in some cases, serve as an important founda-tion for these chapters. Some of these predictions are quite easy to make, and we are confident enough in them to consider them "no-brainers." Others are more compli-cated and stem from a confluence of where we think the evidence is pointing and where we think it "ought" to point. As we acknowledge the limitations in any prognostication process, we also believe that the following prognostications represent the future of the field of school psychology.

- *School psychologists will serve an increasingly diverse population.* As we have shown in Chapter 3, the population of students and families who are served by school psycholo-gists will continue to reflect increased diversity with regard to race or ethnicity, lan-guage, cultural background, and familial composition. The state of California is often considered to be a cultural barometer for future social trends in the United States. Pres-ently, no single racial/ethnic group constitutes more than 50% of the population of the schools in that state. The website for the Languages for Los Angeles project at UCLA (www.humnet.ucla.edu/languagesofla/default.htm, retrieved April 8, 2004) indicates that more than 50 major primary languages are spoken by residents of Los Angeles, and there have been some estimates that the students served by the Los Angeles Unified School District speak an even greater number of primary or native languages. We believe that these figures represent unmistakable trends that will ultimately spread to some extent to all regions of the United States and Canada. Stated simply, school psy-chologists in the future will be expected to have the skills and technology to provide educational and mental health services to an increasingly diverse population.
- *The diversity of school psychologists will increasingly lag behind that of the populations they serve.* Although the population of students and their families served by school psy-chologists will continue to increase in an unprecedented manner in the 21st century, the diversity of school psychologists will continue to lag behind that of the general pop-ulation and is destined to become even more disparate in this regard, at least for the next quarter of the century. At the 2002 Futures Conference, a presentation by Curtis, Grier, and Hunley (2003, 2004) demonstrated convincingly that, despite some overall increases in ethnic/racial diversity of school psychologists in recent years (and a gener-ally strong desire for more diversity within the field), school psychology has become dis-tinctly "Caucasian and female." Expected increases in racial/ethnic diversity among school psychologists will be more than offset by larger increases in all forms of diversity among constituent populations served, causing even greater disparity between typical practitioners and clients. We believe that a major challenge in this regard is that the increased disparity in diversity representation between school psychologists and the populations they serve may foster increased perceptions of a "credibility gap."
- *School psychologists will continue to be in short supply.* At least through the first quar-ter of the 21st century, all indications are that there will continue to be a smaller supply than demand for school psychologists in the United States. These personnel shortages will continue to be especially problematic in rural and urban school systems and in selected regions. As a result, employment prospects for school psychologists will con-tinue to be quite favorable, and the NASP-recommended ratio of 1 school psychologist per 1,000 students in a school system will be unattainable in many school systems, par-

ticularly in poorer districts and in regions in which shortages are most notable. Related to this issue, we foresee a continued strong need not only for school psychology practitioners but also for school psychology educators or trainers as well, such as University of Southern Mississippi faculty member Heather Sterling-Turner, whose vignette appears in Chapter 1. The emerging generation of school psychology educators will need to develop increasingly responsive and innovative ways to make school psychology training available to graduate students, sometimes in nontraditional ways.

• *Public-sector financial stress will further inhibit growth and will require innovative service delivery approaches.* Since about 1980, public services in the United States, especially public education and mental health services, have been operating under increasing economic and political duress, due to a complicated result of unfunded federal and state mandates, tax cuts at the federal level shifting financial burdens to local governments, changes in social and economic conditions, and the advent of a political climate in which many politicians and citizens have fostered a distrust in the public sector and a great desire to reduce its size and increase its efficiency. School psychology services have traditionally been almost exclusively connected to the public sector, and the larger political and economic trends have and will continue to greatly shape and affect the field. On the negative side, many school psychologists will be asked to do "more with less" and will experience higher caseloads and less availability of internal and external support services for the students they serve. On the positive side, these trends will necessitate a climate in which many school psychologists will seize the challenge as an opportunity to deliver services in nontraditional ways, such as moving away from a model of solving one student problem at a time and toward developing systems-level orientations and preventive approaches (Shapiro, 2000). We believe that a move away from targeting services exclusively at the individual student level is inevitable and that the 21st century will see a significant expansion in efforts by school psychologists to engage in prevention activities and to affect entire classrooms, schools, and systems through their services.

• *Role expansion in school psychology will increase.* Despite (or perhaps because of) the staffing shortages and economic challenges that will be faced by the field, many school psychologists will continue to advocate effectively for role expansion and will increasingly distance themselves from the traditional gatekeeper or sorter roles in which static psychometric classification activities are *de rigueur*. Consider the vignette about Trina Spencer from Chapter 1, for example. Her work in parent training and in providing services in a nontraditional setting is but one case of a school psychologist who has effectively moved beyond some of the rigid boundaries of traditional practice and who has been instrumental in helping children and their families as a result. Although some educational systems (and school psychologists) will refuse to extricate the school psychologist from the traditional test-and-place role, innovative school psychologists will successfully negotiate ways to provide meaningful solutions to educational, social, and behavioral problems, and the successes of these efforts will spawn support for role expansion by administrators and teachers who recognize what their school psychologist can do for them. Furthermore, a growing number of school psychology training programs will develop innovative curricula and mission statements that will facilitate such continued role expansion and intervention and problem-solving orientations. We have already witnessed some of this transition taking place. Although it is true that some systems are highly resistant to progressive changes, educational systems that historically have used the psychologist almost exclusively in the sorter role are often more than willing to modify their expectations and place the psychologist in a consultation, training, and intervention role once they see how well a progressively trained practitioner can help them solve big problems within the system. To borrow a phrase, once the genie is out of the bottle, it's hard to get it back in.

• *School psychologists will have increased access to new and effective technologies and tools.* As we have witnessed in recent years with the advent of new models for effective behavioral and academic supports in schools, school psychologists in the 21st century will continue to have increasing access to exciting new tools for providing effective services. In fact, we believe that there will be an almost exponential increase in the availability of such effective new tools. The oft-repeated proverb "necessity is of the mother of invention" will certainly come into play here, because the very big and very real problems faced by children and their families in this century will absolutely necessitate better solutions. Furthermore, the maturing research base in the fields of psychology and education and the increasingly innovative technology by which this information is accessed (instant Internet-based access, for example) will make the availability of new information and tools almost immediate. Consider our vignettes about Margaret McGlinchey and Marty Ikeda from Chapter 1. Here are two examples of school psychologists whose work has evolved and taken on incredibly rich dimensions in helping children and their families through the use of innovative methods and technologies, such as making systems-level changes to improve student referral processes and the use of data-based problem-solving methods to improve student outcomes. We anticipate that exciting innovations such as these will continue to shape the practice of school psychology and the fields of education and psychology in general as we move increasingly in the direction of being a science-based profession.

• *Significant new federal initiatives will continue to affect the practice of school psychology.* This prediction easily fits in the "no-brainer" category of prediction. Looking forward to the middle and end of the 21st century, none of us can possibly imagine the specific social, political, and economic conditions that will result in changes to federal education laws, but if the past is a guide, we can be assured that such changes will indeed happen. In fact, you should be able to safely bet your paycheck on this prediction. The 20th century federal legislation in the United States that most clearly affected school psychology was the passage of the original IDEA in 1975. The 1990, 1997, and 2004 reauthorizations of this law also resulted in immediate responses in some aspects of school psychology practice and training. It takes no stretch of the imagination to believe that some new federal law, similar or greater in impact on school psychology as was IDEA, will become reality later in the 21st century. Although the U.S. federal government does not have the primary responsibility for public education (it is considered a "creature of the states"), presidential administrations have increasingly used federal education initiatives (many of them unfunded or only partially funded) to shape or mandate state policies, and the U.S. Congress has likewise demonstrated similar propensities. It is quite possible that a future 21st-century federal law will even dwarf IDEA and the current No Child Left Behind Act in terms of impact on education and the practice of school psychology. Will publicly funded tuition vouchers for private education become a widespread reality? Will new federal laws bring the special education census to 25% of the student population nationally? Will individual education plans become an entitlement of all students, and not just those identified as having disabilities? Will IDEA be abolished or replaced by something entirely different? These are only a handful of examples of possible future legislation that would affect education, and school psychology, in a dramatic way.

• *An increasing percentage of children and youths in schools will be "at risk."* This prediction is one that we wish we didn't feel compelled to make, but it nonetheless is on the horizon. According to varied social, economic, and health indicators, children born in the United States during the 21st century will face unprecedented new challenges and opportunities, and for an increasing percentage of these children, the result will be increased exposure to circumstances that place them at risk for academic, social, behavioral, health, or economic problems, which are often intertwined (Children's Defense Fund, 2001; Crockett, 2003, 2004). We see these probable developments as having a clear impact on the field of school psychology. Consider the vignette about school psychologist Deanna Sanders from Chapter 1. Throughout her career, she has worked in the forefront of providing services to children and their families who are faced with serious disadvantages and for whom the term "at risk" does not seem to be sufficient. If Deanna's experience is a harbinger of things to come—and we think that it is—then more students will need to become the focus of concern for school teams, and the result will be more opportunities for school psychologists to play a role in developing appropriate, effective programs to support these children. This eventuality will not only require more involvement from school psychologists but will also further enhance the need for practitioners to focus their services in a manner that moves increasingly further away from the "one child at a time"' model of solving educational and social problems.

• *Public schools will become increasingly specialized, unique, focused, and individualized.* Although some individuals may yearn for the perceived "golden age" of public education of the 1950s and early 1960s, when baby boomers nationwide experienced a great deal of perceived similarity or homogeneity among their public schooling curricula and socialization experiences, we believe that the future of public schools will be in the direction of less, not more, uniformity and homogeneity in the schooling experience. Despite some recent federal, state, and provincial initiatives to exert greater control and impose greater accountability among public schools, an interesting social dynamic is evolving that will make the future increasingly diverse. Families in the 21st century want and expect more choice and desire more control over their children's education than was typical in past decades. We anticipate that some of the current fringe or experimental educational innovations will become more common as the 21st century progresses. As a result, a small but steadily increasing percentage of students will receive public education in schools that today represent only a small, experimental component of public schooling. Examples of some of these emerging experimental education innovations include charter schools, smaller and more individualized secondary schools (currently being promoted and funded by the Bill and Melinda Gates Foundation), alternative school offerings, magnet schools, same-gender classrooms and schools, and highly focused specialized schools that emphasize themes such as Afrocentric education, performing arts, science and technology, and international/global education. These trends should not be a surprise—they simply reflect the reality of an increasingly pluralistic society within North America. As a result of this trend away from homogeneity, school psychologists of the 21st century will increasingly be expected to provide more individualized services, assist in making more individual accommodations within mainstream educational environments, and work with school teams that operate under increasingly unique and diverse mission statements.

• *Assessment will continue to be important and will become more useful for intervention.* Think back to our vignette about veteran school psychologist Bob Green in Chapter 1, which we euphemistically titled "surviving the assessment marathon" to reflect the great pressures he has been under throughout his career to process extremely high numbers of assessment referrals. Also consider our discussions of the assessment process in Chapters 7 and 8. In reading this volume you likely have sensed two somewhat contrasting themes: that we view psychological and educational assessment of students to be a critically important activity for school psychologists and that we dislike exceedingly the past and current models of school psychology which are rigidly focused on a gatekeeper or sorter role, or a test-and-place paradigm. We don't actually see a contradiction here. The problem, in our view, is not that school psychologists focus much of their work on assessment. Rather, the problem is that so much of the traditional assessment enterprise is not particularly helpful for solving children's educational and mental health concerns and that so many of these tasks have kept school psychologists out of the intervention planning and delivery role. We believe that assessment will continue to be an important role for school psychologists throughout the 21st century, although this role will become increasingly expanded beyond the assessment and classification niche. Moreover, we believe that over time there will continue to be improvements in the quality and usefulness of assessment methods and tools, both for classification purposes and for intervention planning purposes. The 21st century will see the much discussed but seldom implemented notion of effectively linking assessment to intervention become more a part of routine practice for school psychologists. In addition, if the field moves increasingly toward prevention and systems change, perhaps assessment will include more formative measures for all students. It is feasible that school psychologists might have a role in the development, management, and implementation of such formative or schoolwide assessments.

• *The 21st century includes a bright future for school psychologists.* Although some of our prognostications may be frightening—they certainly are premised on the idea that changes are inevitable and not always desirable—we are "bullish" on the future of the field of school psychology. We believe that the 21st century will see the fruits of the maturation of school psychology and that school psychologists will become increasingly important players in the education and mental health fields. The 20th century witnessed the maturation of the field of school psychology, with its symbolic move from adolescence to adulthood. We have no reservations recommending a career in school psychology to prospective professionals who possess the requisite skills, commitment, and adaptability to be successful and who are motivated by a desire to help shape the future of children and their families through innovative education and mental health service delivery.

## MAPPING OUR FUTURE: A VISION FOR SCHOOL PSYCHOLOGY

We see the 21st century as being ripe for a major positive impact from the field of school psychology if the field sees and seizes the opportunity in a proactive manner. As Sheridan and D'Amato stated in the parallel special issues of *School Psychology Review* and *School Psychology Quarterly* devoted to the proceedings of the 2002 Future of School Psychology Conference:

> Although many visionaries have offered frameworks to advance a new identity for school psychology, one thing is very clear. . . . To realize even the smallest dream for the future of school psychology, it is absolutely essential that all major players—professional organizations, trainers, practitioners—take active steps to make it happen. These steps must be taken

proactively, strategically, and assertively. They must be taken with confidence in one's own skill and expertise but more importantly, they must be taken in cooperation and coordination with others in related fields and disciplines. (2003, p. 354; 2004, p. 8)

We agree that steps toward positive change in the field of school psychology must be taken in cooperation and coordination with our partners in other fields and disciplines. We also believe that the necessity for such coordinated efforts and partnerships should not discourage individual school psychologists from taking small positive steps on their own. As we have stated previously, changes in practice can precede changes in policy. Although top-down change that results from strong and coordinated leadership efforts at the national and state or provincial levels is certainly a model with substantial precedent, bottom-up efforts at the "grassroots" level is also a viable pattern for change. It has been our observation—something we have tried to emphasize within this volume— that individual initiative and efforts of school psychology practitioners, researchers, and trainers, particularly those efforts that are firmly grounded in good theory, science, and practice, are likely to make a significant impact. The "power of one" should not be underestimated.

Although grassroots efforts of individuals and groups can have an enormous positive impact, they also frequently fall by the wayside. Why is this? There are several possible explanations. One possibility we have tried to emphasize is that our efforts to solve problems through the framework of school psychology must be grounded in good theory and science. Efforts that are not built on this solid framework are bound to eventually fail, because no matter how much popularity they attain, they lack the substance to sustain themselves. A somewhat contrasting explanation for failure of efforts within the field of school psychology to make the positive impact that is sought is that, although the scientific base behind our efforts may be solid, these efforts may be misguided in other ways. In other words, we sometimes have situations in which we enlist our considerable scientific, technological, and theoretical resources but focus on unimportant, irrelevant, or ill-considered problems and issues. As Conoley and Gutkin (1995) have stated in their widely cited article on the failure of school psychology to realize its potential:

> School psychology does not suffer from a lack of good science. It suffers from a science that is devoted almost exclusively to answering the wrong sets of questions. It is a science that is preoccupied with the problems of individuals rather than understanding the ecologies in which people function. (p. 210)

We emphatically agree with this criticism. Even if our efforts to enact positive change in delivering educational and mental health services to children and youths are girded by strong theory and scientific rigor, they will ultimately fail if they are focused on the wrong questions, issues, or focal points. An almost obsessive search for within-child psychopathology, preoccupation with descriptive assessment tools that do not inform intervention, and failure to take into account the complex environments and ecological systems in which children exist are but three examples of using theory and science to focus on the wrong issues. For the record, we acknowledge that within-child deficits or dysfunctions do exist and that individually focused assessment and intervention efforts are often necessary. Our concern is that these realities have become the only truth for many practitioners and researchers in our field and that this focus has obscured the more expansive, context-driven view of helping children succeed. For the field of school psychology to move forward in an effective and powerful manner, the major interests and inquiry points of our practitioners, researchers, and trainers must focus on the important issues that are most likely to result in our services influencing positively and in a major way the educational and mental health needs of children and youths.

## Priority Goals and Outcomes from the 2002 Futures Conference

Clearly, efforts to move the field of school psychology forward in achieving its full potential to help serve the educational and mental health needs of children, adolescents, their families, and learning environments must be guided by a strong scientific foundation and must focus on the most critical and functional variables. Successful efforts in this regard must also be guided by a cohesive vision or action plan that articulates clearly the essential goals, outcomes, and domains that will result in the quantity and quality of positive impact we seek. In this regard, we are particularly enthusiastic about the priority goals that emerged from the 2002 Future of School Psychology Conference. Although these goals cannot possibly take into consideration every possible concern, situation, or solution that we must seek in the 21st century, they provide a cohesive road map for moving the field forward over the next several decades. Table 13.1 lists the five general outcome goals identified as critical by conference participants and work-group leaders broken down by subgoals and various types of efforts needed. These outcome goals include improved academic competence for all children (Outcome 1), improved social–emotional functioning for all children (Outcome 2), enhanced family–school partnerships and parental involvement in schools (Outcome 3), more effective education and instruction for all learners (Outcome 4), and increased child and family services in schools that promote health and mental health and are integrated with community services (Outcome 5). According to Dawson, Cummings, Harrison, Short, Gorin, and Palomares (2003, 2004), the 15 priority strategies outlined in Table 13.1 resulted from analyses by work-group chairs at the Futures conference and were later tied to action plans (which are available on the Futures Conference website at www.indiana.edu/~futures). We believe that priority goals and strategies are an example of using a solid scientific-theoretical base to focus on the right issues and that this template can serve as a positive guide to helping the field of school psychology more fully achieve its promise.

## Concluding Comments: Another Look at the "Triangle of Support"

In reviewing the priority goals and outcomes from the 2002 Futures conference (presented in Table 13.1 and in the previous section of this chapter), it is striking to note the strong focus on prevention and early intervention, as well as the explicit emphasis on public health models of service delivery. Each of the five outcome areas includes some emphasis on the need for primary prevention of academic or social–emotional problems, the necessity of early intervention, and/or the importance of using public health models in school psychology service delivery. We emphatically agree that these emphasis areas must be an essential part of the future of school psychology. In several previous chapters of this volume, we have strongly emphasized various models of prevention and early intervention and the need for affecting whole systems, as well as individual children and adolescents. That said, we believe it is appropriate to conclude this final chapter of *School Psychology for the 21st Century* with some additional comments regarding the necessity of moving school psychology practice in this direction.

**TABLE 13.1. Priority Goals and Outcomes from the 2002 Future of School Psychology Conference**

| Outcome | Goal |
| --- | --- |
| *Outcome 1: Improved academic competence for all children* | |
| Advocacy and public policy | Goal A: Advocate for universal early prevention and intervention programs that emphasize language, cognitive, and social–emotional development and are placed in the context of ethnicity, socioeconomic status, gender, and language. |
| Practice | Goal B: Ensure that assessment practices of school psychologists are linked to strategies to improve academic performance and that those assessment practices account for the influence of ethnicity, SES, gender, and language on learning outcomes. |
| Preservice and inservice | Goal C: Develop and implement preservice and inservice training for school psychologists related to universal early prevention and intervention programs. |
| *Outcome 2: Improved social–emotional functioning for all children* | |
| Advocacy and public policy | Goal A: Promote the availability of a comprehensive range of services, from supportive and inclusive placements through interim alternative placements, for students with severe emotional and behavioral disorders. |
| Collaboration and communication | Goal B: Educate all stakeholders about the importance of social–emotional competencies for children. |
| Practice | Goal C: Ensure that school psychologists develop a systematic plan in all schools to reduce social–emotional barriers to learning. |
| *Outcome 3: Enhanced family–school partnerships and parental involvement in schools* | |
| Research and knowledge base | Goal A: Identify evidence-based models of effective family–school partnerships. |
| Practice | Goal B: Ensure that school psychologists engage in activities to change the culture of schooling by making families integral partners in the educational process of children. |
| Preservice training | Goal C: Change preservice education and training of school psychologists candidates to infuse a focus on families as integral partners in the educational process. |
| *Outcome 4: More effective education and instruction for all learners* | |
| Research and knowledge base | Goal A: Identify key components of effective instruction for all learners, including evidence-based approaches to prevention and early intervention for learning problems. |
| Inservice training | Goal B: Provide in-service training for school psychologists in the use of a data-based problem-solving model to implement evidence-based instruction and interventions. |

*(continued)*

**TABLE 13.1.** (*continued*)

| | |
|---|---|
| Preservice and in-service training | Goal C: Implement a national preservice and in-service training initiative for school psychologists regarding effective instruction. |

<u>Outcome 5: Increased child and family services in schools that promote health and mental health and that are integrated with community services</u>

| | |
|---|---|
| Practice | Goal A: Define and promote population-based service delivery in schools and school psychology. |
| In-service training | Goal B: Prepare current practitioners to implement a public health model. |
| Preservice training | Goal C: Prepare future practitioners to implement a public health model. |

*Note.* From Dawson et al. (2003). Copyright 2003 by The Guilford Press. Reprinted by permission.

Figure 13.1 provides another look at the triangle of academic and behavior support model for delivery of school psychology services that has been discussed in prior chapters of this volume. This model is built on the premise that school psychology services should reach all students at all levels of an educational or mental health system. It is also based on the public health model of disease prevention, in which prevention efforts are divided into three distinct areas reflected in the three levels of the triangle (see Adams et al., 1997; Edelstein & Michelson, 1986; Cowen et al., 1996, for more information on public health prevention models). This model is very consistent with the recent trend toward emphasizing positive behavioral and academic supports for stu-

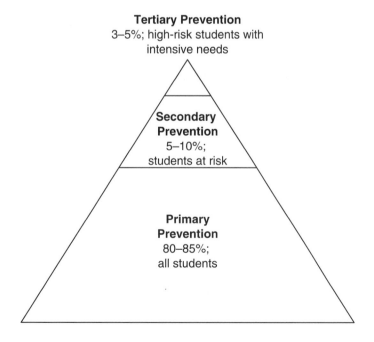

**FIGURE 13.1.** Triangle of support model with levels of prevention from public health model.

dents, as illustrated by the work that has been promoted by the U.S. Department of Education's OSEP Technical Assistance Center on Positive Behavior Supports (see www.pbis.org for more information) and the work of researchers and school systems that is highlighted through this center.

To conclude this final chapter, it is useful to once again consider this "triangle" model and its implications for the practice of school psychology. The bottom of the triangle represents *primary prevention*, the prevention of the occurrence or expression of a particular problem or promotion of universal supports designed to enable, strengthen, or increase likelihood of success. In this model, primary prevention efforts are directed at the 80–85% "typical" students, but in reality, addressing all students—with the understanding that some students will need additional supports. Such efforts are systems- and group-based and involve brief universal screening procedures and the delivery of educational and mental health services within entire classrooms or schools. The middle of the triangle represents *secondary prevention*, or the prevention of side effects or a worsening of an existing problem. Secondary prevention is also conceptualized as early intervention—identifying the early onset of a problem and taking proactive steps to keep the problem from worsening. In the triangle model, secondary prevention services are directed at the 5–15% of students in typical school systems who are beginning to show the signs of academic, behavioral, and/or social–emotional problems or who have significant risk factors that make them vulnerable to such problems. Secondary prevention efforts may involve brief, individual screening and assessment procedures and services delivered within classrooms, within small "pull-out" groups, and, to a limited extent, with individual students identified as at risk. The top of the triangle represents *tertiary prevention*, a concept similar to *rehabilitation*—specific efforts are needed to reduce the serious problem symptoms and to increase the assets of individuals who have severe academic, behavioral, and social–emotional problems with very intense needs. Such services should typically be limited to a small percentage of the entire school population—approximately 3–5% of students whose problems are so serious that they require high-intensity efforts. At this level, assessment efforts are individualized, based on a multi-method design, and comprehensive. Interventions are often delivered individually (such as intense academic tutoring, individual skill training, or mental health counseling). However, in some cases, interventions at the top of the triangle may be delivered in small groups or in classrooms. Special program participation is a given for individual children and youths who require tertiary prevention services to help alleviate their intensive problems. Finally, those students whose intensive needs place them at the very top of the triangle must often receive educational and mental health services in a coordinated manner across school and community settings, using a *wrap-around* model of service in which services are complementary and coordinated and address the full spectrum of needs.

Our view is that the best model of school psychology practice takes into account each of the three levels of the triangle, based on the underlying premises of public health models. In most situations, school psychologists should devote a portion of their time to providing services at each level, thus reaching all students. The desired or optimum distribution of services across each of the three levels will vary with specific assignments and with specific populations, but in general, progressive school psychology services should address all areas—not just the "top of the triangle," as has so often been the case in typical practice. By distributing their expertise across all levels of service delivery needs, school psychologists will ultimately make a larger impact on systems and will prevent many students from "moving up" to a higher level of the triangle.

Public health models of prevention and systems-based "triangle" models of service delivery are nothing new. These models have existed in various stages of refinement within the fields of public health, disease prevention, and community psychology for many years. What is new is the explicit application of these models to the fields of education and children's mental health services in recent years. More specifically, the articulation of these models as a guide to providing effective school psychology services is a new and innovative development. Given the challenges that appear to be looming in the 21st century for children and their families, educational systems, the field of school psychology, and society and culture in general, we believe that these models represent the best hope for the practice of school psychology in the next several decades. Status quo models of school psychology practice that continue the obsession with seeking and identifying pathology, within-child etiologies for learning and social–emotional problems, solving problems exclusively "one child at a time," and providing interventions without considering systemic or ecological contexts are doomed to hinder the progress of the field. We believe that such models, which are unfortunately still very prevalent within school psychology, are ultimately futile and will ultimately be consigned to the junkyard of our professional history. Our optimistic view of the field of school psychology in the 21st century is that it will reach its full promise for positively affecting the educational and mental health needs of children and adolescents. The 20th century evidenced the development and maturation of the field. In the 21st century, school psychologists have a tremendous opportunity and obligation to fulfill the promises that are now within reach.

# DISCUSSION QUESTIONS AND ACTIVITIES

1. Some previous efforts to prognosticate or predict the future of school psychology have been wildly incorrect. Why is the task of prognostication regarding this field so difficult, and what are some of the events that have moved the field in ways that were never previously envisioned?

2. Go the Future of School Psychology website at www.indiana.edu/~futures and review some of the essays, presentation outlines, and conference summary information. After doing so, list what you believe are the two or three most compelling or important things to come out of the Futures conference and why you see these things as so important.

3. We have made some projections or predictions regarding what we believe will be important trends and developments in the near future of the field of school psychology. After reviewing our list of predictions, what things would you, based on your own experiences and conditions in your own area, add to or delete from this list?

4. One of the predictions we have reluctantly made is that the diversity of school psychologists (in terms of gender, ethnicity, and language orientation) will increasingly lag behind the diversity of American society in general. Although numerous efforts have been made to increase the diversity of the field, these efforts have not resulted in making the field more like the population that it serves. Discuss some of the challenges to diversifying the field of school psychology. Brainstorm to develop some innovative ideas on novel ways to more successfully address this issue.

## Appendix A

# The American Psychological Association's Ethical Principles of Psychologists and Code of Conduct (Revised 2002)

# CONTENTS

## 9. Assessment

## 10. Therapy

## INTRODUCTION AND APPLICABILITY

The American Psychological Association's (APA's) Ethical Principles of Psychologists and Code of Conduct (hereinafter referred to as the Ethics Code) consists of an Introduction, a Preamble, five General Principles (A–E), and specific Ethical Standards. The Introduction discusses the intent, organization, procedural considerations, and scope of application of the Ethics Code. The Preamble and General Principles are aspirational goals to guide psychologists toward the highest ideals of psychology. Although the Preamble and General Principles are not themselves enforceable rules, they should be considered by psychologists in arriving at an ethical course of action. The Ethical Standards set forth enforceable rules for conduct as psychologists. Most of the Ethical Standards are written broadly, in order to apply to psychologists in varied roles, although the application of an Ethical Standard may vary depending on the context. The Ethical Standards are not exhaustive. The fact that a given conduct is not specifically addressed by an Ethical Standard does not mean that it is necessarily either ethical or unethical.

This Ethics Code applies only to psychologists' activities that are part of their scientific, educational, or professional roles as psychologists. Areas covered include but are not limited to the clinical, counseling, and school practice of psychology; research; teaching; supervision of trainees; public service; policy development; social intervention; development of assessment instruments; conducting assessments; educational counseling; organizational consulting; forensic activities; program design and evaluation; and administration. This Ethics Code applies to these activities across a variety of contexts, such as in person, postal, telephone, internet, and other electronic transmissions. These activities shall be distinguished from the purely private conduct of psychologists, which is not within the purview of the Ethics Code.

Membership in the APA commits members and student affiliates to comply with the standards of the APA Ethics Code and to the rules and procedures used to enforce them. Lack of awareness or misunderstanding of an Ethical Standard is not itself a defense to a charge of unethical conduct.

The procedures for filing, investigating, and resolving complaints of unethi
cal conduct are described in the current Rules and Procedures of the APA Ethics Committee. APA may impose sanctions on its members for violations of the standards of the Ethics Code, including termination of APA membership, and may notify other bodies and individuals of its actions. Actions that violate the standards of the Ethics Code may also lead to the imposition of sanctions on psychologists or students whether or not they are APA members by bodies other than APA, including state psychological associations, other professional groups, psychology boards, other state or federal agencies, and payors for health services. In addition, APA may take action against a member after his or her conviction of a felony, expulsion or suspension from an affiliated state psychological association, or suspension or loss of licensure. When the sanction to be imposed by APA is less than expulsion, the 2001 Rules and Procedures do not guarantee an opportunity for an in-person hearing, but generally provide that complaints will be resolved only on the basis of a submitted record.

The Ethics Code is intended to provide guidance for psychologists and standards of professional conduct that can be applied by the APA and by other bodies that choose to adopt them. The Ethics Code is not intended to be a basis of civil liability. Whether a psychologist has violated the Ethics Code standards does not by itself determine whether the psychologist is legally liable in a court action, whether a contract is enforceable, or whether other legal consequences occur.

The modifiers used in some of the standards of this Ethics Code (e.g., *reasonably, appropriate, potentially*) are included in the standards when they would (1) allow professional judgment on the part of psychologists, (2) eliminate injustice or inequality that would occur without the modifier, (3) ensure applicability across the broad range of activities conducted by psychologists, or (4) guard against a set of rigid rules that might be quickly outdated. As used in this Ethics Code, the term *reasonable* means the prevailing professional judgment of psychologists engaged in similar activities in similar circumstances, given the knowledge the psychologist had or should have had at the time.

In the process of making decisions regarding their professional behavior, psychologists must consider this Ethics Code in addition to applicable laws and psychology board regulations. In applying the Ethics Code to their professional work, psychologists may consider other materials and guidelines that have been adopted or endorsed by scientific and professional psychological organizations and the dictates of their own conscience, as well as consult with others within the field. If this Ethics Code establishes a higher standard of conduct than is required by law, psychologists must meet the higher ethical standard. If psychologists' ethical responsibilities conflict with law, regulations, or other governing legal authority, psychologists make known their commitment to this Ethics Code and take steps to resolve the conflict in a responsible manner. If the conflict is unresolvable via such means, psychologists may adhere to the requirements of the law, regulations, or other governing authority in keeping with basic principles of human rights.

# PREAMBLE

Psychologists are committed to increasing scientific and professional knowledge of behavior and people's understanding of themselves and others and to the use of such knowledge to improve the condition of individuals, organizations, and society. Psychologists respect and protect civil and human rights and the central importance of freedom of inquiry and expression in research, teaching, and publication. They strive to help the public in developing informed judgments and choices concerning human behavior. In doing so, they perform many roles, such as researcher, educator, diagnostician, therapist, supervisor, consultant, administrator, social interventionist, and expert witness. This Ethics Code provides a common set of principles and standards upon which psychologists build their professional and scientific work.

This Ethics Code is intended to provide specific standards to cover most situations encountered by psychologists. It has as its goals the welfare and protection of the individuals and groups with whom psychologists work and the education of members, students, and the public regarding ethical standards of the discipline.

The development of a dynamic set of ethical standards for psychologists' work-related conduct requires a personal commitment and lifelong effort to act ethically; to encourage ethical behavior by students, supervisees, employees, and colleagues; and to consult with others concerning ethical problems.

# GENERAL PRINCIPLES

This section consists of General Principles. General Principles, as opposed to Ethical Standards, are aspirational in nature. Their intent is to guide and inspire psychologists toward the very highest ethical ideals of the profession. General Principles, in contrast to Ethical Standards, do not represent obligations and should not form the basis for imposing sanctions. Relying upon General Principles for either of these reasons distorts both their meaning and purpose.

## Principle A: Beneficence and Nonmaleficence

Psychologists strive to benefit those with whom they work and take care to do no harm. In their professional actions, psychologists seek to safeguard the welfare and rights of those with whom they interact professionally and other affected persons, and the welfare of animal subjects of research. When conflicts occur among psychologists' obligations or concerns, they attempt to resolve these conflicts in a responsible fashion that avoids or minimizes harm. Because psychologists' scientific and professional judgments and actions may affect the lives of others, they are alert to and guard against personal, financial, social, organizational, or political factors that might lead to misuse of their influence. Psychologists strive to be aware of the possible effect of their own physical and mental health on their ability to help those with whom they work.

## Principle B: Fidelity and Responsibility

Psychologists establish relationships of trust with those with whom they work. They are aware of their professional and scientific responsibilities to society and to the specific communities in which they work. Psychologists uphold professional standards of conduct, clarify their professional roles and obligations, accept appropriate responsibility for their behavior, and seek to manage conflicts of interest that could lead to exploitation or harm. Psychologists consult with, refer to, or cooperate with other professionals and institutions to the extent needed to serve the best interests of those with whom they work. They are concerned about the ethical compliance of their colleagues' scientific and professional conduct. Psychologists strive to contribute a portion of their professional time for little or no compensation or personal advantage.

## Principle C: Integrity

Psychologists seek to promote accuracy, honesty, and truthfulness in the science, teaching, and practice of psychology. In these activities psychologists do not steal, cheat, or engage in fraud, subterfuge, or intentional misrepresentation of fact. Psychologists strive to keep their promises and to avoid unwise or unclear commitments. In situations in which deception may be ethically justifiable to maximize benefits and minimize harm, psychologists have a serious obligation to consider the need for, the possible consequences of, and their responsibility to correct any resulting mistrust or other harmful effects that arise from the use of such techniques.

## Principle D: Justice

Psychologists recognize that fairness and justice entitle all persons to access to and benefit from the contributions of psychology and to equal quality in the processes, procedures, and services being conducted by psychologists. Psychologists exercise reasonable judgment and take precautions to ensure that their potential biases, the boundaries of their competence, and the limitations of their expertise do not lead to or condone unjust practices.

## Principle E: Respect for People's Rights and Dignity

Psychologists respect the dignity and worth of all people, and the rights of individuals to privacy, confidentiality, and self-determination. Psychologists are aware that special safeguards may be necessary to protect the rights and welfare of persons or communities whose vulnerabilities impair autonomous decision making. Psychologists are aware of and respect cultural, individual, and role differences, including those based on age, gender, gender identity, race, ethnicity, culture, national origin, religion, sexual orientation, disability, language, and socioeconomic status and consider these factors when working with members of such groups. Psychologists try to eliminate the effect on their work of biases based on those factors, and they do not knowingly participate in or condone activities of others based upon such prejudices.

## ETHICAL STANDARDS

### 1. Resolving Ethical Issues

*1.01 Misuse of Psychologists' Work*

If psychologists learn of misuse or misrepresentation of their work, they take reasonable steps to correct or minimize the misuse or misrepresentation.

*1.02 Conflicts between Ethics and Law, Regulations, or Other Governing Legal Authority*

If psychologists' ethical responsibilities conflict with law, regulations, or other governing legal authority, psychologists make known their commitment to the Ethics Code and take steps to resolve the conflict. If the conflict is unresolvable via such means, psychologists may adhere to the requirements of the law, regulations, or other governing legal authority.

*1.03 Conflicts between Ethics and Organizational Demands*

If the demands of an organization with which psychologists are affiliated or for whom they are working conflict with this Ethics Code, psychologists clarify the nature of the conflict, make known their commitment to the Ethics Code, and to the extent feasible, resolve the conflict in a way that permits adherence to the Ethics Code.

*1.04 Informal Resolution of Ethical Violations*

When psychologists believe that there may have been an ethical violation by another psychologist, they attempt to resolve the issue by bringing it to the attention of that individual, if an informal resolution appears appropriate and the intervention does not violate any confidentiality rights that may be involved. (See also Standards 1.02, Conflicts Between Ethics and Law, Regulations, or Other Governing Legal Authority, and 1.03, Conflicts Between Ethics and Organizational Demands.)

*1.05 Reporting Ethical Violations*

If an apparent ethical violation has substantially harmed or is likely to substantially harm a person or organization and is not appropriate for informal resolution under Standard 1.04, Informal Resolution of Ethical Violations, or is not resolved properly in that fashion, psychologists take further action appropriate to the situation. Such action might include referral to state or national committees on professional ethics, to state licensing boards, or to the appropriate institutional authorities. This standard does not apply when an intervention would violate confidentiality rights or when psychologists have been retained to review the work of another psychologist whose professional conduct is in question. (See also Standard 1.02, Conflicts Between Ethics and Law, Regulations, or Other Governing Legal Authority.)

*1.06 Cooperating with Ethics Committees*

Psychologists cooperate in ethics investigations, proceedings, and resulting requirements of the APA or any affiliated state psychological association to which they belong. In doing so, they address any confidentiality issues. Failure to cooperate is itself an ethics violation. However, making a request for deferment of adjudication of an ethics complaint pending the outcome of litigation does not alone constitute noncooperation.

## 1.07 Improper Complaints

Psychologists do not file or encourage the filing of ethics complaints that are made with reckless disregard for or willful ignorance of facts that would disprove the allegation.

## 1.08 Unfair Discrimination against Complainants and Respondents

Psychologists do not deny persons employment, advancement, admissions to academic or other programs, tenure, or promotion, based solely upon their having made or their being the subject of an ethics complaint. This does not preclude taking action based upon the outcome of such proceedings or considering other appropriate information.

## 2. Competence

### 2.01 Boundaries of Competence

(a) Psychologists provide services, teach, and conduct research with populations and in areas only within the boundaries of their competence, based on their education, training, supervised experience, consultation, study, or professional experience.

(b) Where scientific or professional knowledge in the discipline of psychology establishes that an understanding of factors associated with age, gender, gender identity, race, ethnicity, culture, national origin, religion, sexual orientation, disability, language, or socioeconomic status is essential for effective implementation of their services or research, psychologists have or obtain the training, experience, consultation, or supervision necessary to ensure the competence of their services, or they make appropriate referrals, except as provided in Standard 2.02, Providing Services in Emergencies.

(c) Psychologists planning to provide services, teach, or conduct research involving populations, areas, techniques, or technologies new to them undertake relevant education, training, supervised experience, consultation, or study.

(d) When psychologists are asked to provide services to individuals for whom appropriate mental health services are not available and for which psychologists have not obtained the competence necessary, psychologists with closely related prior training or experience may provide such services in order to ensure that services are not denied if they make a reasonable effort to obtain the competence required by using relevant research, training, consultation, or study.

(e) In those emerging areas in which generally recognized standards for preparatory training do not yet exist, psychologists nevertheless take reasonable steps to ensure the competence of their work and to protect clients/patients, students, supervisees, research participants, organizational clients, and others from harm.

(f) When assuming forensic roles, psychologists are or become reasonably familiar with the judicial or administrative rules governing their roles.

### 2.02 Providing Services in Emergencies

In emergencies, when psychologists provide services to individuals for whom other mental health services are not available and for which psychologists have not obtained the necessary training, psychologists may provide such services in order to ensure that services are not denied. The services are discontinued as soon as the emergency has ended or appropriate services are available.

### 2.03 Maintaining Competence

Psychologists undertake ongoing efforts to develop and maintain their competence.

### 2.04 Bases for Scientific and Professional Judgments

Psychologists' work is based upon established scientific and professional knowledge of the discipline. (See also Standards 2.01e, Boundaries of Competence, and 10.01b, Informed Consent to Therapy.)

### 2.05 Delegation of Work to Others

Psychologists who delegate work to employees, supervisees, or research or teaching assistants or who use the services of others, such as interpreters, take reasonable steps to (1) avoid delegating such work to persons who have a multiple relationship with those being served that would likely lead to exploitation or loss of objectivity; (2) authorize only those responsibilities that such persons can be expected to perform competently on the basis of their education, training, or experience, either independently or with the level of supervision being provided; and (3) see that such persons perform these services competently. (See also Standards 2.02, Providing Services in Emergencies; 3.05, Multiple Relationships; 4.01, Maintaining Confidentiality; 9.01, Bases for Assessments; 9.02, Use of Assessments; 9.03, Informed Consent in Assessments; and 9.07, Assessment by Unqualified Persons.)

### 2.06 Personal Problems and Conflicts

(a) Psychologists refrain from initiating an activity when they know or should know that there is a substantial likelihood that their personal problems will prevent them from performing their work-related activities in a competent manner.

(b) When psychologists become aware of personal problems that may interfere with their performing work-related duties adequately, they take appropriate measures, such as obtaining professional consultation or assistance, and determine whether they should limit, suspend, or terminate their work-related duties. (See also Standard 10.10, Terminating Therapy.)

## 3. Human Relations

### 3.01 Unfair Discrimination

In their work-related activities, psychologists do not engage in unfair discrimination based on age, gender, gender identity, race, ethnicity, culture, national origin, religion, sexual orientation, disability, socioeconomic status, or any basis proscribed by law.

### 3.02 Sexual Harassment

Psychologists do not engage in sexual harassment. Sexual harassment is sexual solicitation, physical advances, or verbal or nonverbal conduct that is sexual in nature, that occurs in connection with the psychologist's activities or roles as a psychologist, and that either (1) is unwelcome, is offensive, or creates a hostile workplace or educational environment, and the psychologist knows or is told this or (2) is sufficiently severe or intense to be abusive to a reasonable person in the context. Sexual harassment can consist of a single intense or severe act or of multiple persistent or pervasive acts. (See also Standard 1.08, Unfair Discrimination Against Complainants and Respondents.)

### 3.03 Other Harassment

Psychologists do not knowingly engage in behavior that is harassing or demeaning to persons with whom they interact in their work based on factors such as those persons' age, gender, gender identity, race, ethnicity, culture, national origin, religion, sexual orientation, disability, language, or socioeconomic status.

### 3.04 Avoiding Harm

Psychologists take reasonable steps to avoid harming their clients/patients, students, supervisees, research participants, organizational clients, and others with whom they work, and to minimize harm where it is foreseeable and unavoidable.

### 3.05 Multiple Relationships

(a) A multiple relationship occurs when a psychologist is in a professional role with a person and (1) at the same time is in another role with the same person, (2) at the same time is in a relationship with a person closely associated with or related to the person with whom the psychologist has the professional relationship, or (3) promises to enter into another relationship in the future with the person or a person closely associated with or related to the person.

A psychologist refrains from entering into a multiple relationship if the multiple relationship could reasonably be expected to impair the psychologist's objectivity, competence, or effectiveness in performing his or her functions as a psychologist, or otherwise risks exploitation or harm to the person with whom the professional relationship exists.

Multiple relationships that would not reasonably be expected to cause impairment or risk exploitation or harm are not unethical.

(b) If a psychologist finds that, due to unforeseen factors, a potentially harmful multiple relationship has arisen, the psychologist takes reasonable steps to resolve it with due regard for the best interests of the affected person and maximal compliance with the Ethics Code.

(c) When psychologists are required by law, institutional policy, or extraordinary circumstances to serve in more than one role in judicial or administrative proceedings, at the outset they clarify role expectations and the extent of confidentiality and thereafter as changes occur. (See also Standards 3.04, Avoiding Harm, and 3.07, Third-Party Requests for Services.)

### 3.06 Conflict of Interest

Psychologists refrain from taking on a professional role when personal, scientific, professional, legal, financial, or other interests or relationships could reasonably be expected to (1) impair their objectivity, competence, or effectiveness in performing their functions as psychologists or (2) expose the person or organization with whom the professional relationship exists to harm or exploitation.

## 3.07 Third-Party Requests for Services

When psychologists agree to provide services to a person or entity at the request of a third party, psychologists attempt to clarify at the outset of the service the nature of the relationship with all individuals or organizations involved. This clarification includes the role of the psychologist (e.g., therapist, consultant, diagnostician, or expert witness), an identification of who is the client, the probable uses of the services provided or the information obtained, and the fact that there may be limits to confidentiality. (See also Standards 3.05, Multiple Relationships, and 4.02, Discussing the Limits of Confidentiality.)

## 3.08 Exploitative Relationships

Psychologists do not exploit persons over whom they have supervisory, evaluative, or other authority such as clients/patients, students, supervisees, research participants, and employees. (See also Standards 3.05, Multiple Relationships; 6.04, Fees and Financial Arrangements; 6.05, Barter With Clients/Patients; 7.07, Sexual Relationships With Students and Supervisees; 10.05, Sexual Intimacies With Current Therapy Clients/Patients; 10.06, Sexual Intimacies With Relatives or Significant Others of Current Therapy Clients/Patients; 10.07, Therapy With Former Sexual Partners; and 10.08, Sexual Intimacies With Former Therapy Clients/Patients.)

## 3.09 Cooperation with Other Professionals

When indicated and professionally appropriate, psychologists cooperate with other professionals in order to serve their clients/patients effectively and appropriately. (See also Standard 4.05, Disclosures.)

## 3.10 Informed Consent

(a) When psychologists conduct research or provide assessment, therapy, counseling, or consulting services in person or via electronic transmission or other forms of communication, they obtain the informed consent of the individual or individuals using language that is reasonably understandable to that person or persons except when conducting such activities without consent is mandated by law or governmental regulation or as otherwise provided in this Ethics Code. (See also Standards 8.02, Informed Consent to Research; 9.03, Informed Consent in Assessments; and 10.01, Informed Consent to Therapy.)

(b) For persons who are legally incapable of giving informed consent, psychologists nevertheless (1) provide an appropriate explanation, (2) seek the individual's assent, (3) consider such persons' preferences and best interests, and (4) obtain appropriate permission from a legally authorized person, if such substitute consent is permitted or required by law. When consent by a legally authorized person is not permitted or required by law, psychologists take reasonable steps to protect the individual's rights and welfare.

(c) When psychological services are court ordered or otherwise mandated, psychologists inform the individual of the nature of the anticipated services, including whether the services are court ordered or mandated and any limits of confidentiality, before proceeding.

(d) Psychologists appropriately document written or oral consent, permission, and assent. (See also Standards 8.02, Informed Consent to Research; 9.03, Informed Consent in Assessments; and 10.01, Informed Consent to Therapy.)

### 3.11 Psychological Services Delivered to or through Organizations

(a) Psychologists delivering services to or through organizations provide information before-hand to clients and when appropriate those directly affected by the services about (1) the nature and objectives of the services, (2) the intended recipients, (3) which of the individuals are clients, (4) the relationship the psychologist will have with each person and the organization, (5) the probable uses of services provided and information obtained, (6) who will have access to the information, and (7) limits of confidentiality. As soon as feasible, they provide information about the results and conclusions of such services to appropriate persons.

(b) If psychologists will be precluded by law or by organizational roles from providing such information to particular individuals or groups, they so inform those individuals or groups at the outset of the service.

### 3.12 Interruption of Psychological Services

Unless otherwise covered by contract, psychologists make reasonable efforts to plan for facilitating services in the event that psychological services are interrupted by factors such as the psychologist's illness, death, unavailability, relocation, or retirement or by the client's/patient's relocation or financial limitations. (See also Standard 6.02c, Maintenance, Dissemination, and Disposal of Confidential Records of Professional and Scientific Work.)

## 4. Privacy and Confidentiality

### 4.01 Maintaining Confidentiality

Psychologists have a primary obligation and take reasonable precautions to protect confidential information obtained through or stored in any medium, recognizing that the extent and limits of confidentiality may be regulated by law or established by institutional rules or professional or scientific relationship. (See also Standard 2.05, Delegation of Work to Others.)

### 4.02 Discussing the Limits of Confidentiality

(a) Psychologists discuss with persons (including, to the extent feasible, persons who are legally incapable of giving informed consent and their legal representatives) and organizations with whom they establish a scientific or professional relationship (1) the relevant limits of confidentiality and (2) the foreseeable uses of the information generated through their psychological activities. (See also Standard 3.10, Informed Consent.)

(b) Unless it is not feasible or is contraindicated, the discussion of confidentiality occurs at the outset of the relationship and thereafter as new circumstances may warrant.

(c) Psychologists who offer services, products, or information via electronic transmission inform clients/patients of the risks to privacy and limits of confidentiality.

### 4.03 Recording

Before recording the voices or images of individuals to whom they provide services, psychologists obtain permission from all such persons or their legal representatives. (See also Standards 8.03, Informed Consent for Recording Voices and Images in Research; 8.05, Dispensing with Informed Consent for Research; and 8.07, Deception in Research.)

## 4.04 Minimizing Intrusions on Privacy

(a) Psychologists include in written and oral reports and consultations, only information germane to the purpose for which the communication is made.

(b) Psychologists discuss confidential information obtained in their work only for appropriate scientific or professional purposes and only with persons clearly concerned with such matters.

## 4.05 Disclosures

(a) Psychologists may disclose confidential information with the appropriate consent of the organizational client, the individual client/patient, or another legally authorized person on behalf of the client/patient unless prohibited by law.

(b) Psychologists disclose confidential information without the consent of the individual only as mandated by law, or where permitted by law for a valid purpose such as to (1) provide needed professional services; (2) obtain appropriate professional consultations; (3) protect the client/patient, psychologist, or others from harm; or (4) obtain payment for services from a client/patient, in which instance disclosure is limited to the minimum that is necessary to achieve the purpose. (See also Standard 6.04e, Fees and Financial Arrangements.)

## 4.06 Consultations

When consulting with colleagues, (1) psychologists do not disclose confidential information that reasonably could lead to the identification of a client/patient, research participant, or other person or organization with whom they have a confidential relationship unless they have obtained the prior consent of the person or organization or the disclosure cannot be avoided, and (2) they disclose information only to the extent necessary to achieve the purposes of the consultation. (See also Standard 4.01, Maintaining Confidentiality.)

## 4.07 Use of Confidential Information for Didactic or Other Purposes

Psychologists do not disclose in their writings, lectures, or other public media, confidential, personally identifiable information concerning their clients/patients, students, research participants, organizational clients, or other recipients of their services that they obtained during the course of their work, unless (1) they take reasonable steps to disguise the person or organization, (2) the person or organization has consented in writing, or (3) there is legal authorization for doing so.

## 5. Advertising and Other Public Statements

### 5.01 Avoidance of False or Deceptive Statements

(a) Public statements include but are not limited to paid or unpaid advertising, product endorsements, grant applications, licensing applications, other credentialing applications, brochures, printed matter, directory listings, personal resumes or curricula vitae, or comments for use in media such as print or electronic transmission, statements in legal proceedings, lectures and public oral presentations, and published materials. Psychologists do not knowingly make public statements that are false, deceptive, or fraudulent concerning their research, practice, or other work activities or those of persons or organizations with which they are affiliated.

(b) Psychologists do not make false, deceptive, or fraudulent statements concerning (1) their training, experience, or competence; (2) their academic degrees; (3) their credentials; (4) their institutional or association affiliations; (5) their services; (6) the scientific or clinical basis for, or results or degree of success of, their services; (7) their fees; or (8) their publications or research findings.

(c) Psychologists claim degrees as credentials for their health services only if those degrees (1) were earned from a regionally accredited educational institution or (2) were the basis for psychology licensure by the state in which they practice.

## 5.02 Statements by Others

(a) Psychologists who engage others to create or place public statements that promote their professional practice, products, or activities retain professional responsibility for such statements.

(b) Psychologists do not compensate employees of press, radio, television, or other communication media in return for publicity in a news item. (See also Standard 1.01, Misuse of Psychologists' Work.)

(c) A paid advertisement relating to psychologists' activities must be identified or clearly recognizable as such.

## 5.03 Descriptions of Workshops and Non-Degree-Granting Educational Programs

To the degree to which they exercise control, psychologists responsible for announcements, catalogs, brochures, or advertisements describing workshops, seminars, or other non-degree-granting educational programs ensure that they accurately describe the audience for which the program is intended, the educational objectives, the presenters, and the fees involved.

## 5.04 Media Presentations

When psychologists provide public advice or comment via print, internet, or other electronic transmission, they take precautions to ensure that statements (1) are based on their professional knowledge, training, or experience in accord with appropriate psychological literature and practice; (2) are otherwise consistent with this Ethics Code; and (3) do not indicate that a professional relationship has been established with the recipient. (See also Standard 2.04, Bases for Scientific and Professional Judgments.)

## 5.05 Testimonials

Psychologists do not solicit testimonials from current therapy clients/patients or other persons who because of their particular circumstances are vulnerable to undue influence.

## 5.06 In-Person Solicitation

Psychologists do not engage, directly or through agents, in uninvited in-person solicitation of business from actual or potential therapy clients/patients or other persons who because of their particular circumstances are vulnerable to undue influence. However, this prohibition does not preclude (1) attempting to implement appropriate collateral contacts for the purpose of benefiting an already engaged therapy client/patient or (2) providing disaster or community outreach services.

## 6. Record Keeping and Fees

### 6.01 Documentation of Professional and Scientific Work and Maintenance of Records

Psychologists create, and to the extent the records are under their control, maintain, disseminate, store, retain, and dispose of records and data relating to their professional and scientific work in order to (1) facilitate provision of services later by them or by other professionals, (2) allow for replication of research design and analyses, (3) meet institutional requirements, (4) ensure accuracy of billing and payments, and (5) ensure compliance with law. (See also Standard 4.01, Maintaining Confidentiality.)

### 6.02 Maintenance, Dissemination, and Disposal of Confidential Records of Professional and Scientific Work

(a) Psychologists maintain confidentiality in creating, storing, accessing, transferring, and disposing of records under their control, whether these are written, automated, or in any other medium. (See also Standards 4.01, Maintaining Confidentiality, and 6.01, Documentation of Professional and Scientific Work and Maintenance of Records.)

(b) If confidential information concerning recipients of psychological services is entered into databases or systems of records available to persons whose access has not been consented to by the recipient, psychologists use coding or other techniques to avoid the inclusion of personal identifiers.

(c) Psychologists make plans in advance to facilitate the appropriate transfer and to protect the confidentiality of records and data in the event of psychologists' withdrawal from positions or practice. (See also Standards 3.12, Interruption of Psychological Services, and 10.09, Interruption of Therapy.)

### 6.03 Withholding Records for Nonpayment

Psychologists may not withhold records under their control that are requested and needed for a client's/patient's emergency treatment solely because payment has not been received.

### 6.04 Fees and Financial Arrangements

(a) As early as is feasible in a professional or scientific relationship, psychologists and recipients of psychological services reach an agreement specifying compensation and billing arrangements.

(b) Psychologists' fee practices are consistent with law.

(c) Psychologists do not misrepresent their fees.

(d) If limitations to services can be anticipated because of limitations in financing, this is discussed with the recipient of services as early as is feasible. (See also Standards 10.09, Interruption of Therapy, and 10.10, Terminating Therapy.)

(e) If the recipient of services does not pay for services as agreed, and if psychologists intend to use collection agencies or legal measures to collect the fees, psychologists first inform the person that such measures will be taken and provide that person an opportunity to make prompt payment. (See also Standards 4.05, Disclosures; 6.03, Withholding Records for Nonpayment; and 10.01, Informed Consent to Therapy.)

### 6.05 Barter with Clients/Patients

Barter is the acceptance of goods, services, or other nonmonetary remuneration from clients/ patients in return for psychological services. Psychologists may barter only if (1) it is not clinically contraindicated, and (2) the resulting arrangement is not exploitative. (See also Standards 3.05, Multiple Relationships, and 6.04, Fees and Financial Arrangements.)

### 6.06 Accuracy in Reports to Payors and Funding Sources

In their reports to payors for services or sources of research funding, psychologists take reasonable steps to ensure the accurate reporting of the nature of the service provided or research conducted, the fees, charges, or payments, and where applicable, the identity of the provider, the findings, and the diagnosis. (See also Standards 4.01, Maintaining Confidentiality; 4.04, Minimizing Intrusions on Privacy; and 4.05, Disclosures.)

### 6.07 Referrals and Fees

When psychologists pay, receive payment from, or divide fees with another professional, other than in an employer-employee relationship, the payment to each is based on the services provided (clinical, consultative, administrative, or other) and is not based on the referral itself. (See also Standard 3.09, Cooperation with Other Professionals.)

## 7. Education and Training

### 7.01 Design of Education and Training Programs

Psychologists responsible for education and training programs take reasonable steps to ensure that the programs are designed to provide the appropriate knowledge and proper experiences, and to meet the requirements for licensure, certification, or other goals for which claims are made by the program. (See also Standard 5.03, Descriptions of Workshops and Non-Degree-Granting Educational Programs.)

### 7.02 Descriptions of Education and Training Programs

Psychologists responsible for education and training programs take reasonable steps to ensure that there is a current and accurate description of the program content (including participation in required course- or program-related counseling, psychotherapy, experiential groups, consulting projects, or community service), training goals and objectives, stipends and benefits, and requirements that must be met for satisfactory completion of the program. This information must be made readily available to all interested parties.

### 7.03 Accuracy in Teaching

(a) Psychologists take reasonable steps to ensure that course syllabi are accurate regarding the subject matter to be covered, bases for evaluating progress, and the nature of course experiences. This standard does not preclude an instructor from modifying course content or requirements when the instructor considers it pedagogically necessary or desirable, so long as students are made aware of these modifications in a manner that enables them to fulfill course requirements. (See also Standard 5.01, Avoidance of False or Deceptive Statements.)

(b) When engaged in teaching or training, psychologists present psychological information accurately. (See also Standard 2.03, Maintaining Competence.)

## 7.04 Student Disclosure of Personal Information

Psychologists do not require students or supervisees to disclose personal information in course- or program-related activities, either orally or in writing, regarding sexual history, history of abuse and neglect, psychological treatment, and relationships with parents, peers, and spouses or significant others except if (1) the program or training facility has clearly identified this requirement in its admissions and program materials or (2) the information is necessary to evaluate or obtain assistance for students whose personal problems could reasonably be judged to be preventing them from performing their training- or professionally related activities in a competent manner or posing a threat to the students or others.

## 7.05 Mandatory Individual or Group Therapy

(a) When individual or group therapy is a program or course requirement, psychologists responsible for that program allow students in undergraduate and graduate programs the option of selecting such therapy from practitioners unaffiliated with the program. (See also Standard 7.02, Descriptions of Education and Training Programs.)

(b) Faculty who are or are likely to be responsible for evaluating students' academic performance do not themselves provide that therapy. (See also Standard 3.05, Multiple Relationships.)

## 7.06 Assessing Student and Supervisee Performance

(a) In academic and supervisory relationships, psychologists establish a timely and specific process for providing feedback to students and supervisees. Information regarding the process is provided to the student at the beginning of supervision.

(b) Psychologists evaluate students and supervisees on the basis of their actual performance on relevant and established program requirements.

## 7.07 Sexual Relationships with Students and Supervisees

Psychologists do not engage in sexual relationships with students or supervisees who are in their department, agency, or training center or over whom psychologists have or are likely to have evaluative authority. (See also Standard 3.05, Multiple Relationships.)

## 8. Research and Publication

## 8.01 Institutional Approval

When institutional approval is required, psychologists provide accurate information about their research proposals and obtain approval prior to conducting the research. They conduct the research in accordance with the approved research protocol.

## 8.02 Informed Consent to Research

(a) When obtaining informed consent as required in Standard 3.10, Informed Consent, psychologists inform participants about (1) the purpose of the research, expected duration, and procedures; (2) their right to decline to participate and to withdraw from the research once participation has begun; (3) the foreseeable consequences of declining or withdrawing; (4) reasonably foreseeable factors that may be expected to influence their willingness to participate such as potential risks, discomfort, or adverse effects; (5) any prospective research benefits; (6) limits of confidentiality; (7) incentives for participation; and (8) whom to contact for questions about the research and research participants' rights. They provide opportunity for the prospective participants to ask questions and receive answers. (See also Standards 8.03, Informed Consent for Recording Voices and Images in Research; 8.05, Dispensing with Informed Consent for Research; and 8.07, Deception in Research.)

(b) Psychologists conducting intervention research involving the use of experimental treatments clarify to participants at the outset of the research (1) the experimental nature of the treatment; (2) the services that will or will not be available to the control group(s) if appropriate; (3) the means by which assignment to treatment and control groups will be made; (4) available treatment alternatives if an individual does not wish to participate in the research or wishes to withdraw once a study has begun; and (5) compensation for or monetary costs of participating including, if appropriate, whether reimbursement from the participant or a third-party payor will be sought. (See also Standard 8.02a, Informed Consent to Research.)

## 8.03 Informed Consent for Recording Voices and Images in Research

Psychologists obtain informed consent from research participants prior to recording their voices or images for data collection unless (1) the research consists solely of naturalistic observations in public places, and it is not anticipated that the recording will be used in a manner that could cause personal identification or harm, or (2) the research design includes deception, and consent for the use of the recording is obtained during debriefing. (See also Standard 8.07, Deception in Research.)

## 8.04 Client/Patient, Student, and Subordinate Research Participants

(a) When psychologists conduct research with clients/patients, students, or subordinates as participants, psychologists take steps to protect the prospective participants from adverse consequences of declining or withdrawing from participation.

(b) When research participation is a course requirement or an opportunity for extra credit, the prospective participant is given the choice of equitable alternative activities.

## 8.05 Dispensing with Informed Consent for Research

Psychologists may dispense with informed consent only (1) where research would not reasonably be assumed to create distress or harm and involves (a) the study of normal educational practices, curricula, or classroom management methods conducted in educational settings; (b) only anonymous questionnaires, naturalistic observations, or archival research for which disclosure of responses would not place participants at risk of criminal or civil liability or damage their financial standing, employability, or reputation, and confidentiality is protected; or (c) the study of factors related to job or organization effectiveness conducted in organizational settings for which there is no risk to participants' employability, and confidentiality is protected or (2) where otherwise permitted by law or federal or institutional regulations.

## 8.06 Offering Inducements for Research Participation

(a) Psychologists make reasonable efforts to avoid offering excessive or inappropriate financial or other inducements for research participation when such inducements are likely to coerce participation.

(b) When offering professional services as an inducement for research participation, psychologists clarify the nature of the services, as well as the risks, obligations, and limitations. (See also Standard 6.05, Barter With Clients/Patients.)

## 8.07 Deception in Research

(a) Psychologists do not conduct a study involving deception unless they have determined that the use of deceptive techniques is justified by the study's significant prospective scientific, educational, or applied value and that effective nondeceptive alternative procedures are not feasible.

(b) Psychologists do not deceive prospective participants about research that is reasonably expected to cause physical pain or severe emotional distress.

(c) Psychologists explain any deception that is an integral feature of the design and conduct of an experiment to participants as early as is feasible, preferably at the conclusion of their participation, but no later than at the conclusion of the data collection, and permit participants to withdraw their data. (See also Standard 8.08, Debriefing.)

## 8.08 Debriefing

(a) Psychologists provide a prompt opportunity for participants to obtain appropriate information about the nature, results, and conclusions of the research, and they take reasonable steps to correct any misconceptions that participants may have of which the psychologists are aware.

(b) If scientific or humane values justify delaying or withholding this information, psychologists take reasonable measures to reduce the risk of harm.

(c) When psychologists become aware that research procedures have harmed a participant, they take reasonable steps to minimize the harm.

## 8.09 Humane Care and Use of Animals in Research

(a) Psychologists acquire, care for, use, and dispose of animals in compliance with current federal, state, and local laws and regulations, and with professional standards.

(b) Psychologists trained in research methods and experienced in the care of laboratory animals supervise all procedures involving animals and are responsible for ensuring appropriate consideration of their comfort, health, and humane treatment.

(c) Psychologists ensure that all individuals under their supervision who are using animals have received instruction in research methods and in the care, maintenance, and handling of the species being used, to the extent appropriate to their role. (See also Standard 2.05, Delegation of Work to Others.)

(d) Psychologists make reasonable efforts to minimize the discomfort, infection, illness, and pain of animal subjects.

(e) Psychologists use a procedure subjecting animals to pain, stress, or privation only when an alternative procedure is unavailable and the goal is justified by its prospective scientific, educational, or applied value.

(f) Psychologists perform surgical procedures under appropriate anesthesia and follow techniques to avoid infection and minimize pain during and after surgery.

(g) When it is appropriate that an animal's life be terminated, psychologists proceed rapidly, with an effort to minimize pain and in accordance with accepted procedures.

### 8.10 Reporting Research Results

(a) Psychologists do not fabricate data. (See also Standard 5.01a, Avoidance of False or Deceptive Statements.)

(b) If psychologists discover significant errors in their published data, they take reasonable steps to correct such errors in a correction, retraction, erratum, or other appropriate publication means.

### 8.11 Plagiarism

Psychologists do not present portions of another's work or data as their own, even if the other work or data source is cited occasionally.

### 8.12 Publication Credit

(a) Psychologists take responsibility and credit, including authorship credit, only for work they have actually performed or to which they have substantially contributed. (See also Standard 8.12b, Publication Credit.)

(b) Principal authorship and other publication credits accurately reflect the relative scientific or professional contributions of the individuals involved, regardless of their relative status. Mere possession of an institutional position, such as department chair, does not justify authorship credit. Minor contributions to the research or to the writing for publications are acknowledged appropriately, such as in footnotes or in an introductory statement.

(c) Except under exceptional circumstances, a student is listed as principal author on any multiple-authored article that is substantially based on the student's doctoral dissertation. Faculty advisors discuss publication credit with students as early as feasible and throughout the research and publication process as appropriate. (See also Standard 8.12b, Publication Credit.)

### 8.13 Duplicate Publication of Data

Psychologists do not publish, as original data, data that have been previously published. This does not preclude republishing data when they are accompanied by proper acknowledgment.

### 8.14 Sharing Research Data for Verification

(a) After research results are published, psychologists do not withhold the data on which their conclusions are based from other competent professionals who seek to verify the substantive claims through reanalysis and who intend to use such data only for that purpose, provided that the confidentiality of the participants can be protected and unless legal rights concerning proprietary data preclude their release. This does not preclude psychologists from requiring that such individuals or groups be responsible for costs associated with the provision of such information.

(b) Psychologists who request data from other psychologists to verify the substantive claims through reanalysis may use shared data only for the declared purpose. Requesting psychologists obtain prior written agreement for all other uses of the data.

## 8.15 Reviewers

Psychologists who review material submitted for presentation, publication, grant, or research proposal review respect the confidentiality of and the proprietary rights in such information of those who submitted it.

## 9. Assessment

### 9.01 Bases for Assessments

(a) Psychologists base the opinions contained in their recommendations, reports, and diagnostic or evaluative statements, including forensic testimony, on information and techniques sufficient to substantiate their findings. (See also Standard 2.04, Bases for Scientific and Professional Judgments.)

(b) Except as noted in 9.01c, psychologists provide opinions of the psychological characteristics of individuals only after they have conducted an examination of the individuals adequate to support their statements or conclusions. When, despite reasonable efforts, such an examination is not practical, psychologists document the efforts they made and the result of those efforts, clarify the probable impact of their limited information on the reliability and validity of their opinions, and appropriately limit the nature and extent of their conclusions or recommendations. (See also Standards 2.01, Boundaries of Competence, and 9.06, Interpreting Assessment Results.)

(c) When psychologists conduct a record review or provide consultation or supervision and an individual examination is not warranted or necessary for the opinion, psychologists explain this and the sources of information on which they based their conclusions and recommendations.

### 9.02 Use of Assessments

(a) Psychologists administer, adapt, score, interpret, or use assessment techniques, interviews, tests, or instruments in a manner and for purposes that are appropriate in light of the research on or evidence of the usefulness and proper application of the techniques.

(b) Psychologists use assessment instruments whose validity and reliability have been established for use with members of the population tested. When such validity or reliability has not been established, psychologists describe the strengths and limitations of test results and interpretation.

(c) Psychologists use assessment methods that are appropriate to an individual's language preference and competence, unless the use of an alternative language is relevant to the assessment issues.

### 9.03 Informed Consent in Assessments

(a) Psychologists obtain informed consent for assessments, evaluations, or diagnostic services, as described in Standard 3.10, Informed Consent, except when (1) testing is mandated by law or governmental regulations; (2) informed consent is implied because testing is conducted as a routine educational, institutional, or organizational activity (e.g., when participants voluntarily agree to assessment when applying for a job); or (3) one purpose of the testing is to evaluate decisional capacity. Informed consent includes an explanation of the nature and purpose of the assessment, fees, involvement of third parties, and limits of confidentiality and sufficient opportunity for the client/patient to ask questions and receive answers.

(b) Psychologists inform persons with questionable capacity to consent or for whom testing is mandated by law or governmental regulations about the nature and purpose of the proposed assessment services, using language that is reasonably understandable to the person being assessed.

(c) Psychologists using the services of an interpreter obtain informed consent from the client/patient to use that interpreter, ensure that confidentiality of test results and test security are maintained, and include in their recommendations, reports, and diagnostic or evaluative statements, including forensic testimony, discussion of any limitations on the data obtained. (See also Standards 2.05, Delegation of Work to Others; 4.01, Maintaining Confidentiality; 9.01, Bases for Assessments; 9.06, Interpreting Assessment Results; and 9.07, Assessment by Unqualified Persons.)

### 9.04 Release of Test Data

(a) The term *test data* refers to raw and scaled scores, client/patient responses to test questions or stimuli, and psychologists' notes and recordings concerning client/patient statements and behavior during an examination. Those portions of test materials that include client/patient responses are included in the definition of *test data*. Pursuant to a client/patient release, psychologists provide test data to the client/patient or other persons identified in the release. Psychologists may refrain from releasing test data to protect a client/patient or others from substantial harm or misuse or misrepresentation of the data or the test, recognizing that in many instances release of confidential information under these circumstances is regulated by law. (See also Standard 9.11, Maintaining Test Security.)

(b) In the absence of a client/patient release, psychologists provide test data only as required by law or court order.

### 9.05 Test Construction

Psychologists who develop tests and other assessment techniques use appropriate psychometric procedures and current scientific or professional knowledge for test design, standardization, validation, reduction or elimination of bias, and recommendations for use.

### 9.06 Interpreting Assessment Results

When interpreting assessment results, including automated interpretations, psychologists take into account the purpose of the assessment as well as the various test factors, test-taking abilities, and other characteristics of the person being assessed, such as situational, personal, linguistic, and cultural differences, that might affect psychologists' judgments or reduce the accuracy of their interpretations. They indicate any significant limitations of their interpretations. (See also Standards 2.01b and c, Boundaries of Competence, and 3.01, Unfair Discrimination.)

### 9.07 Assessment by Unqualified Persons

Psychologists do not promote the use of psychological assessment techniques by unqualified persons, except when such use is conducted for training purposes with appropriate supervision. (See also Standard 2.05, Delegation of Work to Others.)

### 9.08 Obsolete Tests and Outdated Test Results

(a) Psychologists do not base their assessment or intervention decisions or recommendations on data or test results that are outdated for the current purpose.

(b) Psychologists do not base such decisions or recommendations on tests and measures that are obsolete and not useful for the current purpose.

### 9.09 Test Scoring and Interpretation Services

(a) Psychologists who offer assessment or scoring services to other professionals accurately describe the purpose, norms, validity, reliability, and applications of the procedures and any special qualifications applicable to their use.

(b) Psychologists select scoring and interpretation services (including automated services) on the basis of evidence of the validity of the program and procedures as well as on other appropriate considerations. (See also Standard 2.01b and c, Boundaries of Competence.)

(c) Psychologists retain responsibility for the appropriate application, interpretation, and use of assessment instruments, whether they score and interpret such tests themselves or use automated or other services.

### 9.10 Explaining Assessment Results

Regardless of whether the scoring and interpretation are done by psychologists, by employees or assistants, or by automated or other outside services, psychologists take reasonable steps to ensure that explanations of results are given to the individual or designated representative unless the nature of the relationship precludes provision of an explanation of results (such as in some organizational consulting, preemployment or security screenings, and forensic evaluations), and this fact has been clearly explained to the person being assessed in advance.

### 9.11. Maintaining Test Security

The term *test materials* refers to manuals, instruments, protocols, and test questions or stimuli and does not include *test data* as defined in Standard 9.04, Release of Test Data. Psychologists make reasonable efforts to maintain the integrity and security of test materials and other assessment techniques consistent with law and contractual obligations, and in a manner that permits adherence to this Ethics Code.

## 10. Therapy

### 10.01 Informed Consent to Therapy

(a) When obtaining informed consent to therapy as required in Standard 3.10, Informed Consent, psychologists inform clients/patients as early as is feasible in the therapeutic relationship about the nature and anticipated course of therapy, fees, involvement of third parties, and limits of confidentiality and provide sufficient opportunity for the client/patient to ask questions and receive answers. (See also Standards 4.02, Discussing the Limits of Confidentiality, and 6.04, Fees and Financial Arrangements.)

(b) When obtaining informed consent for treatment for which generally recognized techniques and procedures have not been established, psychologists inform their clients/patients of the developing nature of the treatment, the potential risks involved, alternative treatments that may be available, and the voluntary nature of their participation. (See also Standards 2.01e, Boundaries of Competence, and 3.10, Informed Consent.)

(c) When the therapist is a trainee and the legal responsibility for the treatment provided resides with the supervisor, the client/patient, as part of the informed consent procedure, is informed that the therapist is in training and is being supervised and is given the name of the supervisor.

## 10.02 Therapy Involving Couples or Families

(a) When psychologists agree to provide services to several persons who have a relationship (such as spouses, significant others, or parents and children), they take reasonable steps to clarify at the outset (1) which of the individuals are clients/patients and (2) the relationship the psychologist will have with each person. This clarification includes the psychologist's role and the probable uses of the services provided or the information obtained. (See also Standard 4.02, Discussing the Limits of Confidentiality.)

(b) If it becomes apparent that psychologists may be called on to perform potentially conflicting roles (such as family therapist and then witness for one party in divorce proceedings), psychologists take reasonable steps to clarify and modify, or withdraw from, roles appropriately. (See also Standard 3.05c, Multiple Relationships.)

## 10.03 Group Therapy

When psychologists provide services to several persons in a group setting, they describe at the outset the roles and responsibilities of all parties and the limits of confidentiality.

## 10.04 Providing Therapy to Those Served by Others

In deciding whether to offer or provide services to those already receiving mental health services elsewhere, psychologists carefully consider the treatment issues and the potential client's/patient's welfare. Psychologists discuss these issues with the client/patient or another legally authorized person on behalf of the client/patient in order to minimize the risk of confusion and conflict, consult with the other service providers when appropriate, and proceed with caution and sensitivity to the therapeutic issues.

## 10.05 Sexual Intimacies with Current Therapy Clients/Patients

Psychologists do not engage in sexual intimacies with current therapy clients/patients.

## 10.06 Sexual Intimacies with Relatives or Significant Others of Current Therapy Clients/Patients

Psychologists do not engage in sexual intimacies with individuals they know to be close relatives, guardians, or significant others of current clients/patients. Psychologists do not terminate therapy to circumvent this standard.

## 10.07 Therapy with Former Sexual Partners

Psychologists do not accept as therapy clients/patients persons with whom they have engaged in sexual intimacies.

## 10.08 Sexual Intimacies with Former Therapy Clients/Patients

(a) Psychologists do not engage in sexual intimacies with former clients/patients for at least two years after cessation or termination of therapy.

(b) Psychologists do not engage in sexual intimacies with former clients/patients even after a two-year interval except in the most unusual circumstances. Psychologists who engage in such activity after the two years following cessation or termination of therapy and of having no sexual contact with the former client/patient bear the burden of demonstrating that there has been no exploitation, in light of all relevant factors, including (1) the amount of time that has passed since therapy terminated; (2) the nature, duration, and intensity of the therapy; (3) the circumstances of termination; (4) the client's/patient's personal history; (5) the client's/patient's current mental status; (6) the likelihood of adverse impact on the client/patient; and (7) any statements or actions made by the therapist during the course of therapy suggesting or inviting the possibility of a posttermination sexual or romantic relationship with the client/patient. (See also Standard 3.05, Multiple Relationships.)

### 10.09 Interruption of Therapy

When entering into employment or contractual relationships, psychologists make reasonable efforts to provide for orderly and appropriate resolution of responsibility for client/patient care in the event that the employment or contractual relationship ends, with paramount consideration given to the welfare of the client/patient. (See also Standard 3.12, Interruption of Psychological Services.)

### 10.10 Terminating Therapy

(a) Psychologists terminate therapy when it becomes reasonably clear that the client/patient no longer needs the service, is not likely to benefit, or is being harmed by continued service.

(b) Psychologists may terminate therapy when threatened or otherwise endangered by the client/patient or another person with whom the client/patient has a relationship.

(c) Except where precluded by the actions of clients/patients or third-party payors, prior to termination psychologists provide pretermination counseling and suggest alternative service providers as appropriate.

## History and Effective Date Footnote

This version of the APA Ethics Code was adopted by the American Psychological Association's Council of Representatives during its meeting, August 21, 2002, and is effective beginning June 1, 2003. Inquiries concerning the substance or interpretation of the APA Ethics Code should be addressed to the Director, Office of Ethics, American Psychological Association, 750 First Street, NE, Washington, DC 20002-4242. The Ethics Code and information regarding the Code can be found on the APA website, www.apa.org/ethics. The standards in this Ethics Code will be used to adjudicate complaints brought concerning alleged conduct occurring on or after the effective date. Complaints regarding conduct occurring prior to the effective date will be adjudicated on the basis of the version of the Ethics Code that was in effect at the time the conduct occurred.

The APA has previously published its Ethics Code as follows:

American Psychological Association. (1953). *Ethical standards of psychologists*. Washington, DC: Author.

American Psychological Association. (1959). Ethical standards of psychologists. *American Psychologist, 14*, 279–282.

American Psychological Association. (1963). Ethical standards of psychologists. *American Psychologist, 18*, 56–60.

American Psychological Association. (1968). Ethical standards of psychologists. *American Psychologist, 23*, 357–361.

American Psychological Association. (1977, March). Ethical standards of psychologists. *APA Monitor*, 22–23.

American Psychological Association. (1979). *Ethical standards of psychologists.* Washington, DC: Author.

American Psychological Association. (1981). Ethical principles of psychologists. *American Psychologist, 36*, 633–638.

American Psychological Association. (1990). Ethical principles of psychologists (Amended June 2, 1989). *American Psychologist, 45*, 390–395.

American Psychological Association. (1992). Ethical principles of psychologists and code of conduct. *American Psychologist, 47*, 1597–1611.

Request copies of the APA's Ethical Principles of Psychologists and Code of Conduct from the APA Order Department, 750 First Street, NE, Washington, DC 20002-4242, or phone (202) 336-5510.

# National Association of School Psychologists Professional Conduct Manual

## Principles for Professional Ethics

## Guidelines for the Provision of School Psychological Services

# National Association of School Psychologists

## *Professional Conduct Manual*

*Principles for Professional Ethics*
*Guidelines for the Provision of School Psychological Services*

The contents of this booklet are standards documents that
were approved by the Delegate Assembly of the Association
on July 15, 2000, in Durham, New Hampshire.

This document was prepared by the
Professional Standards Revision Committee

Additional copies are available from
NASP Publications
4340 East West Highway, Suite 402
Bethesda, MD 20814

Or can be found on the NASP website: www.naspweb.org

# TABLE OF CONTENTS

# NATIONAL ASSOCIATION OF SCHOOL PSYCHOLOGISTS PROFESSIONAL CONDUCT MANUAL

## Preface

The National Association of School Psychologists (NASP), founded in 1969 as a not-for-profit organization, is the world's largest association of school psychologists. The mission of NASP is to promote educationally and psycho-logically healthy environments for all children and youth by implementing research-based, effective programs that prevent problems, enhance independence, and promote optimal learning. This is accomplished through state-of-the-art research and train-ing, advocacy, ongoing program evaluation, and caring professional service. Consistent with its mission, NASP has adopted and pro-motes an integrated set of comprehensive standards for prep-aration, credentialing, and professional practice in school psychology.

- *Guidelines for the Provision of School Psychological Services*
- *Principles for Professional Ethics*
- *Standards for the Credentialing of School Psychologists*
- *Standards for Training and Field Placement Programs in School Psychology*

The first of these policy documents appeared in 1972, with the adoption of *Guidelines for Training Programs in School Psychology*. Ethical principles were first adopted in 1974. In1978, NASP adopted "standards" for credentialing, the provision of services, and training.

In addition to serving as a model for individual states, *Standards for the Credentialing of School Psychologists* serve as the foundation for the National School Psychology Certification System (NSPCS), established by NASP on January 1, 1989. Of necessity, national credentialing standards for school psychologists must be consistent with national training standards.

NASP training standards were initially approved by the National Council for the Accredita-tion of Teacher Education(NCATE) in 1982 for the review and accreditation of school psychology programs at the sixth-year/specialist and doctoral levels. In 1988, NCATE began to accredit edu-cation "units"(i.e., the administrative unit that houses professional education programs, typically the college of education), rather than programs. Concurrently, NCATE authorized the review of programs by professional member associations such as NASP for whom standards had been approved by NCATE. Consequently, only programs reviewed by NASP since 1988 can be identi-fied as being "NASP Approved."

Ethical principles articulate the standards of NASP regard-ing the conduct expected of a professional school psychologist. Guidelines for the provision of services are intended to inform both the profession and the public of the hallmark of quality services that should be the goal of every school psychologist and every school psychological services delivery unit. Consequently, both documents are of major importance in defining the field and in promoting excellence in the services provided by school psychologists.

Standards for training and for credentialing, ethical principles, and guidelines for practice have undergone review and revision several times since their initial adoption. The policy docu-ments included here represent the most recent revision and were adopted by the Delegate Assem-bly of NASP on July 15, 2000.

### Procedures for Revision and Adoption of Standards

In accordance with NASP policy, all NASP standards are reviewed every five years. The most recent review and revision was initiated in January, 1998, with a strategic planning process relative to all association standards. Because of their interrelatedness, all NASP standards (Hereafter, for ease of communication, if the phrase "all standards" is used, it will refer not only to standards for credentialing and training, but to ethical principles and guidelines for practice as well.) were revised concurrently. To ensure consistency, as well as participation by a broad range of interested constituencies, all four sets of standards were revised using a three-tiered structure.

Level I consisted of a 15-member Professional Standards Revision Committee that was responsible for soliciting and considering recommendations for revision of the standards, as well as reactions to drafts of revised standards. Although primary responsibility for the actual drafting of language was assigned to subgroups, all 15 members of the Committee were responsible for deciding what revisions were to be incorporated into each set of standards. The following persons served on the Professional Standards Revision Committee:

| | |
|---|---|
| Rhonda Armistead | Sawyer Hunley |
| George Batsche | Cornell Lane |
| Steven Coolahan | Joseph Prus |
| Michael Curtis | Daniel Reschly |
| Margaret Dawson | Jean Tanous |
| Fred Grossman | Nancy Waldron |
| Patti Harrison | Gordon Wrobel |
| Patricia Howard | |

Level II was titled the Development Group and included 43members who were asked to critically review each draft of the revised standards and to provide the Committee with reactions and recommendations for further modification. The Development Group was carefully constituted to provide representation from a wide range of interested constituencies. The membership reflected gender and geographical balance, as well as representation for members of minority groups, university faculty, practicing school psychologists, state consultants, parents, and students. Membership also included representation based upon roles within NASP (e.g., state delegate, delegate representative, officer, program manager, committee or board chair/editor)and roles in other relevant organizations (e.g., Division of School Psychology of the American Psychological Association [APA], Council of Directors of School Psychology Programs [CDSPP], Trainers of School Psychologists [TSP], parent advocacy organizations, and state school psychology associations). The following persons served in the Development Group:

| | |
|---|---|
| Eric Andreassen | Josephine McCall |
| Leigh Armistead | Jeffrey McNish |
| James Batts | Deborah McVey |
| Travis Bonner | Kathleen Minke |
| Philip Bowser | Leslie Munson |
| Lakeisha Bush | Jack Naglieri |
| Andrea Canter | Karen O'Brien |
| Deborah Crockett | Pamela Oksman |
| Beth Doll | Lynda Thompson Palacek |
| William Donelson | Joseph Perry |
| Ruth Fodness | Fred Provenzano |
| Michael Forcade | Mary Jo Quinlan |
| Ginger Gates | Robert Rhodes |
| Jerrold Harrenstein | Deborah Rose |
| Arthur Hernandez | Susan Safranski |

| | |
|---|---|
| Lee Huff | Anastasia Skalski |
| John Jones | Julie Staresnick |
| Jack Kamins | James Tallmadge |
| Judith Kaufman | Lynn Thies |
| Richard Mainzer | Caroline Wandle |
| Antigo Martin | Barbara Bole Williams |
| Michael Martin | |

Level III was titled the Reaction Group and included the entire leadership of NASP, as well as that of several other interested constituencies (Division of School Psychology of the APA, CDSPP, TSP) from whom input, reactions, and recommendations were solicited. The faculty of every identifiable school psychology training program were included in this group.

Following the strategic planning process, the Committee formulated a set of directions for proposed revisions. Those directions and potential revisions were presented to, discussed and approved by the NASP Delegate Assembly in July 1998.

Subsequently, all members of the NASP leadership and all members of the Development Group were invited to submit recommendations for revision of all standards. Announcement of the revision of standards and an invitation to provide recommendations for revision were published in the NASP *Communiqué*, which has a circulation of more than 21,000, including all association members, as well as a large number of interested constituencies. Recommendations for revision also were formally solicited from NCATE.

Based on input received, consideration of the school psychology literature, and national studies of demographic characteristics and professional practices in school psychology, drafts of revised standards were completed and disseminated to all members of both the Development Group and the entire NASP leadership. In addition, drafts of revised standards were posted on NASP's website and commentary was invited. Reactions and implications for further revision were discussed with the NASP Executive Council in January 1999.

A subsequent draft of each of the revised standards was again disseminated to the Development Group. Reactions were used to further refine the revised standards. Furthermore, in order to solicit and consider the perspectives of any interested person, the draft revisions of standards were announced and input solicited through NASP's website and also announced in the *Communiqué*. Open sessions were held at the 1999 NASP convention for the purpose of soliciting recommendations regarding the revisions. In addition to announcement in the convention program, a letter was mailed to all university training program directors/coordinators notifying them of the revision of training standards and inviting them and their faculty to the open session at the convention. The proposed revisions also were discussed by the NASP Executive Council and Delegate Assembly in April 1999.

Using all input received, another draft of revised standards was developed and disseminated in July 1999. In addition to commentary, each respondent was invited to also indicate agreement or disagreement with each specific standard. Widespread support for the proposed standards was received.

Despite strong support for the proposed standards, every comment and recommendation received was considered by the committee. Some suggestions led to further refinement of the standards. For example, the development of expanded descriptions of domains of school psychology training and practice were developed and included with the training standards in an appendix.

The most recent drafts of the revised standards were again disseminated and posted on the Association's webpage. Respondents were invited to comment and to express agreement or disagreement, as well as to provide recommendations for change. Proposed standards were again presented to he NASP Executive Council in January 2000 for discussion.

Having received widespread support, the proposed standards ere presented to the NASP Delegate Assembly in April2000 for the first formal reading prior to consideration of adoption (NASP policy requires that standards be presented o the Delegate Assembly for two formal readings in order to be adopted). The proposed standards were presented to the NASP Delegate Assembly for the second formal reading in July 2000. *Guidelines for the Provision of School Psychological Services, Principles for Professional Ethics, Standards for the Credentialing of School Psychologists,* and *Standards for Training and Field Placement Programs in School Psychology* were each adopted by unanimous vote of the Delegate Assembly on July 15, 2000. The following dates should be used for implementation of the standards: *Guidelines for the Provision of School Psychological Services,* effective July 15, 2000; *Principles for Professional Ethics,* effective January 1, 2001; *Standards for the Credentialing of School Psychologists,* effective January 1, 2005; *Standards for Training and Field Placement Programs in School Psychology,* effective January 1, 2002

# NATIONAL ASSOCIATION OF SCHOOL PSYCHOLOGISTS PRINCIPLES FOR PROFESSIONAL ETHICS

## I. Introduction

The formal principles that elucidate the proper conduct of a professional school psychologist are known as Ethics. By virtue of joining the Association, each NASP member agrees to abide by the Ethics, acting in a manner that shows respect for human dignity and assuring a high quality of professional service. Although ethical behavior is an individual responsibility, it is in the interest of an association to adopt and enforce a code of ethics. If done properly, members will be guided toward appropriate behavior, and public confidence in the profession will be enhanced. Additionally, a code of ethics should provide due process procedures to protect members from potential abuse of the code. The NASP *Principles for Professional Ethics* have been written to accomplish these goals.

The principles in this manual are based on the assumptions that 1) school psychologists will act as advocates for their students/clients, and 2) at the very least, school psychologists will do no harm. These assumptions necessitate that school psychologists "speak up" for the needs and rights of their students/clients even at times when it may be difficult to do so. School psychologists also are constrained to provide only those services for which they have acquired an acknowledged level of experience, training, and competency. Beyond these basic premises, judgment is required to apply the ethical principles to the fluid and expanding interactions between school and community.

There are many different sources of advice for the proper way to behave; local policies, state laws, federal laws, credentialing standards, professional association position statements, and books that recommend "Best Practices" are just a few. Given one's employment situation and the array of recommendations, events may develop in which the ethical course of action is unclear.

The Association will seek to enforce the Ethical Principles with its members. NASP's *Guidelines for the Provision of School Psychological Services* are typically not enforced, al-though all members should work toward achieving the hallmarks of quality services delivery that are described therein. Similarly, "position statements" and "best practices" documents are not adjudicated. The guidance of the *Ethical Principles* is intentionally broad to make it more enduring than other documents that reflect short-term opinions about specific actions shaped by local events, popular trends, o recent developments in the field. The member must use judgment to infer the situation-specific rule from the general ethical principle. The lack of a specific reference to a particular action does not indicate permission or provide a defense against a charge of unethical practice. (For example, the document frequently refers to a school psychologist's relationships with a hypothetical "student/client." Because school psychologists work in a wide variety of settings, there is no single term that neatly identifies the "other" individual in the professional relationship. Therefore, one should apply *Ethical Principles* in all professional situations, realizing that one is not released from responsibility simply because another individual is not strictly a "student" or a "client.")

The principles in this manual are organized into several sections as a result of editorial judgment. Therefore, principles discussed in one section may also apply to other sections. Every school psychologist, regardless of position (e.g., practitioner, researcher, university trainer, supervisor, state or federal consultant, administrator of psychological services) or setting (e.g., public or private school, community agency, hospital, university, private practice) should reflect upon the theme represented in each ethical principle to determine its application to her or his individual situation. For example, although a given principle may specifically discuss responsibilities toward "clients," the intent is that the standards would also apply to supervisees, trainees, and research participants. At times, the *Ethics* may require a higher standard of behavior than the prevailing policies and pertinent laws. Under such conditions, members should adhere to the *Ethics*. Ethical behavior may occasionally be forbidden by policy or law, in which case members are expected to declare their dilemma and work to bring the discrepant regulations into compliance with the *Ethics*. To obtain additional assistance in applying these principles to a particular setting, a school psychologist should consult with experienced school psychologists and seek advice from the National Association of School Psychologists or the state school psychology association.

Throughout the *Principles for Professional Ethics*, it is assumed that, depending on the role and setting of the school psychologist, the client could include children, parents, teachers and other school personnel, other professionals, trainees, or supervisees.

Procedural guidelines for filing an ethical complaint and the adjudication of ethical complaints are available from the NASP office or website (www.naspweb.org)

## II. Professional Competency

### A. General

1. School psychologists recognize the strengths and limitations of their training and experience, engaging only in practices for which they are qualified. They enlist the assistance of other specialists in supervisory, consultative, or referral roles as appropriate in providing services. They must continually obtain additional training and education to provide the best possible services to children, families, schools, communities, trainees, and supervisees.

2. Competence levels, education, training, and experience are declared and accurately represented to clients in a professional manner.

3. School psychologists do not use affiliations with persons, associations, or institutions to imply a level of professional competence that exceeds that which has actually been achieved.

4. School psychologists engage in continuing professional development. They remain current regarding developments in research, training, and professional practices that benefit children, families, and schools.

5. School psychologists refrain from any activity in which their personal problems or conflicts may interfere with professional effectiveness. Competent assistance is sought to alleviate conflicts in professional relationships.

6. School psychologists know the *Principles for Professional Ethics* and thoughtfully apply them to situations within their employment setting or practice. Ignorance or misapplication of an ethical principle is not a reasonable defense against a charge of unethical behavior.

## III. Professional Relationships

### A. General

1. School psychologists are committed to the application of their professional expertise for the purpose of promoting improvement in the quality of life for children, their families, and the school community. This objective is pursued in ways that protect the dignity and rights of those involved. School psychologists accept responsibility for the appropriateness of their professional practices.

2. School psychologists respect all persons and are sensitive to physical, mental, emotional, political, economic, social, cultural, ethnic and racial characteristics, gender, sexual orientation, and religion.

3. School psychologists in all settings maintain professional relationships with children, parents, and the school community. Consequently, parents and children are to be fully informed about all relevant aspects of school psychological services in advance. The explanation should take into account language and cultural differences, cognitive capabilities, developmental level, and age so that it may be understood by the child, parent, or guardian.

4. School psychologists attempt to resolve situations in which there are divided or conflicting interests in a manner that is mutually beneficial and protects the rights of all parties involved.

5. School psychologists are responsible for the direction and nature of their personal loyalties or objectives. When these commitments may influence a professional relationship, school psychologists inform all concerned persons of relevant issues in advance, including, when applicable, their direct supervisor for consideration of reassignment of responsibilities.

6. School psychologists do not exploit clients through professional relationships or condone these actions in their colleagues. No individuals, including children, clients, employees, colleagues, trainees, parents, supervisees, and research participants, will be exposed to deliberate comments, gestures, or physical contacts of asexual nature. School psychologists do not harass or demean others based on personal characteristics. School psychologists do not engage in sexual relation-ships with their students, supervisees, trainees, or pastor present clients.

7. Dual relationships with clients are avoided. Namely, personal and business relations with clients may cloud one's judgment. School psychologists are aware of these situations and avoid them whenever possible.

8. School psychologists attempt to resolve suspected detrimental or unethical practices on an informal level. If informal efforts are not productive, the appropriate professional organization is contacted for assistance, and procedures established for questioning ethical practice are followed:

   a. The filing of an ethical complaint is a serious matter. It is intended to improve the behavior of a colleague that is harmful to the profession and/or the public. Therefore, school psychologists make every effort to discuss the ethical principles with other professionals who may be in violation.

   b. School psychologists enter into the complaint process thoughtfully and with concern for the well-being of all parties involved. They do not file or encourage the filing of an ethics complaint that is frivolous or motivated by revenge.

   c. Some situations may be particularly difficult to analyze from an ethical perspective. School psychologists consult ethical standards from related fields and seek assistance from knowledgeable, experienced school psychologists and relevant state/national associations to ascertain an appropriate course of action.

   d. School psychologists document specific instances of suspected ethical violations (i.e., date, time, relevant details) as well as attempts to resolve these violations.

9. School psychologists respect the confidentiality of information obtained during their professional work. Information is revealed only with the informed consent of the child, or the child's parent or legal guardian, except in those situations in which failure to release information would result in clear danger to the child or others. Obsolete confidential information will be shredded or otherwise destroyed before placement in recycling bins or trash receptacles.

10. School psychologists discuss confidential information only for professional purposes and only with persons who have a legitimate need to know.

11. School psychologists inform children and other clients of the limits of confidentiality at the outset of establishing a professional relationship.

## B. Students

1. School psychologists understand the intimate nature of consultation, assessment, and direct service. They engage only in professional practices that maintain the dignity and integrity of children and other clients.

2. School psychologists explain important aspects of their professional relationships in a clear, understandable manner that is appropriate to the child's or other client's age and ability to understand. The explanation includes the reason why services were requested, who will receive information about the services provided, and the possible outcomes.

3. When a child initiates services, school psychologists understand their obligation to respect the rights of a child to initiate, participate in, or discontinue services voluntarily (See III-C-2 for further clarification). When another party initiates services, the school psychologist will make every effort to secure voluntary participation of the child.

4. Recommendations for program changes or additional services will be discussed with appropriate individuals, including any alternatives that may be available.

## C. Parents, Legal Guardians, and Appointed Surrogates

1. School psychologists explain all services to parents in a clear, understandable manner. They strive to propose a set of options that takes into account the values and capabilities of each parent. Service provision by interns, practicum students, or other trainees should be explained and agreed to in advance.

2. School psychologists recognize the importance of parental support and seek to obtain that support by assuring that there is direct parent contact prior to seeing the child on an ongoing basis. (Emergencies and "drop-in" self-referrals will require parental notification as soon as possible. The age and circumstances under which children may seek services without parental consent varies greatly; be certain to comply with III-D-5.) School psychologists secure continuing parental involvement by a frank and prompt reporting to the parent of findings and progress that conforms to the limits of previously determined confidentiality.

3. School psychologists encourage and promote parental participation in designing services provided to their children. When appropriate, this includes linking interventions between the school and the home, tailoring parental involvement to the skills of the family, and helping parents gain the skills needed to help their children.

4. School psychologists respect the wishes of parents who object to school psychological services and attempt to guide parents to alternative community resources.

5. School psychologists discuss with parents the recommendations and plans for assisting their children. The discussion includes alternatives associated with each set of plans, which show

respect for the ethnic/cultural values of the family. The parents are informed of sources of help available at school and in the community.

6. School psychologists discuss the rights of parents and children regarding creation, modification, storage, and disposal of confidential materials that will result from the provision of school psychological services.

## D. Community

1. School psychologists also are citizens, thereby accepting the same responsibilities and duties as any member of society. They are free to pursue individual interests, except to the degree that those interests compromise professional responsibilities.

2. School psychologists may act as individual citizens to bring about social change in a lawful manner. Individual actions should not be presented as, or suggestive of, representing the field of school psychology or the Association.

3. As employees or employers, in public or independent practice domains, school psychologists do not engage in or condone practices that discriminate against children, other clients, or employees (if applicable) based on race, disability, age, gender, sexual orientation, religion, national origin, economic status, or native language.

4. School psychologists avoid any action that could violate or diminish the civil and legal rights of children and other clients.

5. School psychologists adhere to federal, state, and local laws and ordinances governing their practice and advocacy efforts. If regulations conflict with ethical guide-lines, school psychologists seek to resolve such conflict through positive, respected, and legal channels, including advocacy efforts involving public policy.

## E. Other Professionals

1. To best meet the needs of children and other clients, school psychologists cooperate with other professional disciplines in relationships based on mutual respect.

2. School psychologists recognize the competence of other professionals. They encourage and support the use of all resources to best serve the interests of children and other clients.

3. School psychologists should strive to explain their field and their professional competencies, including roles, assignments, and working relationships to other professionals.

4. School psychologists cooperate and coordinate with other professionals and agencies with the rights and needs of children and other clients in mind. If a child or other client is receiving similar services from another professional, school psychologists promote coordination of services.

5. The child or other client is referred to another professional for services when a condition or need is identified which is outside the professional competencies or scope of the school psychologist.

6. When transferring the intervention responsibility for a child or other client to another professional, school psychologists ensure that all relevant and appropriate individuals, including the child/client when appropriate, are notified of the change and reasons for the change.

7. When school psychologists suspect the existence of detrimental or unethical practices by a member of another profession, informal contact is made with that person to express the concern. If the situation cannot be resolved in this manner, the appropriate professional organization is contacted for assistance in determining the procedures established by that profession for examining the practices in question.

8. School psychologists who employ, supervise, or train other professionals, accept the obligation to provide continuing professional development. They also provide appropriate working conditions, fair and timely evaluation, and constructive consultation.

### F. School Psychologist Trainees and Interns

1. School psychologists who supervise interns are responsible for all professional practices of the supervisees. They assure children and other clients and the profession that the intern is adequately supervised as designated by the practice guidelines and training standards for school psychologists.

2. School psychologists who conduct or administer training programs provide trainees and prospective trainees with accurate information regarding program sponsorships/endorsements/accreditation, goals/objectives, training processes and requirements, and likely outcomes and benefits.

3. School psychologists who are faculty members in colleges or universities or who supervise clinical or field placements apply these ethical principles in all work with school psychology trainees. In addition, they promote the ethical practice of trainees by providing specific and comprehensive instruction, feedback, and mentoring.

4. School psychology faculty members and clinical or field supervisors uphold recognized standards of the profession by providing training related to high quality, responsible, and research-based school psychology services. They provide accurate and objective information in their teaching and training activities; identify any limitations in information; and acknowledge disconfirming data, alternative hypotheses, and explanations.

5. School psychology faculty members and clinical or field supervisors develop and use evaluation practices for trainees that are objective, accurate, and fair.

## IV. Professional Practices—General Principles

### A. Advocacy

1. School psychologists typically serve multiple clients including children, parents, and systems. When the school psychologist is confronted with conflicts between client groups, the primary client is considered to be the child. When the child is not the primary client, the individual or group of individuals who sought the assistance of the school psychologist is the primary client.

2. School psychologists consider children and other clients to be their primary responsibility, acting as advocates for their rights and welfare. If conflicts of interest between clients are present, the school psychologist supports conclusions that are in the best interest of the child. When choosing a course of action, school psychologists take into account the rights of each individual involved and the duties of school personnel.

3. School psychologists' concerns for protecting the rights and welfare of children are communicated to the school administration and staff as the top priority in determining services.

4. School psychologists understand the public policy process to assist them in their efforts to advocate for children, parents, and systems.

### B. Service Delivery

1. School psychologists are knowledgeable of the organization, philosophy, goals, objectives, and methodologies of the setting in which they are employed.

2. School psychologists recognize that an understanding of the goals, processes, and legal requirements of their particular workplace is essential for effective functioning within that setting.

3. School psychologists attempt to become integral members of the client service systems to which they are assigned. They establish clear roles for themselves within that system.

4. School psychologists who provide services to several different groups may encounter situations in which loyalties are conflicted. As much as possible, the stance of the school psychologist is made known in advance to all parties to prevent misunderstandings.

5. School psychologists promote changes in their employing agencies and community service systems that will benefit their clients.

## C. Assessment and Intervention

1. School psychologists maintain the highest standard for educational and psychological assessment and direct and indirect interventions.

a. In conducting psychological, educational, or behavioral evaluations or in providing therapy, counseling, or consultation services, due consideration is given to individual integrity and individual differences.

b. School psychologists respect differences in age, gender, sexual orientation, and socioeconomic, cultural, and ethnic backgrounds. They select and use appropriate assessment or treatment procedures, techniques, and strategies. Decision-making related to assessment and subsequent interventions is primarily data-based.

2. School psychologists are knowledgeable about the validity and reliability of their instruments and techniques, choosing those that have up-to-date standardization data and are applicable and appropriate for the benefit of the child.

3. School psychologists use multiple assessment methods such as observations, background information, and information from other professionals, to reach comprehensive conclusions.

4. School psychologists use assessment techniques, counseling and therapy procedures, consultation techniques, and other direct and indirect service methods that the profession considers to be responsible, research-based practice.

5. School psychologists do not condone the use of psycho-logical or educational assessment techniques, or the misuse of the information these techniques provide, by unqualified persons in any way, including teaching, sponsorship, or supervision.

6. School psychologists develop interventions that are appropriate to the presenting problems and are consistent with data collected. They modify or terminate the treatment plan when the data indicate the plan is not achieving the desired goals.

7. School psychologists use current assessment and intervention strategies that assist in the promotion of mental health in the children they serve.

## D. Reporting Data and Conference Results

1. School psychologists ascertain that information about children and other clients reaches only authorized persons.

a. School psychologists adequately interpret information so that the recipient can better help the child or other clients.

b. School psychologists assist agency recipients to establish procedures to properly safeguard confidential material.

2. School psychologists communicate findings and recommendations in language readily understood by the intended recipient. These communications describe potential consequences associated with the proposals.

3. School psychologists prepare written reports in such form and style that the recipient of the report will be able to assist the child or other clients. Reports should emphasize recommendations and interpretations; unedited computer-generated reports, pre-printed "check-off" or "fill-in-the-blank" reports, and reports that present only test scores or global statements regarding eligibility for special education without specific recommendations for intervention are seldom useful. Reports should include an appraisal of the degree of confidence that could be assigned to the information. Alterations of previously released reports should be done only by the original author.

4. School psychologists review all of their written documents for accuracy, signing them only when correct. Interns and practicum students are clearly identified as such, and their work is co-signed by the supervising school psychologist. In situations in which more than one professional participated in the data collection and reporting process, school psychologists assure that sources of data are clearly identified in the written report.

5. School psychologists comply with all laws, regulations, and policies pertaining to the adequate storage and disposal of records to maintain appropriate confidentiality of information.

## E. Use of Materials and Technology

1. School psychologists maintain test security, preventing the release of underlying principles and specific content that would undermine the use of the device. School psychologists are responsible for the security requirements specific to each instrument used.

2. School psychologists obtain written prior consent or they remove identifying data presented in public lectures or publications.

3. School psychologists do not promote or encourage inappropriate use of computer-generated test analyses or reports. In accordance with this principle, a school psychologist would not offer an unedited computer report as his or her own writing or use a computer-scoring system for tests in which he or she has no training. They select scoring and interpretation services on the basis of accuracy and professional alignment with the underlying decision rules.

4. School psychologists maintain full responsibility for any technological services used. All ethical and legal principles regarding confidentiality, privacy, and responsibility for decisions apply to the school psychologist and cannot be transferred to equipment, software companies, or data-processing departments.

5. Technological devices should be used to improve the quality of client services. School psychologists will resist applications of technology that ultimately reduce the quality of service.

6. To ensure confidentiality, student/client records are not transmitted electronically without a guarantee of privacy. In line with this principle, a receiving FAX machine must be in a secure location and operated by employees cleared to work with confidential files, and e-mail messages must be encrypted or else stripped of all information that identifies the student/client.

7. School psychologists do not accept any form of remuneration in exchange for data from their client data base without informed consent.

## F. Research, Publication, and Presentation

1. When designing and implementing research in schools, school psychologists choose topics and employ research methodology, subject selection techniques, data-gathering methods, and

analysis and reporting techniques that ar grounded in sound research practice. School psychologists clearly identify their level of training and graduate degree on all communications to research participants.

2. Prior to initiating research, school psychologists working in agencies without review committees should have at least one other colleague, preferably a school psychologist, review the proposed methods.

3. School psychologists follow all legal procedures when conducting research, including following procedures related to informed consent, confidentiality, privacy, protection from harm or risks, voluntary participation, and disclosure of results to participants. School psychologists demonstrate respect for the rights of and well-being of research participants.

4. In publishing reports of their research, school psychologists provide discussion of limitations of their data and acknowledge existence of disconfirming data, as well as alternate hypotheses and explanations of their findings.

5. School psychologists take particular care with information presented through various impersonal media (e.g., radio, television, public lectures, popular press articles, promotional materials.). Recipients should be informed that the information does not result from or substitute for a professional consultation. The information should be based on research and experience within the school psychologist's recognized sphere of competence. The statements should be consistent with these ethical principles and should not mistakenly represent the field of school psychology or the Association.

6. School psychologists uphold copyright laws in their publications and presentations and obtain permission from authors and copyright holders to reproduce other publications or materials. School psychologists recognize that federal law protects the rights of copyright holders of published works and authors of non-published materials.

7. When publishing or presenting research or other work, school psychologists do not plagiarize the works or ideas of others and acknowledge sources and assign credit to those whose ideas are reflected.

8. School psychologists do not publish or present fabricated or falsified data or results in their publications and presentations.

9. School psychologists make available data or other information upon which conclusions and claims reported in publications and presentations are based, provided that the data are needed to address a legitimate concern or need and that the confidentiality and other rights of all research participants are protected.

10. If errors are discovered after the publication or presentation of research and other information, school psychologists make efforts to correct errors by publishing errata, retractions, or corrections.

11. School psychologists accurately reflect the contributions of authors and other individuals in publications and presentations. Authorship credit and the order in which authors are listed are based on the relative contributions of the individual authors. Authorship credit is given only to individuals who have made substantial professional contributions to the research, publication, or presentation.

12. School psychologists only publish data or other information that make original contributions to the professional literature. School psychologists do not publish the same findings in two or more publications and do not duplicate significant portions of their own previous publications without permission of copyright holders.

13. School psychologists who participate in reviews of manuscripts, proposals, and other materials for consideration for publication and presentation respect the confidentiality and proprietary rights of the authors. School psychologists who review professional materials limit their use of the materials to the activities relevant to the purposes of the professional review. School

psychologists who review professional materials do not communicate the identity of the author, quote from the materials, or duplicate or circulate copies of the materials without the author's permission.

## V. Professional Practice Settings—Independent Practice

### A. Relationship with Employers

1. Some school psychologists are employed in a variety of settings, organizational structures, and sectors and, as such, may create a conflict of interest. School psychologists operating in these different settings recognize the importance of ethical standards and the separation of roles and take full responsibility for protecting and completely informing the consumer of all potential concerns.

2. School psychologists dually employed in independent practice and in a school district may not accept any form of remuneration from clients who are entitled to the same service provided by the school district employing the school psychologist. This includes children who attend the non-public schools within the school psychologist's district.

3. School psychologists in independent practice have an obligation to inform parents of any school psychological services available to them at no cost from the public or private schools prior to delivering such services for remuneration.

4. School psychologists working in both independent practice and employed by school districts conduct all independent practice outside of the hours of contracted public employment.

5. School psychologists engaged in independent practice do not use tests, materials, equipment, facilities, secretarial assistance, or other services belonging to the public sector employer unless approved in advance by the employer.

### B. Service Delivery

1. School psychologists conclude a financial agreement in advance of service delivery.
    a. School psychologists ensure to the best of their ability that the client clearly understands the agreement.
    b. School psychologists neither give nor receive any remuneration for referring children and other clients for professional services.

2. School psychologists in independent practice adhere to the conditions of a contract until service there under has been performed, the contract has been terminated by mutual consent, or the contract has otherwise been legally terminated.

3. School psychologists in independent practice prevent misunderstandings resulting from their recommendations, advice, or information. Most often, direct consultation between the school psychologist in private practice and the school psychologist responsible for the student in the public sector will resolve minor differences of opinion without unnecessarily confusing the parents, yet keep the best interests of the student or client in mind.

4. Personal diagnosis and therapy are not given by means of public lectures, newspaper columns, magazine articles, radio and television programs, or mail. Any information shared through mass media activities is general in nature and is openly declared to be so.

### C. Announcements/Advertising

1. Appropriate announcement of services, advertising, and public media statements may be necessary for school psychologists in independent practice. Accurate representations of training,

experience, services provided, and affiliation are done in a restrained manner. Public statements must be based on sound and accepted theory, research, and practice.

2. Listings in telephone directories are limited to the following: name/names, highest relevant degree, state certification/licensure status, national certification status, address, telephone number, brief identification of major areas of practice, office hours, appropriate fee information, foreign languages spoken, policy regarding third-party payments, and license number.

3. Announcements of services by school psychologists in independent practice are made in a formal, professional manner using the guidelines of V-C-2. Clear statements of purposes with unequivocal descriptions of the experiences to be provided are given. Education, training, and experience of all staff members are appropriately specified.

4. School psychologists in independent practice may use brochures in the announcement of services. The brochures may be sent to other professionals, schools, business firms, governmental agencies, and other similar organizations.

5. Announcements and advertisements of the availability of publications, products, and services for sale are professional and factual.

6. School psychologists in independent practice do not directly solicit clients for individual diagnosis, therapy, and for the provision of other school psychological services.

7. School psychologists do not compensate in any manner a representative of the press, radio, or television in return for personal professional publicity in a news item.

# NATIONAL ASSOCIATION OF SCHOOL PSYCHOLOGISTS GUIDELINES FOR THE PROVISION OF SCHOOL PSYCHOLOGICAL SERVICES

## Introduction

The *Guidelines for the Provision of School Psychological Services* represent the position of the National Association of School Psychologists (NASP) regarding the delivery of appropriate and comprehensive school psychological services. First written in 1978, revised in 1984, 1992, 1997, and 2000, the *Guidelines* serve as a guide to the organization and delivery of school psychological services at the federal, state, and local levels. The *Guidelines* provide direction to school psychologists, students, and trainers in school psychology, administrators of school psychological services, and consumers of school psychological services regarding excellence in professional school psychology. They also delineate what services might reasonably be expected to be available from most school psychologists and, thus, should help to further define the field. In addition, they are intended to educate the profession and the public regarding appropriate professional practices and, hopefully, will stimulate the continued development of the profession.

A principal objective of the *Guidelines* is to inform policy and decision-makers of the major characteristics of comprehensive school psychological services. The first section presents the responsibilities of the individual school psychologist. The second section outlines responsibilities that should be assumed by the unit responsible for providing psychological services within an organization (e.g., school district, community agency) that employs school psychologists. The "unit" is defined as the entity (e.g., the single school psychologist in a small district, a psychological services unit in a large district, a district that contracts with an agency for psycho-logical services) that is responsible for ensuring that schools, students, and families receive comprehensive psychological services.

Not all school psychologists or school psychological service units will be able to meet every standard contained within this document. Nevertheless, it is anticipated that these guidelines will serve as a model of "good practice" for pro-gram development and professional practice on a federal, state, and local level.

School psychologists will perceive that it is in their own best interest—and that of the agencies, parents, and children they serve—to adhere to and support these *Guidelines*. NASP encourages state and federal legislators, local school boards, and the administrative leaders of federal, state, and local education agencies to support the concepts contained within these *Guidelines*.

NASP acknowledges that the *Guidelines* set requirements for services not presently mandated by federal law or regulation and not always mandated in state laws and administrative rules. Future amendments of such statutes and rules, and the state and local plans resulting from them, should incorporate the suggestions contained in this document. Furthermore, NASP understands that school psychological services are provided within the context of ethical and legal mandates. Nothing in these *Guidelines* should be construed as superseding such relevant rules and regulations.

The *Guidelines* provide flexibility, permitting agencies and professionals to develop procedures, polices, and administrative organizations that meet both the needs of the agency and the professional's desire to operate within recognized professional standards of practice. At the same time, the *0* have sufficient specificity to insure that services will be provided appropriately and adequately.

## Practice Guidelines

### Practice Guideline 1

School psychologists use a decision-making process in collaboration with other team members to (a) identify academic and behavior problems, (b) collect and analyze information to understand the problems, (c) make decisions about service delivery, and (d) evaluate the outcomes of the service delivery.

School psychologists must (a) utilize current professional literature on various aspects of education and child development, (b) translate research into practice through the problem-solving process, and (c) use research design and statistics skills to conduct investigations to develop and facilitate effective services.

1.1 School psychologists define problems in ways that(a)identify desired goals (e.g., academic/behavioral),(b) are measurable, (c) are agreed upon by those involved, and (d) are linked appropriately to assessment strategies.

1.2 School psychologists select assessment method(s) that are validated for the problem area under consideration including formal and informal assessment procedures, as appropriate, and include data collected from all settings and persons necessary and appropriate to complete the problem-solving process.

1.3 School psychologists develop and implement effective interventions that are based upon the data collected and related directly to the desired outcomes of those interventions.

1.4 School psychologists use appropriate assessment information to evaluate interventions to determine their effectiveness, their need for modification, or their need for redevelopment. Effectiveness is determined by the relationship between the actual outcome of the intervention and the desired goal articulated in the problem solving process.

1.5 School psychologists apply the problem-solving process to broader research and systems-level problems that result in the identification of factors that influence learning and behavior, the evaluation of the outcomes of classroom, building, and system initiatives and the implementation of decision-making practices designed to meet general public accountability responsibilities.

## Practice Guideline 2

School psychologists must have the ability to listen well, participate in discussions, convey information, and work together with others at an individual, group, and systems level. School psychologists must understand the degree to which policy influences systems, systems influence pro-grams, programs and interventions impact consumers, and the methods to facilitate organizational development through strategic change.

2.1 School psychologists use decision-making skills and are proficient in systems consultation to facilitate communication and collaboration with students and school personnel, community professionals, agencies, and families/schools.

2.2 School psychologists participate in public policy discussions and understand the process by which public policy influences systems. By applying decision-making methods to public policy determination, school psychologists facilitate organization development and change.

2.3 School psychologists must be able to present and disseminate information to diverse communities, such as parents, teachers, school boards, policy makers, business leaders, and fellow school psychologists in a variety of contexts, in an organized and meaningful manner.

2.4 School psychologists facilitate the development of healthy learning environments and reduce divisiveness through the use of conflict resolution and negotiation nskills.

2.5 School psychologists function as change agents, using their skills in communication, collaboration, and consultation to promote necessary change at the individual student, classroom, building, and district local, state, and federal levels.

## Practice Guideline 3

School psychologists (in collaboration with others) develop challenging but achievable cognitive and academic goals for all students, provide information about ways in which students can achieve these goals, and monitor student progress towards these goals.

3.1 School psychologists apply current empirically based theory and knowledge of learning theory and cognitive processes to the development of effective instructional strategies to promote student learning and social and emotional development.

3.2 School psychologists incorporate assessment information to the development of instructional strategies to meet the individual learning needs of children.

3.3 School psychologists use appropriate and applicable assessment techniques to assess progress toward academic goals and assist in revising instructional methodology as necessary.

3.4 School psychologists assist in facilitating and implementing a variety of research-based instructional methods (e.g., cooperative learning, class-wide peer tutoring, cognitive strategy training) to enhance learning of students at the individual, group, and systems level.

3.5 School psychologists assist in the design and delivery of curriculum to help students develop behaviors to support effective learning such as study skills, self-regulation and self-monitoring, planning/organization, time management skills, and making choices that maintain physical and mental health.

3.6 School psychologists promote the principles of student-centered learning to help students develop (when appropriate) their individual ability to be self-regulated learners, including the ability to set individual learning goals, design a learning process to achieve those goals, and assess outcomes to determine whether the goals were achieved.

3.7 School psychologists are informed about advances in curriculum and instruction and share this knowledge with educators, parents, and the community at large to promote improvement in instruction, student achievement, and healthy lifestyles.

## Practice Guideline 4

School psychologists make decisions based on multiple theoretical perspectives and translate current scientific information to develop effective behavioral, affective, or adaptive goals for all students, facilitate the implementation of programs/interventions to achieve these goals, and monitor progress towards these goals.

4.1 School psychologists use decision-making models (e.g., functional behavioral assessment) that consider the antecedents, consequences, functions, and potential causes of behavioral problems experienced by students with disabilities, which may impair learning or socialization.

4.2 School psychologists identify factors that facilitate the development of optimal learning environments. Optimal learning environments are characterized as settings where all members of the school or agency community treat one another with respect and dignity. Optimal learning environments are characterized as settings where students' basic needs are assured so that learning can occur and health and mental health are systematically evaluated.

4.3 School psychologists facilitate the development and implementation of strategies that result in instructional environments which foster learning and high rates of academic engaged time and reduce the presence of factors that promote alienation and impact learning and behavioral progress.

4.4 School psychologists demonstrate appropriate knowledge of treatment acceptability and treatment integrity by including these principles in the development, implementation, and evaluation of interventions.

4.5 School psychologists apply the principles of generalization and transfer of training in the development of interventions in such a way that, when appropriate, interventions can be implemented across settings—school, home, and community.

4.6 School psychologists develop and implement behavior change programs (individual, group, classroom) that demonstrate the use of alternative, appropriate approaches (e.g., positive reinforcement, social skills training, academic interventions) to student discipline, ecological and behavioral approaches to classroom management, and awareness of classroom climate.

4.7 School psychologists assist parents and other adult caregivers in the development, implementation, and evaluation of behavior change programs in the home in order to facilitate the learning and behavioral growth of their child.

4.8 School psychologists incorporate appropriate strategies when developing and delivering intervention programs to facilitate successful transitions of students from one environment to another environment. These programs include program to program, early childhood to school, school to school, and school to work transitions.

4.9 School psychologists evaluate interventions (learning/behavioral) for individuals and groups. These include the skills necessary both to evaluate the extent to which the intervention contributed to the outcome and to identify what constitutes a "successful" outcome.

## Practice Guideline 5

School psychologists have the sensitivity, knowledge, and skills to work with individuals and groups with a diverse range of strengths and needs from a variety of racial, cultural, ethnic, experiential, and linguistic backgrounds.

5.1 School psychologists develop academic and behavioral interventions. They recognize that interventions most likely to succeed are those which are adapted to the individual needs and characteristics of the student(s)for whom they are being designed.

5.2 School psychologists recognize (in themselves and others and in the techniques and instruments that they use for assessment and intervention) the subtle racial, class, gender, and cultural biases they may bring to their work and the way these biases influence decision-making, instruction, behavior, and long-term outcomes for students. School psychologists work to reduce and eliminate these biases where they occur.

5.3 School psychologists promote practices that help children of all backgrounds feel welcome and appreciated in the school and community.

5.4 School psychologists incorporate their understanding of the influence of culture, background, and individual learning characteristics when designing and implementing interventions to achieve learning and behavioral outcomes.

## Practice Guideline 6

School psychologists demonstrate their knowledge of schools (or other institutional settings) as systems when they work with individuals and groups to facilitate structure and public policies that create and maintain schools and other systems as safe, caring, and inviting places for all persons in that system.

6.1 School psychologists use their knowledge of development, learning, family, and school systems to assist schools and communities to develop policies and practices related to discipline, decision-making, instructional support, staff training, school improvement plans, program evaluation, transition plans, grading, retention, and home-school partnerships.

6.2 School psychologists use their knowledge of organizational development and systems theory to assist in creating climates that result in mutual respect and caring for all individuals in the system, an atmosphere of decision-making and collaboration, and a commitment to quality services.

6.3 School psychologists regularly participate in the development of policies and procedures that advocate for effective programs and services.

6.4 School psychologists are actively involved in the development of systems change plans (such as school improvement plans) that directly impact the programs and services available to children, youth, and their families and that directly impact the ways in which school psychologists deliver their services.

6.5 School psychologists assist in the development of policies and procedures to ensure that schools are safe and violence free. School psychologists participate in the implementation and evaluation of programs that result in safe and violence free schools and communities.

6.6 School psychologists are actively involved in public policy at the local, state, and federal levels as a means of creating systems of effective educational services.

6.7 School psychologists are aware of funding mechanisms that are available to school and communities that support health and mental health services. School psychologists participate in the development of funding strategies to assure that needed services are available to students and their families.

## Practice Guideline 7

School psychologists shall appropriately utilize prevention, health promotion, and crisis intervention methods based on knowledge of child development, psychopathology, diversity, social stressors, change, and systems.

7.1 School psychologists shall apply knowledge of child development, psychopathology, diversity, social stressors, change, and systems to the identification and recognition of behaviors that are precursors to school dropouts or the development of mental health disorders such as conduct disorders or internalizing disorders.

7.2 School psychologists shall provide direct counseling and indirect interventions through consultation for students with disabilities and suspected disabilities who experience mental health problems that impair learning and/or socialization.

7.3 School psychologists shall develop, implement, and evaluate prevention and intervention programs based on recognized factors that are precursors to development of severe learning and behavioral problems.

7.4 School psychologists shall collaborate with school personnel, parents, students, and the community to provide competent mental health support during and after crises (for example, suicide, death, natural disasters, murder, bombs or bomb threats, extraordinary violence, and sexual harassment).

7.5 School psychologists promote wellness by (a) collaborating with other health care professionals to provide a basic knowledge of behaviors that lead to good health for children; (b) facilitating environmental changes conducive to good health and adjustment of children; and (c)accessing resources to address a wide variety of behavioral, learning, mental, and physical needs.

### Practice Guideline 8

School psychologists have knowledge of family influences that affect students' wellness, learning, and achievement and are involved in public policy that promotes partner-ships between parents, educators, and the community.

8.1 School psychologists design and implement and evaluate programs to promote school–family partnerships for the purpose of enhancing academic and behavioral goals for students. These might include (but are not limited to)developing parent education programs, establishing drop-in centers for parents, establishing homework hotlines, or providing other supports for parents to help them parent successfully and to help them enhance the academic and psychological development of their children.

8.2 School psychologists help parents feel comfortable participating in school functions or activities. These might include providing support for them when participating on special education and I.E.P. teams, encouraging parental involvement in school-wide committees such as school improvement teams, *and* facilitating home-school communication when problems arise and includes assisting parents in accessing community-based services for their family.

8.3 School psychologists educate the school community regarding the influence of family involvement on school achievement and advocate for parent involvement in school governance and policy development whenever feasible.

8.4 School psychologists help create linkages between schools, families, and community agencies and help coordinate services when programming for children involves multiple agencies.

8.5 School psychologists are knowledgeable about the local system of care and related community services available to support students and their families.

8.6 School psychologists work with parent organizations to promote public policy that empowers parents to be competent consumers of the local system of services.

8.7 School psychologists are active participants in public policy by serving on committees, participating in workgroups and task forces, and in responding to proposed legislation and rules.

### Guidelines for the Organization and Operation of the Unit

#### Unit Guideline 1: Organization of Service Delivery

School psychological services are provided in a coordinated, organized fashion and are delivered in a manner that ensures the provision of a comprehensive and seamless continuum of services. Services are delivered following the completion of a strategic planning process based on the needs of the consumers and an empirically supported program evaluation model.

1.1 School psychological services are available and accessible to all students and clients served by the agency and are in proportion to the needs of the client.

1.2 School psychological services are available to all students on an equal basis and are not determined by a specific funding source. Services are provided to students based on their need, not based on their eligibility to generate specific funding.

1.3 School psychological services are integrated with other school and community services. Students and their families should not be responsible for the integration of these services based on funding, setting, or program location. Therefore, school psychological and mental health services are provided through a "seamless" system of care.

1.4 School psychological services units ensure that the services delivered by the unit and provided directly by the school psychologist to consumers are based on a strategic plan. The plan is developed based on the collective needs of the district and community with the primary focus being the specific needs of the population served by individual practitioners.

1.5 School psychological services units conduct regular evaluations of the collective services provided by the unit as well as those services provided by individual practitioners. The evaluation process focuses on both the nature and extent of the services provided (process) and the student/family focused outcomes of those services (product).

1.6 The school psychological services unit provides a range of services to their clients. These consist of direct and indirect services that require involvement with the entire educational system as well as other services systems in the community. The consumers of and participants in these services include: students, teachers, administrators, other school personnel, families, caretakers, other community and regional agencies, and resources that support the educational process.

## Unit Guideline 2: Climate

It is the responsibility of the unit to create a climate in which school psychological services can be delivered with mutual respect for all parties. Employees of the unit have the freedom to advocate for the services that are necessary to meet the needs of consumers and are free from artificial, administrative, or political constraints that might hinder or alter the provision of appropriate services.

2.1 Providers of school psychological services maintain a cooperative relationship with colleagues and co-workers in the best mutual interests of clients. Conflicts are resolved in a professional manner.

2.2 The potential negative impact of administrative constraints on effective services is kept to a minimum. The school psychologist will advocate for administrative policies that support the school psychologist in seeking the needed services and will provide mechanisms for referral and consultation regarding unmet health and mental health needs.

2.3 Members of the unit advocate in a professional manner for the most appropriate services for their clients without fear of reprisal from supervisors or administrators.

2.4 School psychological service units are aware of the impact of work environment on the job satisfaction of unit employees and on the quality of services provided to consumers. Measures of work climate are included when the unit conducts self-evaluations.

2.5 School psychological service units promote and advocate for balance between professional and personal lives of unit employees. Unit supervisors monitor work and stress levels of employees and take steps to reduce pressure when the well-being of the employee is at risk. Supervisors are available to employees to problem solve when personal factors may adversely affect job performance and when job expectations may adversely affect the personal life of the employee.

## Unit Guideline 3: Physical, Personnel, and Fiscal Support Systems

School psychological services units ensure that (a) an adequate recruitment and retention plan for employees exists to ensure adequate personnel to meet the needs of the system; (b) all sources of funding, both public and private, are used and maximized to ensure the fiscal support necessary to provide adequate services; (c) all employees have adequate technology, clerical services, and a physical work environment; and (d) employees have adequate personnel benefits necessary to support the work of the unit including continuing educational professional development.

3.1 School psychological services units assume the professional responsibility and accountability for services provided through the recruitment of qualified and diverse staff and the assurance that staff members function only in their areas of competency.

3.2 School psychological services units support recruitment and retention of qualified staff by advocating for appropriate ratios of school psychology services staff to students. The ratio of staff to students should not exceed one staff person for every 1000 students.

3.3 School psychological services units utilize advanced technologies (e.g., computer-assisted) in time management, communication systems, data management systems, and service delivery.

3.4 School psychological services unit have access to adequate clerical assistance, appropriate professional work materials, sufficient office and work space, adequate technology support (e.g., e-mail, computer) and general working conditions that enhance the delivery of effective services. Included are test materials, access to private telephone and office, secretarial services, therapeutic aids, and professional literature.

## Unit Guideline 4: Communication and Technology

The school psychological services unit ensures that policies and practices exist which result in positive, proactive communication and technology systems both within the unit, its central organizational structure, and those organizational structures with which the unit interacts.

4.1 School psychological service units provide opportunities for members of the unit to communicate with each other about issues of mutual professional interest on a regular basis.

4.2 School psychological services units maintain a formal system of communication channels with other units within the parent organization and between the unit and other agencies with whom it interacts on behalf of clients. The unit engages in decision-making and strategic planning with other units and agencies in order to ensure optimal services are provided to mutual clients.

4.3 School psychological services units ensure that staff members have access to the technology necessary to perform their jobs adequately and to maintain communication with service providers and clients within and outside the unit. The requirement for confidentiality is respected, with adequate resources available to service providers to ensure confidential communication.

4.4 School psychological services units' policy on student records is consistent with state and federal rules and laws and ensures the protection of the confidentiality of the student and his or her family. The policy specifies the types of data developed by the school psychologist that are classified as school or pupil records. The policy gives clear guidance regarding which documents belong (consistent with FERPA or similar state/court regulations) to the school and the student/

guardian and which documents (such as clinical notes) are the personal property of the school psychologist.

4.5 Parents may inspect and review any personally identifiable data relating to their children that were collected, maintained, or used in his/her evaluation. Although test protocols are part of the student's record, school psychologists protect test security and observe copyright restrictions. Release of records and protocols is done consistent with state/federal regulations.

## Unit Guideline 5: Supervision

The school psychological services unit ensures that all personnel have levels and types of supervision adequate to ensure the provision of effective and accountable services. Supervision is provided through an ongoing, positive, systematic, collaborative process between the school psychologist and the school psychology supervisor. This process focuses on promoting professional growth and exemplary professional practice leading to improved performance by all concerned including the school psychologist, supervisor, students, and the entire schoolcommunity.

5.1 A supervisor of a school psychological services unit holds or meets the criteria for the Nationally Certified School Psychologist (NCSP) credential and has been identified by an employing agency and/or school psychological service unit as a supervisor responsible for school psychology services in the agency or unit. Supervisors hold a state school psychologist credential and have a minimum of three years of experience as a practicing school psychologist. Training and/or experience in the supervision of school personnel are desirable.

5.2 When supervision is required for interns, beginning school psychologists, or others for whom supervision is necessary, such supervision will be provided at least 2hours per week for persons employed full-time.

5.3 Supervisors lead school psychological services units in developing, implementing, and evaluating a coordinated plan for accountability and evaluation of all services provided in order to maintain the highest level of effectiveness. Such plans include specific, measurable objectives pertaining to the planned effects of services. Evaluation is both formative and summative. Supervisors provide leadership by promotion of innovative service delivery systems that reflect best practices in the field of school psychology.

5.4 Supervisors lead school psychological services units in developing, implementing, and evaluating a coordinated plan for accountability and evaluation of all services provided by individual staff members and by the unit as a whole in order to maintain the highest level of services. Such plans include specific, measurable objectives pertaining to the planned effects of services on all relevant elements of the system and the students it serves. Evaluation is both formative and summative.

5.5 The school psychological services unit continues to provide supervision or peer review for its school psychologists after their first year of employment to ensure continued professional growth and development and support for complex or difficult cases.

5.6 Supervisors coordinate the activities of the school psychological services unit with other professional services units through review and discussion of 1) intervention planning and outcomes; 2) comprehensive, systemic procedures and special concerns; and 3) discrepancies among views of various professional service providers or employing agencies.

5.7 Supervisors ensure that practica and internship experiences occur under conditions of appropriate supervision including 1) access to professional school psychologists who will serve as appropriate role models, 2) provision of supervision by an appropriately credentialed school psychologist, and 3) provision of supervision within the guidelines of the training institution and *NASP Standards for Training and Field Placement Programs in School Psychology*.

5.8 Supervisors provide professional leadership through participation in school psychology professional organizations and active involvement in local, state and federal public policy development.

### Unit Guideline 6: Professional Development and Recognition Systems

Individual school psychologists and the school psychological services unit develop professional development plans annually. The school psychological services unit ensures that continuing professional development of its personnel is both adequate for and relevant to the service delivery priorities of the unit and that recognition systems exist to reflect the continuum of professional development activities embraced by its personnel.

6.1 All school psychologists within the unit actively participate in activities designed to continue, enhance, and upgrade their professional training and skills to help ensure quality service provision.

6.2 The school psychological services unit provides support(e.g., funding, time, supervision) to ensure that school psychologists have sufficient access to continuing professional development and supervision activities at a minimal level necessary to maintain the NCSP.

6.3 School psychologists develop a formal professional development plan and update this plan annually. The goals, objectives, and activities of the plan are influenced by the following factors in order of priority: (1) the most pressing needs of the population and community served;(2) the knowledge, skills, and abilities required to implement initiatives sponsored by the unit; and (3) the individual interest areas of the school psychologists employed by the unit.

6.4 School psychologists seek and use appropriate types and levels of supervision as they acquire new knowledge, skills, and abilities through the professional development process.

6.5 School psychologists document the type, level, and intensity of their professional development activities. The school psychological services unit provides technology and personnel resources to assist in these activities.

6.6 School psychologists individually seek appropriate levels of advanced recognition (e.g., advanced degrees, levels established by district, state, or national recognition bodies) to reflect on-going professional development.

6.7 School psychological services units provide levels of recognition (e.g., salary, opportunity to use new skills) within the unit that reflect the professional development of the school psychologists in the unit.

### Unit Guideline 7: Contracted/Independent Provider Services

The school psychological services unit is responsible for providing psychological services. These services can come from district employed school psychologists, from psychologists employed in independent practice, or through other agencies. Regardless of whether personnel are employed or contracted, it is the responsibility of the unit to ensure the same level and quality of services as those provided by personnel from within the unit.

7.1 Contractual school psychological services encompass the same comprehensive continuum of services as is provided by regularly employed school psychologists. These services include opportunities for follow-up and continuing consultation appropriate to the needs of the student. Individual contracts for services may be limited as long as the school psychological services unit ensures comprehensive services overall.

7.2 Contractual school psychological services are not used as a means to decrease the amount and quality of school psychological services provided by an employing agency. They may be used to augment and enhance programs, as in the case of retaining needed expertise, to coordinate with other community health services, and to assure that services are available to students and their families.

7.4 Contracted services may be used as a mechanism to maximize available resources. However, any such models of service must provide comprehensive psychological services and must assure quality services of equal or greater value when compared to services provided by school-based personnel.

7.5 Contractual school psychological services are provided ina manner that protects the due process rights of students and their parents as defined by state and federal laws and regulations.

7.6 Psychologists providing contractual school psychological services provide those services in a manner consistent with these *Guidelines*, *NASP Principles for Professional Ethics*, and other relevant professional guidelines and standards.

7.7 Persons providing contractual psychological services are fully credentialed school psychologists as defined by these or other (e.g., state certification boards) recognized standards. In specific instances, however, services by credentialed psychologists in other specialty areas (e.g., clinical, industrial/organizational, neuropsychology) might be used to supplement school psychological services and should be coordinated with school psychological services.

7.8 Psychologists providing contractual school psychological services will require regular evaluation of the quality of services provided as well as the continued need for contracted services.

7.9 A credentialed school psychologist who has completed a school psychology training program that meets the criteria specified in the NASP *Standards for Training and Field Placement Programs in School Psychology* and two full-time years (one of which may be internship) of satisfactory, properly supervised experience is considered qualified for personally supervised, independent practice with peer review, regardless of work setting. (NOTE: "Independent practice" as used in this paragraph refers to autonomous functioning within the employing school or agency. Contrast this with the licensure rules of various states for "private practice.")

7.10 A credentialed school psychologist or an organized group of credentialed school psychologists may engage in independent practice outside of a school agency or unit pursuant to existing rules regarding the independent practice of psychology within a given state. Units will support public policy that will provide for the independent practice of school psychology.

# References

Abbott, M., Walton, C., Tapia, Y., & Greenwood, C. R. (1999). Research to practice: A "blueprint" for closing the gap in local schools. *Exceptional Children, 65*, 339–352

Abramowitz, A. J., O'Leary, S. G., & Futtersak, M. W. (1988). The relative impact of long and short reprimands on children's off-task behavior in the classroom. *Behavior Therapy, 19*, 243–247.

Abramowitz, A. J., O'Leary, S. G., & Rosen, L. A. (1987). Reducing off-task behavior in the classroom: A comparison of encouragement and reprimands. *Journal of Abnormal Child Psychology, 15*, 153–163.

Achenbach, T. M., & Rescorla, L. A. (2001). *Manual for the ASEBA school-age forms and profiles.* Burlington: University of Vermont.

Acker, M. M., & O'Leary, S. G. (1987). Effects of reprimands and praise on appropriate behavior in the classroom. *Journal of Abnormal Child Psychology, 15*, 549–557.

Adams, G. R., Hampton, R. L., Gullotta, T. P., Weissberg, R. P., & Ryan, B. A. (Eds.). (1997). *Establishing preventative services.* Thousand Oaks, CA: Sage.

Adams, M. J. (1990). *Beginning to read: Thinking and learning about print.* Cambridge, MA: MIT Press.

Adelman, H. S., & Taylor, L. (1997). Toward a scale-up model for replicating new approaches to schooling. *Journal of Educational and Psychological Consultation, 8*, 197–230.

Alessi, G. (1987). Generative strategies and teaching for generalization. *The Analysis of Verbal Behavior, 5*, 15–27.

Alessi, G. (1988). Diagnosis diagnosed: A systemic reaction. *Professional School Psychology, 3*, 145–151.

American Academy of Pediatrics. (2001). Clinical practice guideline: Treatment of the child with attention-deficit/hyperactivity disorder. *Pediatrics, 105*, 1058–1070.

American Educational Research Association, American Psychological Association, & National Council on Measurement in Education. (1999). *Standards for educational and psychological testing.* Washington, DC: American Educational Research Association.

American Psychiatric Association. (1994). *Diagnostic and statistical manual of mental disorders* (4th ed.). Washington, DC: Author

American Psychological Association. (1990). *APA guidelines for providers of psychological services to ethnic, linguistic, and culturally diverse populations.* Retrieved May 3, 2004, from www.apa.org/pi/oema/guide.html.

American Psychological Association. (2002a). *Ethical principles of psychologists and code of conduct.* Washington, DC: Author. Retrieved July 1, 2004, from www.apa.org/ethics/code2002.pdf.

American Psychological Association. (2002b). *Guidelines and principles for accreditation of programs in professional psychology.* Washington, DC: American Psychological Association. Retrieved July 19, 2005, from www.apa.org/ed/accreditation/policies.html.

American Psychological Association. (2002c). *Guidelines on multicultural education, training, research, practice, and organizational change for psychologists.* Retrieved May 3, 2004, from www.apa.org/.html.

American Psychological Association. (2003). *C-18 core faculty in doctoral programs.* Washington, DC: Author.

American Psychological Association Division of School Psychology. (2005). *Archival description of the specialty of school psychology.* Retrieved February 8, 2005, from www.indiana.edu/~div16/G&O.htm.

American School Counselor Association. (2003). *Careers/roles, student to counselor ratios.* Retrieved July 2, 2003, from www.schoolcounselor.org/content.cfm?L1=9.

Angold, A., Costello, E., & Erkanli, A. (1999). Comorbidity. *Journal of Child Psychology and Psychiatry, 40,* 55–87.

Arter, J. A., & Jenkins, J. R. (1977). Examining the benefits and prevalence of modality considerations in special education. *Journal of Special Education, 11,* 281–298.

Arter, J. A., & Jenkins, J. R. (1979). Differential diagnosis-prescriptive teaching: A critical appraisal. *Review of Educational Research, 49,* 517–555.

Atkinson, D. R., Morten, G., & Sue, D. W. (1998). *Counseling American minorities.* Boston: McGraw-Hill.

Baer, D. M., & Bushell, D. (1981). The future of behavior analysis in the schools? Consider its recent past, and then ask a different question. *School Psychology Review, 10,* 259–270.

Bailey, D. S. (2004). Number of psychology PhDs declining. *APA Monitor on Psychology, 35*(2), 18.

Bandura, A. (1978). The self-system in reciprocal determination. *American Psychologist, 33,* 344–358.

Barbe, W. B., & Milone, M. N. (1980). Modality. *Instructor, 89,* 44–47.

Bardon, J. I. (1986). Psychology and schooling: The interrelationships among persons, processes, and products. In S. N. Elliott & J. C. Witt (Eds.), *The delivery of psychological services in schools: Concepts, processes, and issues* (pp. 53–79). Hillsdale, NJ: Erlbaum.

Bardon, J. I., & Bennett, V. C. (1974). *School psychology.* Englewood Cliffs, NJ: Prentice-Hall.

Barkley, R. A. (1997). *Defiant children: A clinician's manual for assessment and parent training* (2nd ed.). New York: Guilford Press.

Barkley, R. A. (2006). *Attention-deficit hyperactivity disorder: A handbook for diagnosis and treatment* (3rd ed.). New York: Guilford Press.

Barkley, R. A., McMurray, M. B., Edelbrock, C. S., & Robbins, K. (1990). Side effects of methylphenidate in children with attention deficit hyperactivity disorder: A systematic, placebo-controlled evaluation. *Pediatrics, 86,* 184–192.

Batsche, G. M., & Curtis, M. J. (2003). The creation of the National School Psychology Certification System. *Communique, 32*(4), 6–7.

Bellak, L., & Bellak. S. (1949). *The Children's Apperception Test.* Larchmont, NY: CPS.

Bennett, F. C., Brown, R. T., Craver, J., & Anderson, D. (1999). Stimulant medication for the child with attention-deficit hyperactivity disorder. *Pediatric Clinics of North America, 46,* 929–944.

Bergan, J. R., & Kratochwill, T. R. (1990). *Behavioral consultation and therapy.* New York: Plenum.

Berlin, I. (1974). *Slaves without masters: The free Negro in the antebellum south.* New York: Pantheon.

Berry, J. W., & Annis, R. C. (1974). Acculturative stress: The role of ecology, culture and differentiation. *Journal of Cross-Cultural Psychology, 5,* 382–406.

Bersoff, D. N. (1995). *Ethical conflicts in psychology*. Washington, DC: American Psychological Association.

Best, J. H., & Sidwell, R. T. (1967). *The American legacy of learning: Readings in the history of education*. Philadelphia: Lippincott.

Biglan, A., Mrazek, P. J., Carnine, D., & Flay, B. R. (2003). The integration of research and practice in the prevention of youth problem behaviors. *American Psychologist, 58*, 433–440.

Bijou, S. W. (1993). *Behavior analysis of child development* (rev. ed.). Reno, NV: Context Press.

Board of Education of the Hendrick Hudson Central School District v. Rowley, 458 U.S. 176 (1982).

Board of Education, Sacramento City Unified School District v. Holland, 786 F. Supp. 874 (E.D. Cal. 1992).

Bracken, B. A., & McCallum, R. S. (1998). *Universal Nonverbal Intelligence Test*. Itasca, IL: Riverside.

Bracken, B. A., & Naglieri, J. A. (2003). Assessing diverse populations with nonverbal tests of general intelligence. In C. R. Reynolds & R. W. Kamphaus (Eds.), *Handbook of psychological and educational assessment of children: Intelligence, aptitude, and achievement* (2nd ed., pp. 243–274). New York: Guilford Press.

Bradley-Johnson, S., & Dean, V. J. (2000). Role change for school psychology: The challenge continues in the new millennium. *Psychology in the Schools, 37*(1), 1–5.

Bramlett, R. K., Murphy, J. J., Johnson, J., Wallingsford, L., & Hall, J. D. (2002). Contemporary practices in school psychology: A national survey of roles and referral problems. *Psychology in the Schools, 39*, 327–335.

Brestan, E. V., & Eyberg, S. M. (1998). Effective psychosocial treatments of conduct-disordered children and adolescents: 29 years, 82 studies, and 5, 272 kids. *Journal of Clinical and Child Psychology, 27*, 180–189.

Brown v. Board of Educ., 347 U.S. 483 (1954).

Brown, R. T., Freeman, W. S., Perrin, J. M., Stein, M. T., Amler, R. W., & Feldman, H. (2001). Prevalence and assessment of attention-deficit/hyperactivity disorder in primary care settings. *Pediatrics, 107*, E43.

Brown, R. T., & Sammons, M. T. (2002). Pediatric psychopharmacology: A review of new developments and recent research. *Professional Psychology: Research and Practice, 33*, 135–147.

Burt, M. K., Dulay, H. C., & Hernandez, Chavez, E. (19760. *Bilingual syntax measure I (BSM)*. New York: The Psychological Corporation.

Butcher, J. N., Williams, C. L., Graham, J. R., Archer, R. P., Tellegen, A., Ben-Porath, Y. S., & Kaemmer, B. (1992). *Minnesota Multiphasic Personality Inventory–Adolescent: Manual for administration, scoring, and interpretation*. Minneapolis: University of Minnesota Press.

Butts, R. F. (1978). *Public education in the United States: From revolution to reform*. New York: Holt, Rinehart & Winston.

Calhoun, D. (Ed.). (1969). *The educating of Americans: A documentary history*. Boston: Houghton Mifflin.

Campbell, D. T. (1988). The experimenting society. In S. Overman (Ed.), *Methodology and epistemology for social science* (pp. 290–314). Chicago: University of Chicago Press.

Carlberg, C., & Kavale, K. (1980). The efficacy of special versus regular class placement for exceptional children: A meta-analysis. *Journal of Special Education, 14*, 295–309.

Carnine, D. (1989). Designing practice activities. *Journal of Learning Disabilities, 22*, 603–607.

Carnine, D. (1997). Bridging the research-to-practice gap. *Exceptional Children, 63*, 513–521.

Carnine, D. (1999). Campaigns for moving research into practice. *Remedial and Special Education, 20*, 2–6, 35.

Carroll, J. B. (1963). A model of school learning. *Teachers College Record, 64*, 723–733.

Cedar Rapids Community School District v. Garrett F., 526 U.S. 66 (1999).

Chafouleas, S. M., Riley-Tillman, T. C., & Eckert, T. L. (2003). A comparison of school psychologists' acceptability, training, and use of norm-referenced, curriculum-based, and brief experimental analysis methods to assess reading. *School Psychology Review, 32*, 272–281.

Chavat, J. L. (2003). The school psychologist shortage: Evidence for effective advocacy. *Communiqué*, *32*(2), 1, 3–4.

Cherry v. Matthews, 419 F. Supp. 922 (D. D.C. 1976).

Children's Defense Fund. (2001). *The state of America's children yearbook 2001*. Washington, DC: Author.

Clark, E. (2002). Working together for a shared vision. *School Psychologist*, *57*, 40.

Cohen, J. (1988). *Statistical power analysis for the behavioral sciences* (2nd ed.). Hillsdale, NJ: Erlbaum.

Colvin, G. (2002). Designing classroom organization and structure. In K. L. Lane, F. M. Gresham, & T. E. O'Shaughnessy (Eds.), *Interventions for children with or at risk for emotional and behavioral disorders* (pp. 159–174). Boston: Allyn & Bacon.

Compton, S. N., March, J. S., Brent, D., Albano, A. M., Weersing, V. R., & Curry, J. (2004). Cognitive-behavioral psychotherapy for anxiety and depressive disorders in children and adolescents: An evidence-based medicine review. *Journal of the American Academy of Child and Adolescent Psychiatry*, *43*, 930–959.

Connolly, A. J. (1988). *KeyMath–Revised: A diagnostic inventory of essential mathematics*. Circle Pines, MN: American Guidance Service.

Connolly, A. J. (1997). *KeyMath–Revised: A diagnostic inventory of essential mathematics–Normative update*. Circle Pines, MN: AGS.

Conoley, J. C., & Gutkin, T. B. (1995). Why didn't–why doesn't–school psychology realize its promise? *Journal of School Psychology*, *33*, 209–217.

Cook, T. D., & Campbell, D. T. (1979). *Quasi-experimentation: Design and analysis issues for field settings*. Boston: Houghton-Mifflin.

Cooper, J. O., Heron, T. E., & Heward, W. L. (1987). *Applied behavior analysis*. Upper Saddle River, NJ: Prentice-Hall.

Council for Exceptional Children. (2004). *No Child Left Behind Act of 2001: Reauthorization of the Elementary and Secondary Education Act. A technical assistance report*. Arlington, VA: Author. Retrieved June 10, 2004, from www.cec.sped.org/pp/OverviewNCLB.pdf.

Cowen, E. L., Hightower, A. D., Pedro-Carroll, J., Work, W. C., Wyman, P. A., & Haffney, W. G. (Eds.). (1996). *School-based prevention for children at risk: The primary mental health project*. Washington, DC: American Psychological Association.

Crockett, D. (2003). Critical issues children face in the 2000s. *School Psychology Quarterly*, *18*, 446–453.

Crockett, D. (2004). Critical issues children face in the 2000s. *School Psychology Review*, *33*, 78–82.

Cronbach, L. J. (1957). The two disciplines of scientific psychology. *American Psychologist*, *1*, 671–684.

Cronbach, L. J. (1975). Beyond the two disciplines of scientific psychology. *American Psychologist*, *30*, 116–127.

Cronbach, L. J., & Snow, R. E. (1977). *Aptitudes and instructional methods: A handbook for research on instruction*. New York: Irvington.

Cullinan, D., Lloyd, J., & Epstein, M. H. (1981). Strategy training: A structured approach to arithmetic instruction. *Exceptional Education Quarterly*, *2*, 41–49.

Cummins, J. (1984). *Bilingualism and special education: Issues in assessment and pedagogy*. San Diego, CA: College Hill.

Cummins, J., Muñoz-Sandoval, A. F., Alvarado, C. G., & Ruef, M. L. (1998). *The Bilingual Verbal Ability Tests*. Itasca, IL: Riverside Publishing.

Curtis, M. J. (2002, November). *The changing face of school psychology: Past, present, and future*. Webcast presentation at the Future of School Psychology Conference, Indianapolis, Indiana. Retrieved March 4, 2004, from www.indiana.edu/~futures/presentations.html.

Curtis, M. J., Grier, J. E. C., & Hunley, S. A. (2003). The changing face of school psychology: Trends in data and projections for the future. *School Psychology Quarterly*, *18*, 409–430.

Curtis, M. J., Grier, J. E. C., & Hunley, S. A. (2004). The changing face of school psychology: Trends in data and projections for the future. *School Psychology Review*, *33*, 49–66.

Curtis, M. J., Hunley, S. A., & Chesno Grier, J. E. (2002). Relationships among the professional practices and demographic characteristics of school psychologists. *School Psychology Review*, *31*, 30–42.

Curtis, M. J., Hunley, S. A., & Grier, E. C. (2004). The status of school psychology: Implications of a major personnel shortage. *Psychology in the Schools*, *41*, 431–442.

Curtis, M. J., Hunley, S. A., Walker, K. J., & Baker, A. C. (1999). Demographic characteristics and professional practices in school psychology. *School Psychology Review*, *28*, 104–116.

Curtis, M. J., & Stollar, S. A. (2002). Best practices in system-level change. In A. Thomas & J. Grimes (Eds.), *Best practices in school psychology: IV* (pp. 223–234). Bethesda, MD: National Association of School Psychologists.

Daly, E. J., III, Lentz, F. E., & Boyer, J. (1996). The instructional hierarchy: A conceptual model for understanding the effective components of reading interventions. *School Psychology Quarterly*, *11*, 369–386.

Daly, E. J., III, Witt, J. C., Martens, B. K., & Dool, E. J. (1997). A model for conducting a functional analysis of academic performance problems. *School Psychology Review*, *26*, 554–574.

Dana, R. H. (1993). *Multicultural assessment perspectives for professional psychology*. Boston: Allyn & Bacon.

Daniel R. R. v. State Board of Education, 874 F. 2d 1035 (5th Cir. 1989).

Dawson, M., Cummings, J. A., Harrison, P. L., Short, R. J., Gorin, S., & Palomares, R. (2003). The 2002 multisite conference on the future of school psychology: Next steps. *School Psychology Quarterly*, *18*, 497–509.

Dawson, M., Cummings, J. A., Harrison, P. L., Short, R. J., Gorin, S., & Palomares, R. (2004). The 2002 multisite conference on the future of school psychology: Next steps. *School Psychology Review*, *33*, 115–125.

De Avila, E., & Duncan, S. (2005). *Language assessment scales*. New York: McGraw-Hill.

deHirsch, K., Jansky, J., & Langford, W. L. (1966). *Predicting reading failure*. New York: Harper & Row.

Demaray, M. K., Carlson, J. S., & Hodgson, K. K. (2003). Assistant professors of school psychology: A national survey of program directors and job applicants. *Psychology in the Schools*, *40*, 691–698.

Deno, S. L. (1985). Curriculum-based measurement: The emerging alternative. *Exceptional children*, *52*, 219–232.

Deno, S. L. (2002). Problem-solving as "best practice." In A. Thomas & J. Grimes (Eds.) *Best practices in school psychology: IV* (Vol. 1, pp. 37–55). Bethesda, MD: National Association of School Psychologists.

Deno, S. L. (2003). Developments in curriculum-based measurement. *Journal of Special Education*, *37*, 184–192.

Deno, S. L., Espin, C. A., & Fuchs, L. S. (2002). Evaluation strategies for preventing and remediating basic skill deficits. In M. R. Shinn, H. M. Walker, & G. Stoner (Eds.), *Interventions for academic and behavior problems: II. Preventive and remedial approaches* (pp. 213–242). Bethesda, MD: National Association of School Psychologists.

Derry, S. J., & Murphy, D. A. (1986). Designing systems that train learning ability: From theory to practice. *Review of Educational Research*, *56*, 1–39.

Deshler, D. D., & Schumaker, J. B. (1986). Learning strategies: An instructional alternative for low-achieving adolescents. *Exceptional Children*, *52*, 583–590.

Dettmer, P., Dyck, N., & Thurston, L. P. (2002). *Consultation, collaboration, and teamwork for students with special needs* (4th ed.). Boston: Allyn & Bacon.

Doll, B., & Lyon, M. A. (1998). Risk and resilience: Implications for the delivery of educational and mental health services in schools. *School Psychology Review*, *27*, 348–363.

Drum, D. J., & Figler, H. E. (1973). *Outreach in counselling: Applying the growth and prevention model in schools and colleges*. Oxford, UK: Intext Educational.

Dunn, R. S. (1979). Learning—A matter of style. *Educational Leadership*, *36*, 430–432.

DuPaul, G. J., Barkley, R. A., & Connor, D. F. (1998). Stimulants. In R. A. Barkley, *Attention-deficit hyperactivity disorder: A handbook for diagnosis and treatment* (2nd ed., pp. 510–551). New York: Guilford Press.

DuPaul, G. J., & Stoner, G. (2003). *ADHD in the schools: Assessment and intervention strategies* (2nd ed.). New York: Guilford Press

Dwyer, K. P. (2004). Is every school psychologist a mental health provider? Yes? *Communiqué, 32*(7), 11–12.

Eckert, T. L., Shapiro, E. S., & Lutz, J. G. (1995). Teachers' acceptability of alternative psychoeducational measures: The acceptability of curriculum-based assessment. *School Psychology Review, 24*, 497–511.

Edelstein, B. A., & Mickelson, L. (Eds.). (1986). *Handbook of prevention.* New York: Plenum.

Egeland, B., Carlson, E., & Sroufe, L. A. (1993). Resilience as process. *Development and Psychopathology, 5*, 517–528.

Elias, M. J., Zins, J. E., Graczyk, P. A., & Weissberg, R. P. (2003). Implementation, sustainability, and scaling up of social-emotional and academic innovations in public schools. *School Psychology Review, 32*, 303–319.

Elliot, C. D. (1990). *Differential Ability Scales.* San Antonio, TX: Psychological Corporation.

Engelman, S. (1997). Theory of mastery and acceleration. In J. W. Lloyd, E. J. Kame'enui, & D. Chard (Eds.), *Issues in educating students with disabilities* (pp. 177–195). Mahwah, NJ: Erlbaum.

Epps, S., Ysseldyke, J., & McGue, M. (1984). Differentiating LD and non-LD students: "I know one when I see one." *Learning Disability Quarterly, 7*, 89–101.

Fagan, T. K. (1995). Trends in the history of school psychology in the United States. In A. Thomas & J. Grimes (Eds.), *Best practices in school psychology: III* (pp. 59–67). Washington, DC: National Association of School Psychologists.

Fagan, T. K. (2002). Trends in the history of school psychology in the United States. In A. Thomas & J. Grimes (Eds.), *Best practices in school psychology: IV* (pp. 209–221). Bethesda, MD: National Association of School Psychologists.

Fagan, T. K., & Wells, P. D. (2000). History and status of school psychology accreditation in the United States. *School Psychology Review, 29*, 28–58.

Fagan, T. K., & Wise, P. S. (1994). *School psychology: Past, present, and future.* White Plains, NY: Longman.

Fagan, T. K., & Wise, P. S. (2000). *School psychology: Past, present, and future* (2nd ed.). Bethesda, MA: National Association of School Psychologists.

Felton, R. H., & Pepper, P. P. (1995). Early identification of phonological deficits in kindergarten and early elementary children at risk for reading disability. *School Psychology Review, 24*, 405–414.

Ferritor, D. C., Buckholt, D., Hamblin, R. L., & Smith, L. (1972). The noneffects of contingent reinforcement for attending behavior on work accomplished. *Journal of Applied Behavior Analysis, 5*, 7–17.

Finger, M. S., & Rand, K. L. (2003). Addressing validity concerns in clinical psychology research. In M. C. Roberts & S. S. Ilardi (Eds.), *Handbook of research methods in clinical psychology* (pp. 13–30). Malden, MA: Blackwell.

Fireoved, R., & Cancelleri, R. (1985). What training programs need to emphasize: Notes from the field. *Trainer's Forum, 5*(1), 4–5.

Flanagan, D. P., & Ortiz, S. O. (2002). Best practices in intellectual assessment: Future directions. In A. Thomas & J. Grimes (Eds.), *Best practices in school psychology: IV* (pp. 1351–1372). Bethesda, MD: National Association of School Psychologists.

Fletcher, J. M., Francis, D. J., Shaywitz, S. E., Lyon, G. R., Foorman, B. R., Stuebing, K. K., & Shaywitz, B. A. (1998). Intelligent testing and the discrepancy model for children with learning disabilities. *Learning Disabilities Research and Practice, 13*, 186–203.

Fletcher, J. M., Shaywitz, S. E., Shankweiler, D. P., Katz, L., Liberman, I. Y., Fowler, A., et al. (1994). Cognitive profiles of reading disability: Comparisons of discrepancy and low achievement definitions. *Journal of Educational Psychology, 85*, 1–23.

Forness, S. T. (1970). Educational prescription for the school psychologist. *Journal of School Psychology, 8*, 96–98.

Forness, S. T. (2003a). Barriers to evidence-based treatment: Developmental psychopathology and the interdisciplinary disconnect in school mental health practice. *Journal of School Psychology*, *41*, 61–67.

Forness, S. T. (2003b). Parting reflections on education of children with emotional or behavioral disorders. *Education and Treatment of Children*, *26*, 320–324.

Forness, S. T., & Kavale, K. A. (2001). Reflections on the future of prevention. *Preventing School Failure*, *45*, 75–81.

Frank, G. (1984). The Boulder Model: History, rationale, and critique. *Professional Psychology: Research and Practice*, *15*, 417–435.

Freeman, K. A. (2003). Single subject designs. In J. C. Thomas & M. Hersen (Eds.), *Understanding research in clinical and counseling psychology* (pp. 181–208). Mahwah, NJ: Erlbaum.

Friedman, R. M. (2003). Improving outcomes for students through the application of a public health model to school psychology: A commentary. *Journal of School Psychology*, *41*, 69–75.

Friman, P. C., & Blum, N. (2002). Primary care behavioral pediatrics. In M. Hersen & W. Sledge (Eds.), *Encyclopedia of psychotherapy* (pp. 379–399) New York: Academic Press.

Fuchs, D., Fuchs, L. S., Harris, A. H., & Roberts, P. H. (1996). Bridging the research-to-practice gap with mainstream assistance teams: A cautionary tale. *School Psychology Quarterly*, *11*, 244–266.

Fuchs, L. S., & Fuchs, D. (1998). Treatment validity: A unifying concept for reconceptualizing the identification of learning disabilities. *Learning Disabilities Research and Practice*, *13*, 204–219.

Fuchs, L. S., Fuchs, D., Hosp, M., & Jenkins, J. (2001). Oral reading fluency as an indicator of reading competence: A theoretical, emprical, and historical analysis. *Scientific Studies in Reading*, *5*, 239–256.

Fuchs, L. S., Fuchs, D., & Speece, D. L. (2002). Treatment validity as a unifying construct for identifying learning disabilities. *Learning Disability Quarterly*, *25*, 33–45.

Fullan, M. (2000). The three stories of education reform. *Phi Delta Kappan*, *8*, 581–584.

Fullan, M., Bertani, A., & Quinn, J. (2004). New lessons for districtwide reform. *Educational Leadership*, *4*, 42–46.

Gayer, H. L., Brown, M. B., Gridley, B. E., & Treloar, J. H. (2003). Predoctoral psychology intern selection: Does program type make a difference? *Social Behavior and Personality*, *31*, 313–322.

Gersten, R., & Chard, D. (1999). Number sense: Rethinking arithmetic instruction for students with mathematical disabilities. *Journal of Special Education*, *33*, 18–28.

Gersten, R., Chard, D., & Baker, S. (2000). Factors enhancing sustained use of research-based instructional practices. *Journal of Learning Disabilities*, *33*(5), 445–457.

Gersten, R., Vaughn, S., Deshler, D., & Schiller, E. (1997). What we know about using research findings: Implications for improving special education practice. *Journal of Learning Disabilities*, *30*, 466–476.

Gettinger, M. (1988). Methods of proactive classroom management. *School Psychology Review*, *17*, 227–242.

Gettinger, M., & Seibert, J. K. (2002). Best practices in increasing academic learning time. In A. Thomas & J. Grimes (Eds.), *Best practices in school psychology: IV* (pp. 773–787). Bethesda, MD: National Association of School Psychologists.

Gimpel, G. A., & Collett, B. R. (2002). Best practices in behavioral parent training. In A. Thomas & J. Grimes (Eds.), *Best practices in school psychology: IV* (pp. 451–466). Bethesda, MD: National Association of School Psychologists.

Glass, G. V. (1983). Effectiveness of special education. *Policy Studies Review*, *2*, 65–78.

Good, R. H., III, Gruba, J., & Kaminski, R. A. (2002). Best practices in using Dynamic Indicators of Basic Early Literacy Skills (DIBELS) in an outcomes-driven model. In A. Thomas & J. Grimes (Eds.), *Best practices in school psychology: IV* (Vol. 1, pp. 699–720). Bethesda, MD: National Association of School Psychologists.

Good, R. H., Simmons, D. C., & Smith, S. B. (1998). Effective academic interventions in the United States: Evaluating and enhancing the acquisition of early reading skills. *School Psychology Review*, *27*, 740–753.

Good, T. L., & Brophy, J. E. (1994). *Looking in classrooms* (6th ed.). New York: HarperCollins.

Gopaul-McNicol, S. A. (1997). A theoretical framework for training monolingual school psychologists to work with multilingual/multicultural children: An exploration of the major competencies. *Psychology in the Schools, 34*, 17–29.

Graham, S., Harris, K. R., MacArthur, C. A., & Schwartz, S. (1991). Writing and writing instruction for students with learning disabilities: Review of a research program. *Learning Disabilities Quarterly, 14*, 89–114.

Gray, S. W. (1963). *The psychologist in the schools.* New York: Holt, Rinehart, & Winston.

Greenberg, M. T., Weissberg, R. P., O'Brien, M. U., Zins, J. E., Fredericks, L., Resnik, H., & Elias, M. J. (2003). Enhancing school-based prevention and youth development through coordinated social, emotional, and academic learning. *American Psychologist, 58*, 466–474.

Greene, M. M. (2003). Program evaluation. In J. C. Thomas & M. Hersen (Eds.), *Understanding research in clinical and counseling psychology* (pp. 209–242). Mahwah, NJ: Erlbaum.

Greenhill, L. L., Halperin, J. M., & Abikoff, H. (1999). Stimulant medications. *Journal of the American Academy of Child and Adolescent Psychiatry, 38*, 503–512.

Greenhill, L. L., Swanson, J. M., Vitiello, B., Davies, M., Clevenger, W., Wu, M., et al. (2001). Impairment and deportment responses to different methylphenidate doses in children with ADHD: The MTA titration trial. *Journal of the American Academy of Child and Adolescent Psychiatry, 40*, 180–187.

Gresham, F. M., & Noell, G. H. (1999). A functional model of assessment and treatment as a foundation of special education. In D. J. Reschly, W. D. Tilly, & J. Grimes (Eds.), *Special education in transition: Functional assessment and noncategorical programming* (pp. 49–80). Longmont, CO: Sopris West.

Gresham, F. M., Watson, T. S., & Skinner, C. H. (2001). Functional behavioral assessment: Principles, procedures, and future directions. *School Psychology Review, 30*, 156–172.

Grimes, J., & Tilly, D. W. (1996). Policy and process: Means to lasting educational change. *School Psychology Review, 25*(4), 465–476.

Grossen, B., Caros, J., Carnine, D., Davis, B., Deshler, D., Schumaker, J., et al. (2002). Big ideas (plus a little effort) produce big results. *Teaching Exceptional Children, 34*, 70–73.

Hall, R. V., Lund, D. E., & Jackson, D. (1968). Effects of teacher attention on study behavior. *Journal of Applied Behavior Analysis, 1*, 1–12.

Halsell, M. A. (2002). Best practices in increasing cross-cultural competence. In A. Thomas & J. Grimes (Eds.), *Best practices in school psychology: IV* (pp. 353–362). Bethesda, MD: National Association of School Psychologists.

Hammill, D. D., Pearson, N. A., & Weiderholt, J. L. (1997). *Comprehensive Test of Nonverbal Intelligence.* Austin, TX: Pro-Ed.

Hanf, C. (1969). *A two-stage program for modifying maternal controlling during mother–child (m-c) interaction.* Paper presented at the annual meeting of the Western Psychological Association, Vancouver, BC.

Haring, N. G., Lovitt, T. C., Eaton, M. D., & Hansen, C. L. (1978). *The fourth R: Research in the classroom.* Columbus, OH: Merrill.

Hart, B., & Risley, T. R. (1995). *Meaningful differences in the everyday experience of young American children.* Baltimore: Brookes.

Harvey, V. (2002). Best practices in teaching study skills. In A. Thomas & J. Grimes (Eds.), *Best practices in school psychology: IV* (pp. 831–849). Bethesda, MD: National Association of School Psychologists.

Hayes, S. C., & Follette, W. C. (1992). Can functional analysis provide a substitute for syndromal classification? *Behavioral Assessment, 14*, 345–365.

Hembree-Kigin, T. L., & McNeil, C. B. (1995). *Parent–child interaction therapy.* New York: Plenum.

Hendry, C. N. (2003). Clinical assessment of children's academic achievement. In C. R. Reynolds & R. W. Kamphaus (Eds.), *Handbook of psychological and educational assessment of children: Intelligence, aptitude, and achievement* (2nd ed., pp. 438–472). New York: Guilford Press.

Herrnstein, R. J., & Murray, C. (1994). *The bell curve: Intelligence and class structure in American life.* New York: Free Press.

Hildreth, G. H. (1930). Psychological service for school problems. Yonkers-on-Hudson, NY: World Book Co.

Hirst, W. E. (1963). Know your school psychologist. *School Psychologist, 33*(4), 1.

History of American Education Web Project. (2004). *Progressive period of American education.* Retrieved October 8, 2004, from www.nd.edu/˜rbarger/www7/.

Hoagwood, K., & Johnson, J. (2003). School psychology: A public health framework: I. From evidence-based policies. *Journal of School Psychology, 41,* 3–21.

Hollingworth, L. S. (1933). Psychological service for public schools. *Teachers College Record, 34,* 368–379.

Hosp, J. L., & Reschly, D. J. (2002). Regional differences in school psychology practice. *School Psychology Review, 31,* 11–29.

Howell, K. W., & Kelley, B. (2002). Curriculum clarification, lesson design, and delivery. In F. M. Gresham, K. L. Lane, & T. O'Shaughnessy (Eds.), *Academic and social–behavioral interventions for students with or at-risk for emotional and behavioral disorders* (pp. 55–73). Boston: Allyn and Bacon.

Howell, K. W., & Nolet, V. (2000). *Curriculum-based evaluation: Teaching and decision making* (3rd ed.). Belmont, CA: Wadsworth.

Hughes, J. N., & Baker, D. B. (1990). *The clinical child interview.* New York: Guilford Press.

Hunley, S. (2004). The NCSP challenge. *Communique, 32*(5), 35.

Hunter, L. (2003). School psychology: A public health framework III: Managing disruptive behavior in schools: The value of a public health and evidence-based perspective. *Journal of School Psychology, 41,* 39–59.

Ibraham, F. A., Roysircar-Sodowsky, G., & Ohnishi, H. (2001). Worldview: Recent developments and needed directions. In J. G. Ponterotto, J. M. Casas, L. A. Suzuki, & C. M. Alexander (Eds.), *Handbook of multicultural counseling* (pp. 425–456). Thousand Oaks, CA: Sage.

Ingraham, C. L. (2000). Consultation through a multicultural lens: Multicultural and cross-cultural consultation in schools. *School Psychology Review, 29,* 320–343.

Irving Independent School District v. Tatro, 468 U.S. 883 (1984).

Jacob, S., & Hartshorne, T. S. (2003). *Ethics and law for school psychologists* (4th ed.). Hoboken, NJ: Wiley.

Jacobson, N. S., & Truax, P. (1991). Clinical significance: A statistical approach to defining meaningful clinical change in psychotherapy research. *Journal of Consulting and Clinical Psychology, 59,* 12–19.

Jacob-Timm, S. (1999). Ethically challenging situations encountered by school psychologists. *Psychology in the Schools, 36,* 205–217.

Jaeger, P. T., & Bowman, C. A. (2002). *Disability matters: Legal and pedagogical issues of disability in education.* Westport, CT: Bergin & Garvey.

Jensen, P., Arnold, L., Richters, J., et al. (1999). 14–month randomized clinical trial of treatment strategies for attention deficit hyperactivity disorder. *Archives of General Psychiatry, 56,* 1073–1086.

Jensen, P. S., Hinshaw, S. P., Kraemer, H. C., Lenora, N., Newcorn, J. H., Abikoff, H. B., et al. (2001). ADHD comorbidity findings from the MTA study: Comparing comorbid subgroups. *Journal of the American Academy of Child and Adolescent Psychiatry, 40,* 147–158.

Johnson, D., & Myklebust, H. (1967). *Learning disabilities: Educational principles and practices.* New York: Grune & Stratton.

Johnson, M. B., Whitman, T. L., & Johnson, M. (1980). Teaching addition and subtraction to mentally retarded children: A self-instructional program. *Applied Research in Mental Retardation, 1,* 141–160.

Joint Committee on Testing Practices. (20040. *Code of fair testing practices in education.* Washington, DC: Author. Retrieved August 6, 2004, from www.apa.org/science/FinalCode.pdf

Juel, C. (1988). Learning to read and write: A longitudinal study of 54 children from first through fourth grades. *Journal of Educational Psychology, 80,* 437–447.

Kame'enui, E., & Carnine, D. (Eds.). (2001). *Effective teaching strategies that accommodate diverse learners.* Columbus, OH: Merrill.

Kamphaus, R. W., Reynolds, C. R., & Imperato-McCammon, C. (1999). Roles of diagnosis and classification in school psychology. In C. R. Reynolds & T. B. Gutkin (Eds.), *Handbook of school psychology* (3rd ed., pp. 292–306). New York: Wiley

Kampwirth, T. J., & Bates, M. (1980). Modality preference and teaching method: A review of research. *Academic Therapy, 15,* 597–605.

Kaslow, N. J., & Thompson, M. P. (1998). Applying the criteria for empirically supported treatments to studies of psychosocial interventions for child and adolescent depression. *Journal of Child Clinical Psychology, 27,* 146–155.

Kaufman, A. S., & Kaufman, N. L. (2004a). *Kaufman Assessment Battery for Children–Second Edition.* Circle Pines, MN: AGS.

Kaufman, A. S., Lichtenberger, E. O., & Naglieri, J. A. (1999). Intelligence testing in the schools. In C. R. Reynolds & T. B. Gutkin (Eds.), *Handbook of school psychology* (3rd ed., pp. 307–349). New York: Wiley

Kavale, K. A., & Forness, S. R. (1987). Substance over style: Assessing the efficacy of modality testing and teaching. *Exceptional Children, 54,* 228–239.

Kazdin, A. E. (1997). Parent management training: Evidence, outcomes, and issues. *Journal of the American Academy of Child and Adolescent Psychiatry, 36,* 1349–1356.

Kazdin, A. E. (1998). *Research design in clinical psychology* (3rd ed.). Boston: Allyn & Bacon.

Kazdin, A. E. (1999). The meanings and measurement of clinical significance. *Journal of Consulting and Clinical Psychology, 67,* 332–339.

Kazdin, A. E. (2000). *Psychotherapy for children and adolescents: Directions for research and practice.* New York: Oxford University Press.

Kazdin, A. E. (2001). *Behavior modification in applied settings* (6th ed.). Belmont, CA: Wadsworth.

Kazdin, A. E. (2003). Psychotherapy for children and adolescents. *Annual Reviews in Psychology, 54,* 253–276.

Kazdin, A. E. (2004). Psychotherapy for children and adolescents. In M. J. Lambert (Ed.), *Bergin and Garfield's handbook of psychotherapy and behavior change* (5th ed., pp. 543–589). New York: Wiley.

Kazdin, A. E., & Weisz, J. R. (Eds.). (2004). *Evidence-based psychotherapies for children and adolescents.* New York: Guilford Press.

Keith, T. Z. (2002). Best practices in applied research. In A. Thomas & J. Grimes (Eds.), *Best practices in school psychology: IV* (pp. 91–102). Bethesda, MD: National Association of School Psychologists.

Kendall, P. C., Aschenbrand, S. G., & Hudson, J. L. (2003). Child-focused treatment of anxiety. In A. E. Kazdin (Ed.), *Evidence-based psychotherapies for children and adolescents* (pp. 81–100). New York: Guilford Press.

Kendall, P. C., Panichelli-Mindel, S. M., Sugarman, A., & Callahan, S. A. (1997). Exposure to child anxiety: Theory, research, and practice. *Clinical Psychology: Science and Practice, 4,* 724–730.

Kenyon, P. (1999). *What would you do? An ethical case workbook for human service professionals.* Pacific Grove, CA: Brooks-Cole.

Kephart, N. C. (1960). *The slow learner in the classroom.* Columbus, OH: Merrill.

Kim, B. S. K., & Abreu, J. M. (2001). Acculturation measurement. In J. G. Ponterotto, J. M. Casas, L. A. Suzuki, & C. M. Alexander (Eds.), *Handbook of multicultural counseling* (pp. 394–424). Thousand Oaks, CA: Sage.

Kimble, G. A. (1984). Psychology's two cultures. *American Psychologist, 39,* 833–839.

Kirk, S. A., McCarthy, J. J., & Kirk, W. D. (1968). *The Illinois Test of Psycholinguistic Abilities* (rev. ed.). Urbana: University of Illinois.

Knoff, H. M. (2002). Best practices in facilitating school reform, organizational change, and strategic planning. In A. Thomas & J. Grimes (Eds.), *Best practices in school psychology: IV* (Vol. 1, pp. 235–253). Bethesda, MD: National Association of School Psychologists.

Kohn, A. (1993). *Punished by rewards: The trouble with gold stars, incentive plans, A's, praise, and other bribes.* Boston: Houghton-Mifflin.

Kovacs, M. (1991). *The Children's Depression Inventory.* North Tonawanda, NY: Multi-Health Systems.

Kounin, J. (1970). *Discipline and group management in classrooms.* New York: Holt, Rinehart,& Winston.

Kratochwill, T. R., & Bergan, J. R. (1990). *Behavioral consultation in applied settings: An individual guide.* New York: Plenum Press.

Kratochwill, T. R., & Shernoff, E. S. (2004). Evidence-based practice: Promoting evidence based interventions in school psychology. *School Psychology Review, 33,* 34–48.

Kratochwill, T. R., & Stoiber, K. C. (2000a). Diversifying theory and science: Expanding boundaries of empirically supported interventions in schools. *Journal of School Psychology, 38,* 349–358.

Kratochwill, T. R., & Stoiber, K. C. (2000b). Empirically supported interventions and school psychology: Conceptual and practical issues: Part II. *School Psychology Quarterly, 15,* 233–253.

Kratochwill, T. R., & Stoiber, K. C. (2002). Evidence-based interventions in school psychology: Conceptual foundations of the Procedural Coding Manual of Division 16 and the Society for the Study of School Psychology Task Force. *School Psychology Quarterly, 17,* 341–389.

Kryzanowski, J., & Carnine, D. W. (1980). Effects of massed versus spaced formats in teaching sound/symbol correspondences to young children. *Journal of Reading Behavior, 12,* 225–230.

LaBerge, D., & Samuels, S. J. (1974). Toward a theory of automatic information processing in reading. *Cognitive Psychology, 6,* 293–323.

Lambert, M. J. (Ed.). (2004). *Bergin and Garfield's handbook of psychotherapy and behavior change* (5th ed.). New York: Wiley.

Lane, K. L., Gresham, F. M., & O'Shaughnessy, T. E. (Eds.). (2002). *Interventions for children with or at risk for emotional and behavioral disorders.* Boston: Allyn & Bacon.

Leahey, T. H. (1987). *A history of modern psychology: Main currents in psychological thought* (2nd ed.). Englewood Cliffs, NJ: Prentice-Hall.

Lentz, B. K. (1992). Self-managed learning strategy systems for children and youth. *School Psychology Review, 21,* 211–228.

Lentz, F. E., & Shapiro, E. S. (1985). Behavioral school psychology: A conceptual model for the delivery of psychological services. In T. Kratochwill (Ed.), *Advances in school psychology* (Vol. 5, pp. 191–221). Hillsdale, NJ: Erlbaum.

Lewinsohn, P. M., & Clarke, G. N. (1999). Psychosocial treatments for adolescent depression. *Clinical Psychology Review, 19,* 329–342.

Little, S. G., & Akin-Little, K. A. (2004). Academic school psychologists: Addressing the shortage. *Psychology in the Schools, 41,* 451–459.

Lloyd, J. W., Forness, S. R., & Kavale, K. A. (1998). Some methods are more effective than others. *Intervention in School and Clinic, 33,* 195–200.

Lloyd, J. W., Hallahan, D. P., Kauffman, J. M., & Keller, C. E. (1998). Academic problems. In R. J. Morris & T. R. Kratochwill (Eds.), *The practice of child therapy* (3rd ed., pp. 167–198). Boston: Allyn & Bacon.

Lopez, E. C. (2002). Best practices in working with school interpreters to deliver psychological services to children and families. In A. Thomas & J. Grimes (Eds.), *Best practices in school psychology: IV* (pp. 1419–1432). Bethesda, MD: National Association of School Psychologists.

Luckey, B. M. (1951, May). Duties of the school psychologist: Past, present and future. *Division of School Psychologists Newsletter,* 4–10.

Lund, A. R., Reschly, D. J., & Martin, L. M. C. (1998). School psychology personnel needs: Correlates of current patterns and historical trends. *School Psychology Review, 27,* 106–120.

Luthar, S. S., & Cichetti, D. (2000). The construct of resilience: Implications for interventions and social policies. *Development and Psychopathology, 12,* 857–885.

Lynam, D. R., Milich, R., Zimmerman, R., Novak, S. P., Logan, T. K., Martin, C., et al. (1999). Project DARE: No effects at 10–year follow-up. *Journal of Consulting and Clinical Psychology, 67,* 590–593.

Maag, J. W. (1990). Social skills training in schools. *Special Services in the Schools, 6,* 1–19.

Magary, J. F. (1967). Emerging viewpoints in school psychological services. In J. F. Magary (Ed.), *School psychological services in theory and practice: A handbook* (pp. 671–755). Englewood Cliffs, NJ: Prentice-Hall.

March, J. S. (1997). *Multidimensional Anxiety Scale for Children.* North Tonawanda, NY: Multi-Health Systems.

Markwardt, F. C. (1989). *Peabody Individual Achievement Test–Revised.* Circle Pines, MN: AGS.

Markwardt, F. C. (1997). *Peabody Individual Achievement Test–Revised: Normative update.* Circle Pines, MN: AGS.

Martines, D. (2003, Fall). Suggestions for training cross-cultural consultant school psychologists. *Trainer's Forum, 23,* 5–13.

Masten, A. S., & Coatsworth, J. D. (1998). The development of competence in favorable and unfavorable environments: Lessons from research on successful children. *American Psychologist, 53,* 205–220.

Mastropieri, M. A., Leinart, A., & Scruggs, T. E. (1999). Strategies to increase reading fluency. *Interventions in School and Clinic, 34,* 278–283.

McArthur, D. S., & Roberts, D. E. (1982). *Roberts Apperception Test for Children.* Los Angeles: Western Psychological Services.

McDougal, J. L., Clonan, S. M., & Martens, B. K. (2000). Using organizational change procedures to promote the acceptability of prereferral intervention services: The school-based intervention team project. *School Psychology Quarterly, 15,* 149–171.

McGrew, K. S., & Woodcock, R. W. (2001). *Technical manual: Woodcock-Johnson III.* Itasca, IL: Riverside.

McMahon, R. J., & Forehand, R. L. (2003). *Helping the noncompliant child: Family-based treatment for oppositional disorder* (2nd ed.). New York: Guilford Press.

Meece, J. L., & Kurtz-Costes, B. (2001). Introduction: The schooling of ethnic minority children and youth. *Educational Psychology, 36,* 1–7.

Meichenbaum, D. H., & Goodman, J. (1971). Training impulsive children to talk to themselves: A means of developing self-control. *Journal of Abnormal Psychology, 77,* 117–126.

Merrell, K. W. (2001). *Helping students overcome depression and anxiety: A practical guide.* New York: Guilford Press.

Merrell, K. W. (2003). *Behavioral, social, and emotional assessment of children and adolescents* (2nd ed.). Mahwah, NJ: Erlbaum.

Messick, S. (1995). Validity of psychological assessment: Validation inferences from persons' responses and performances as scientific inquiry into score meaning. *American Psychologist, 50,* 741–749.

Miller, G., Giovenco, A., & Rentiers, K. A. (1987). Fostering comprehension monitoring in below average readers through self-instruction training. *Journal of Reading Behavior, 19,* 379–394.

Miller, G. E., Brehm, K., & Whitehouse, S. (1998). Reconceptualizing school-based prevention for antisocial behavior within a resiliency framework. *School Psychology Review, 27,* 364–379.

Mills v. Board of Education of the District of Columbia 348 F. Supp. 866 (1972).

MTA Cooperative Group. (1999a). A 14-month randomized clinical trial of treatment strategies for attention-deficit/hyperactivity disorder. *Archives of General Psychiatry, 56,* 1073–1086.

MTA Cooperative Group. (1999b). Moderators and mediators of treatment response for children with attention-deficit/hyperactivity disorder: The multimodal treatment study of children with attention-deficit/hyperactivity disorder. *Archives of General Psychiatry, 56,* 1088–1096.

Nastasi, B. K., Varjas, K., Sarkar, S., & Jayasena, A. (1998). Participatory model of mental health programming: Lessons learned from work in a developing country. *School Psychology Review, 27*(2), 260–276.

National Association of School Psychologists. (2000a). *Professional conduct manual: Principles for professional ethics and guidelines for the provision of school psychological services.* Bethesda, MD: Author.

National Association of School Psychologists. (2000b). *Standards for training and field placement programs in school psychology*. Bethesda, MD: Author.

National Association of School Psychologists. (2003a). *Minority demographics in school psychology*. Retrieved October 15, 2003, from www.nasponline.org/culturalcompetence/minority_demog .html.

National Association of School Psychologists. (2003b). *Position statement on minority recruitment*. Retrieved October 15, 2003, from www.nasponline.org/about_nasp/minority.html.

National Association of School Psychologists. (2004). *National school psychology certification system*. Retrieved February 3, 2004, from www.nasponline.org/certification/ncsp_system.html.

National Association of School Psychologists. (2005). *What is a school psychologist?* Retrieved February 8, 2005, from www.nasponline.org/about_nasp/whatisa.html.

National Reading Council. (1998). *Preventing reading difficulties in young children*. Washington, DC: National Academy Press.

National Reading Panel. (2000). *Teaching children to read: An evidence-based assessment of the scientific research literature on reading and its implications for reading instruction: Reports of the subgroups*. Bethesda, MD: National Institute of Child Health and Human Development.

Neisser, U., Boodoo, G., Bouchard, T. J., Boykin, A. W., Broday, N., Ceci, S. J., et al. (1996). Intelligence: Knowns and unknowns. *American Psychologist, 51*, 77–101.

Nettles, S. M., Mucherah, W., & Jones, D. S. (2000). Understanding resilience: The role of social resources. *Journal of Education for Students Placed At Risk, 5*, 47–60.

Neufeldt, V. (1989). *Webster's New World Dictionary: Third College Edition*. New York: Prentice Hall.

New Mexico Department of Education. (2001). *Technical assistance document for nondiscriminatory assessment of culturally and linguistically diverse school-age children*. Albuquerque, NM: New Mexico Department of Education.

Ninness, H. A. C., & Glenn, S. S. (1988). *Applied behavioral analysis in school psychology: A research guide to principles and procedures*. Westport, CT: Greenwood Press.

Oakland, T. D., & Cunningham, J. (1992). A survey of school psychology in developed and developing countries. *School Psychology International, 13*, 99–129.

Oberti v. Board of Education of the Borough of Clementon School District, 995 F.2d 1204 (3rd Cir. 1993).

Ochoa, S. H., Rivera, B., & Ford, L. (1997). An investigation of school psychology training pertaining to bilingual psycho-educational assessment of primarily Hispanic students: Twenty-five years after Diana v. California. *Journal of School Psychology, 35*, 329–349.

Ollendick, T. H., & King, N. J. (1998). Empirically supported treatments for children with phobic and anxiety disorders: Current status. *Journal of Clinical Child Psychology, 27*, 156–167.

O'Neill, R. E., Horner, R. H., Albin, R. W., Sprague, J. R., Storey, K., & Newton, J. S. (1997). *Functional assessment and program development for problem behavior: A practical handbook* (2nd ed.). Pacific Grove, CA: Brooks/Cole.

Ortiz, S. O. (2002). *Best practices in nondiscriminatory assessment*. In A. Thomas & J. Grimes (Eds.), *Best practices in school psychology: IV* (pp. 1321–1336). Bethesda, MD: National Association of School Psychologists.

Ortiz, S. O., & Flanagan, D. P. (2002). Best practices in working with culturally diverse children and families. In A. Thomas & J. Grimes (Eds.), *Best practices in school psychology: IV* (pp. 337–351). Bethesda, MD: National Association of School Psychologists.

OSEP Center on Positive Behavioral Interventions and Supports. (2000). Applying positive behavior support and functional behavioral assessment in schools. *Journal of Positive Behavior Interventions, 2*, 131–143.

Padilla, A. (2001). Issues in culturally appropriate assessment. In L. A. Suzuki, J. G. Ponterroto, & P. J. Meller (Eds.), *Handbook of multicultural assessment* (2nd ed., pp. 5–28). San Francisco: Wiley.

Paine, S. C., Radicchi, J., Rosellini, L. C., Deutchmann, L., & Darch, C. B. (1983). *Structuring your classroom for academic success*. Champaign, IL: Research Press.

Patterson, G. R. (1982). *Coercive family process.* Eugene, OR: Castalia.

Patterson, G. R., Reid, J. B., & Dishion, T. J. (1992). *Antisocial boys.* Eugene, OR: Castalia.

Pelham, W. E., Wheeler, T. , & Chronis, A. (1998). Empirically supported psychosocial treatments for attention deficit hyperactivity disorder. *Journal of Child Clinical Psychology, 27,* 190–205.

Pellegrino, J. W., & Goldman, S. R. (1987). Information processing and elementary mathematics. *Journal of Learning Disabilities, 20,* 23–32.

Pennsylvania Association for Retarded Children (PARC) v. Commonwealth of Pennsylvania, 334 F. Supp. 1257 (E.D. Pa. 1971), 343 F. Supp. 279 (E.D. Pa. 1972).

Pianta, R. C., & Walsh, D. J. (1998). Applying the construct of resilience in schools: Cautions from a developmental systems perspective. *School Psychology Review, 27,* 407–417.

Polk v. Central Susquehanna Intermediate Unit 16, 853 F. 2d 171 (3rd Cir. 1988).

Power, T. J. (2000). Commentary: The school psychologist as community-focused, public health professional: Emerging challenges and implications for training. *School Psychology Review, 29,* 557–559.

Power, T. J. (2003). Promoting children's mental health: Reform through interdisciplinary and community partnerships. *School Psychology Review, 32,* 3–16.

Power, T. J., DuPaul, G. J., Shapiro, E. S., & Parrish, J. M. (1995). Pediatric school psychology: The emergence of a subspecialty. *School Psychology Review, 24,* 244–257.

Power, T. J., Shapiro, E. S., & DuPaul, G. J. (2003). Preparing psychologists to link systems of care in managing and preventing children's health problems. *Journal of Pediatric Psychology, 28,* 147–155.

Pratt, R., & Rittenhouse, G. (Eds.). (1998). *The condition of education: 1998.* Washington, DC: U.S. Government Printing Office.

President's Commission on Excellence in Special Education. (2002). *A new era: Revitalizing special education for children and their families.* Washington, DC: U.S. Department of Education. Retrieved July 15, 2004, from www.ed.gov/inits/commissionsboards/whspecialeducation/reports/index.html.

Pressley, M. (1996). The challenges of instructional scaffolding: The challenges of instruction that supports student thinking. *Learning Disabilities Research and Practice, 11,* 138–146.

Pressley, M., Woloshyn, V., Burkell, J., Cariglia-Bull, T., Lysynchuk, L., McGoldrick, J. A., et al. (1995). *Cognitive strategy instruction that really improves children's academic performance* (2nd ed.). Cambridge, MA: Brookline.

Prevatt, F. F. (1999). Personality assessment in the schools. In C. R. Reynolds & T. B. Gutkin (Eds), *Handbook of school psychology* (3rd ed., pp. 434–451). New York: Wiley

Pyrczak, F. (1999). *Evaluating research in academic journals: A practical guide to realistic evaluation.* Los Angeles: Author.

Quinn, K. P., & McDougal, J. L. (1998). A mile wide and a mile deep: Comprehensive interventions for children and youth with emotional and behavioral disorders and their families. *School Psychology Review, 27,* 191–203.

Rathvon, N. (1999). *Effective school interventions: Strategies for enhancing academic achievement and social competence.* New York: Guilford Press.

Ravitch, D. (1974). *The great school wars: New York City, 1805–1973: A history of the public schools as battlefield of social change.* New York: Basic Books.

Ravitch, D. (2000). *Left back: A century of failed school reforms.* New York: Simon & Schuster.

Reid, R., Maag, J. W., Vasa, S. F., & Wright, G. (1994). Who are the children with attention deficit-hyperactivity disorder? A school-based survey. *Journal of Special Education, 28,* 117–137.

Reschly, D., & Wilson, M. (1997). Characteristics of school psychology graduate education: Implications for the entry level discussion and doctoral level specialty definition. *School Psychology Review, 26,* 74–92.

Reschly, D. J. (1997). Utility of individual ability measures and public policy choices for the 21st century. *School Psychology Review, 26,* 234–241.

Reschly, D. J. (2000). The present and future status of school psychology in the United States. *School Psychology Review, 29,* 507–522.

Reschly, D. J., & Grimes, J. P. (2002). Best practices in intellectual assessment. In A. Thomas & J. Grimes (Eds.), *Best practices in school psychology: IV* (pp. 1337–1350) Bethesda, MD: National Association of School Psychologists.

Reschly, D. J., Tilly, W. D., III, & Grimes, J. P. (Eds.). (1999). *Special education in transition: Functional assessment and noncategorical programming.* Longmont, CO: Sopris West.

Reschly, D. J., & Wilson, M. S. (1995). School psychology practitioners and faculty: 1986 to 1991–92 trends in demographics, roles, satisfaction, and system reform. *School Psychology Review, 24,* 62–80.

Reschly, D. J., & Ysseldyke, J. E. (2002). Paradigm shift: The past is not the future. In A. Thomas & J. Grimes (Eds.), *Best practices in school psychology: IV* (pp. 3–36). Bethesda, MD: National Association of School Psychologists.

Reynolds, C. R., & Gutkin, T. B. (Eds.). (1999). *Handbook of school psychology* (3rd ed.). New York: Wiley.

Reynolds, C. R., & Kamphaus, R. W. (2004). *Behavior Assessment System for Children* (2nd ed.). Circle Pines, MN: American Guidance Service.

Rhodes, R. L., Ochoa, S., & Ortiz, S. (2005). *Assessing culturally and linguistically diverse students: A practical guide.* New York: Guilford Press.

Rogers, M. R. (2000). Examining the cultural context of consultation. *School Psychology Review, 29,* 414–418.

Roid, G. H. (2003). *Stanford-Binet Intelligence Scales–Fifth Edition.* Itasca, IL: Riverside.

Roid, G. H., & Miller, L. J. (1997). *Leiter International Performance Scale–Revised.* Wood Dale, IL: Stoelting.

Root, R. W., & Resnick, R. J. (2003). An update on the diagnosis and treatment of attention-deficit/hyperactivity disorder in children. *Professional Psychology: Research and Practice, 34,* 34–41.

Rossi, P. H., & Freeman, H. E. (1993). *Evaluation: A systemic approach* (5th ed.). Newbury Park, CA: Sage.

Rothstein, L. F. (2000). *Special education law* (3rd ed.). Boston: Allyn & Bacon.

Rummler, G. A., & Brache, A. P. (1995). *Improving performance: How to manage the white space on the organization chart* (2nd ed.). San Francisco: Jossey-Bass.

Sacramento City School District v. Rachel H., 14 F. 3d 1398 (9th Cir. 1994).

Samuels, S. J., & Flor, R. F. (1997). The importance of automaticity for developing expertise in reading. *Reading and Writing Quarterly: Overcoming Learning Difficulties, 13,* 107–121.

Samuels, S. J., LaBerge, D., & Bremer, C. (1978). Units of word recognition: Evidence for developmental change. *Journal of Verbal Learning and Verbal Behavior, 17,* 715–720.

Sattler, J. M. (2001). *Assessment of children: Cognitive applications* (4th ed.). San Diego, CA: Author.

Savage, T. A., Prout, H. T., & Chard, K. M. (2004). School psychology and issues of sexual orientation: Attitudes, beliefs, and knowledge. *Psychology in the Schools, 41,* 201–210.

Scotti, J. R., Morris, T. L., & Cohen, S. H. (2003). Validity: Making inferences from research outcomes. In J. C. Thomas & M. Hersen (Eds.), *Understanding research in clinical and counseling psychology* (pp. 97–129). Mahwah, NJ: Erlbaum.

Scotti, J. R., Morris, T. L., McNeil, C. B., & Hawkins, R. P. (1996). DSM-IV and disorders of childhood and adolescence: Can structural criteria be functional? *Journal of Consulting and Clinical Psychology, 64,* 1177–1191.

Serna, L., Lambros, K. M., Nielsen, E., & Forness, S. R. (2002). Head Start children at risk for emotional or behavioral disorders: Behavioral profiles and clinical implications of a primary prevention program. *Behavioral Disorders, 27,* 137–141.

Serna, L., Nielson, E., Mattern, N., Schau, C., & Forness, S. R. (2002). Use of different measures to identify preschoolers at risk for emotional or behavioral disorders: Impact on gender and ethnicity. *Education and Treatment of Children, 25,* 243–260.

Shapiro, E. S. (1996). *Academic skill problems: Direct assessment and intervention* (2nd ed.). New York: Guilford Press.

Shapiro, E. S. (2000). School psychology from an instructional perspective: Solving big, not little problems. *School Psychology Review, 29*, 560–572.

Shapiro, E. S. (2004). *Academic skill problems: Direct assessment and intervention* (3rd ed.). New York: Guilford Press.

Shapiro, E. S., Angello, L. M., & Eckert, T. L. (2004). Has curriculum-based assessment become a staple of school psychology practice? An update and extension of knowledge, use, and attitudes from 1990 to 2000. *School Psychology Review, 33*, 249–257.

Shapiro, E. S., & Cole, C. L. (1994). *Behavior change in the classroom: Self-management interventions.* New York: Guilford Press.

Shapiro, E. S., & Eckert, T. L. (1993). Curriculum-based assessment among school psychologists: Knowledge, attitudes, and use. *Journal of School Psychology, 31*, 375–384.

Shapiro, E. S., & Eckert, T. L. (1994). Acceptability of curriculum-based assessment by school psychologists. *Journal of School Psychology, 32*, 167–184.

Shapiro, E. S., & Heick, P. F. (2004). School psychologist assessment practices in the evaluation of students referred for social/behavioral/emotional problems. *Psychology in the Schools, 41*, 551–561.

Shapiro, E. S., & Kratochwill, T. R. (2000). *Behavioral assessment in schools: Theory, research, and clinical foundations* (2nd ed.). New York: Guilford Press.

Shapiro, E. S., & Kratochwill, T. R. (2002). *Conducting school-based assessment of child and adolescent behavior.* New York: Guilford Press.

Sheridan, S. M. (2000). Considerations of multiculturalism and diversity in behavioralconsultation with parents and teachers. *School Psychology Review, 29*, 344–353.

Sheridan, S. M., & D'Amato, R. C. (2003). Partnering to chart our futures. *School Psychology Quarterly, 18*, 352–357.

Sheridan, S. M., & D'Amato, R. C. (2004). Partnering to chart our futures. *School Psychology Review, 33*, 7–11.

Sheridan, S. M., & Gutkin, T. B. (2000). The ecology of school psychology: Examining and changing our paradigm for the 21st century. *School Psychology Review, 29*, 485–502.

Shinn, M. R. (Ed.). (1989). *Curriculum-based measurement: Assessing special populations.* New York: Guilford Press.

Shinn, M. R. (Ed.). (1998). *Advances in curriculum-based measurement.* New York: Guilford Press.

Shinn, M. R. (2002). Best practices in using curriculum-based measurement in a problem-solving model. In A. Thomas & J. Grimes (Eds.), *Best practices in school psychology: IV* (pp. 671–697). Bethesda, MD: National Association of School Psychologists.

Shinn, M. R., Collins, V. L., & Gallagher, S. (1998). Curriculum-based measurement and its use in a problem-solving model with students from minority backgrounds. In M. Shinn (Ed.), *Advanced applications of curriculum-based measurement* (pp. 143–174). New York: Guilford Press.

Shinn, M. R., Walker, H. M., & Stoner, G. (2002). *Interventions for achievement and behavior problems: II* (2nd ed). Bethesda, MD: National Association of School Psychologists.

Short, R. J. (2002). School psychology as a separate profession: An unsupportable direction. *School Psychologist, 56*, 111–117.

Simmons, D. C., & Kame'enui, E. J. (Eds.). (1998). *What reading research tells us about children with diverse learning needs: Bases and basics.* Mahwah, NJ: Erlbaum.

Simmons, D. C., & Kame'enui, E. J. (1998). Introduction. In D. C. Simmons & E. J. Kame'enui (Eds.), *What reading research tells us about children with diverse learning needs: Bases and basics* (p. 1). Mahwah, NJ: Erlbaum.

Simmons, D. C., Kame'enui, E. J., Good, R. H., III, Harn, B. A., Cole, C., & Braun, D. (2002). Building, implementing, and sustaining a beginning reading improvement model school by school and lessons learned. In M. Shinn, G. Stoner, & H. M. Walker (Eds.), *Interventions for academic and behavior problems: II. Preventative and remedial approaches* (pp. 537–569). Bethesda, MD: National Association of School Psychologists.

Simmons, D. C., Kuykendall, K., King, K., Cornachione, C., & Kame'enui, E. J. (2000). Implementation of a schoolwide reading improvement model: "No one ever told us it would be this hard!" *Learning Disabilities Research and Practice, 15*, 92–100.

Skiba, R. J., & Peterson, R. L. (2000). School discipline at a crossroads: From zero tolerance to early response. *Exceptional Children*, *66*, 335–347.

Skinner, C. H., Skinner, A. L., & Sterling-Turner, H. E. (2002). Best practices in contingency management: Application of individual and group contingencies in educational settings. In A. Thomas & J. Grimes (Eds.), *Best practices in school psychology: IV* (pp. 817–830). Bethesda, MD: National Association of School Psychologists.

Smith, C. L., & Freeman, R. L. (2002). Using continuous system level assessment to build school capacity. *American Journal of Evaluation*, *23*(3), 307–319.

Smith, T. L. (1967). Protestant schooling and American nationality, 1800–1850. *Journal of American History*, *53*, 687.

Snider, V. E. (1992). Learning styles and learning to read: A critique. *Remedial and Special Education*, *13*, 6–18.

Sodowsky, G. R., Kwan, K. K., & Pannu, R. (1995). Ethnic identity of Asians in the United States. In J. G. Ponterotto, J. M. Casas, L. A. Suzuki, & C. M. Alexander (Eds.), *Handbook of multicultural counseling* (pp. 123–154). Thousand Oaks, CA: Sage.

Spencer, T. J., Biederman, J., & Wilens, T. (2000). Pharmacotherapy of attention-deficit hyperactivity disorder. *Child Adolescent Psychiatric Clinics of North America*, *9*, 77–97.

Spencer, T. J., Biederman, J., Wilens, T., Harding, M., O'Donnell, D., & Griffen, S. (1996). Pharmacotherapy of attention-deficit hyperactivity disorder across the life cycle. *Journal of the American Academy of Child and Adolescent Psychiatry*, *35*, 409–432.

Spivak, G., & Swift, M. (1973). The classroom behavior of children: A critical review of teacher-administered rating scales. *Journal of Special Education*, *7*, 55–89.

Stanovich, K. E. (1986). Matthew effects in reading: Some consequences of individual differences in the acquisition of early literacy. *Reading Research Quarterly*, *21*, 360–406.

Stanovich, K. E. (2000). *Progress in understanding reading: Scientific foundations and new frontiers*. New York: Guilford Press.

Stein, M., Carnine, D., & Dixon, R. (1998). Direct instruction: Integrating curriculum design and effective teaching practice. *Intervention in School and Clinic*, *33*, 227–234.

Stetson, R., Stetson, E. G., & Sattler, J. M. (2001). Assessment of academic achievement. In J. M. Sattler (Ed.), *Assessment of children: Cognitive applications* (4th ed., pp. 576–609). San Diego, CA: Sattler.

Stokes, T. F., & Baer, D. M. (1977). An implicit technology of generalization. *Journal of Applied Behavior Analysis*, *10*, 349–367.

Stoner, G., Shinn, M. R., & Walker, H. M. (1991). *Interventions for achievement and behavior problems*. Washington, DC: National Association of School Psychologists.

Strein, W., Hoagwood, K., & Cohn, A. (2003). School psychology. A public health perspective I. Prevention, populations, and systems change. *Journal of School Psychology*, *41*, 23–38.

Sue, D. (1981). *Counseling the culturally different: Theory and practice* (3rd ed.). New York: Wiley.

Sue, D. W., & Sue, D. (1999). *Counseling the culturally different: Theory and practice* (3rd ed.). New York: Wiley.

Sugai, G. (2003). Commentary: Establishing efficient and durable systems of school-based support. *School Psychology Review*, *32*(4), 530–535.

Sugai, G., & Horner, R. H. (2002a). The evolution of discipline practices: School-wide positive behavior supports. *Child and Family Behavior Therapy*, *24*, 23–50.

Sugai, G., & Horner, R. H. (2002b). An introduction to the special series on positive behavior support. *Journal of Emotional and Behavioral Disorders*, *10*(3), 130–136.

Sugai, G., Horner, R. H., Dunlap, G. Hieneman, M., Lewis, T. J., Nelson, C. M., et al. (2000). Applying positive behavioral support and functional behavioral assessment in schools. *Journal of Positive Behavioral Interventions*, *2*, 131–143.

Sugai, G., Sprague, J. R., Horner, R. H., & Walker, H. M. (2000). Preventing school violence: The use of office discipline referrals to assess and monitor schoolwide discipline interventions. *Journal of Emotional and Behavioral Disorders*, *8*, 94–101.

Swanson, H. L. (1999). Instructional components that predict treatment outcomes for students with learning disabilities: Support for a combined strategy and direct instruction model. *Learning Disabilities Research*, *14*, 129–140.

Swanson, P. N., & De La Paz, S. (1998). Teaching effective comprehension strategies to students with learning and reading disabilities. *Intervention in School and Clinic, 33,* 209–218.

Szapocznik, J., Kurtines, W. M., & Fernandez, T. (1980). Acculturation, biculturalism, and adjustment among Cuban Americans. In A. M. Padilla (Ed.), *Acculturation: Theory, models and some new findings* (pp. 139–159). Boulder, CO: Westview.

Szapocznik, J., Kurtines, W. M., & Fernandez, T. (1980). Bicultural involvement and adjustment in Hispanic-American youths. *International Journal of Intercultural Relations, 4,* 353–365.

Takushi, R., & Uomoto, J. M. (2001). The clinical interview from a multicultural perspective. In L. A. Suzuki, J. G. Ponterotto, & P. J. Meller (Eds.), *Handbook of multicultural assessment* (pp. 47–66). San Francisco: Jossey-Bass.

Tarasoff v. Regents of the University of California, 529 P.2d 334; 118 Cal. Rptr. 129 (Cal. 1974).

Tarasoff v. Regents of the University of California, 17 Cal. 3d 425, 551 P.2d 334; 131 Cal Rptr. 14 (Cal. 1976).

Tarver, S. G., & Dawson, M. M. (1978). Modality preference and the teaching of reading: A review. *Journal of Learning Disabilities, 11,* 5–17.

Taylor, L., Nelson, P., & Adelman, H. S. (1999). Scaling-up reforms across a school district. *Reading and Writing Quarterly, 15,* 303–325.

Tharinger, D. J., & Palomares, R. S. (2004). An APA-informed perspective on the shortage of school psychologists: Welcome licensed psychologists into the schools (and did we mention xeriscape gardening together?). *Psychology in the Schools, 41,* 461–472.

Thomas, A. (1998). *Directory of school psychology graduate programs.* Bethesda, MD: National Association of School Psychologists.

Thomas, A. (1999). School psychology 2000: Personnel needs in the next millennium. *Communique, 28*(4), 10.

Thomas, A. (2000a). School psychology 2000: Average salary data. *Communiqué, 28*(6), 28

Thomas, A. (2000b). School psychology 2000: Salaries. *Communiqué, 28*(5), 32.

Thomas, A. (2000c). School psychology 2000: What is average? *Communiqué, 28*(8), 34.

Thomas, A., & Grimes, J. (2002). Appendix: University training programs in school psychology. In. A. Thomas & J. Grimes (Eds.), *Best practices in school psychology: IV* (p. 1749). Bethesda, MD: National Association of School Psychologists.

Thurlow, M. L., & Ysseldyke, J. E. (1982). Instructional planning: Information collected by school psychologists vs. information considered useful by teachers. *Journal of School Psychology, 20,* 3–10.

Tilly, D. (2002). Best practices in school psychology as a problem-solving enterprise. In A. Thomas & J. Grimes (Eds.), *Best practices in school psychology: IV* (Vol. 1, pp. 21–36). Bethesda, MD: National Association of School Psychologists.

Tindall, R. H. (1979). School psychology: The development of a profession. In G. Phye & D. J. Reschly (Eds.), *School psychology: Perspectives and issues* (pp. 3–24). New York: Academic Press.

Tyack, D. B. (Ed.). (1967). *Turning points in American educational history.* Waltham, MA: Blaisdell.

U.S. Bureau of the Census. (1992). *United States Census, 1992 Updated.* Washington, DC: U.S. Government Printing Office.

U.S. Bureau of the Census. (1998). *Statistical abstract of the United States* (118th ed.). Washington, DC: U.S. Government Printing Office.

U.S. Bureau of the Census. (1999). *Statistical abstract of the United States* (119th ed.). Washington, DC: U.S. Government Printing Office.

U.S. Bureau of the Census. (2001, March). *Overview of race and Hispanic origin: 2000 census brief* (Publication No. C2KBR/01-1). Washington, DC: U.S. Government Printing Office.

U.S. Bureau of the Census. (2002). *Statistical abstract of the United States* (122nd ed.). Washington, DC: U.S. Government Printing Office.

U.S. Department of Education. (2002). *Twenty-fourth annual report to Congress on the implementation of the Individuals with Disabilities Education Act.* Washington, DC: Author. Retrieved June 15, 2004, from www.ed.gov/about/reports/annual/osep/2002/index.html.

VanDerHeyden, A. M., & Witt, J. C. (2005). Quantifying the context of assessment: Capturing the effect of base rates on screening accuracy. *School Psychology Review, 34,* 161–183.

VanDerHeyden, A. M., Witt, J. C., & Barnett, D. W. (in press). The emergence and possible futures of response to intervention. *Journal of Psychoeducational Assessment.*

Vázquez, L. A. (1997). A systematic multicultural curriculum model: The pedagogical process. In D. B. Pope-Davis & H. L. K. Coleman (Eds.), *Multicultural counseling competencies: Assessment, education and training, and supervision* (pp. 159–179). Thousand Oaks, CA: Sage.

Vázquez, L. A. (2003, September). *Use of interpreters and translators.* Paper presented at the meeting of the New Mexico Association of School Psychologists, Las Cruces.

Walker, H., Colvin, G., & Ramsey, E. (1995). *Antisocial behavior in public school: Strategies and best practices.* Pacific Grove, CA: Brooks/Cole.

Walker, H. M. (2001). Invited commentary on "Preventing mental disorders in school-aged children: Current state of the field." *Prevention and Treatment, 4,* Article 2. Retrieved July 19, 2005, from journals.apa.org/prevention/volume4/pre0040002c.html.

Walker, H. M., Horner, R. H., Sugai, G., Bullis, M., Sprague, J. R., Bricker, D., & Kaufman, M. J. (1996). Integrated approaches to preventing antisocial behavior patterns among school-age children and youth. *Journal of Emotional and Behavioral Disorders, 4,* 193–256.

Watson, T. S., & Steege, M. W. (2003). *Conducting school-based functional behavioral assessments: A practitioner's guide.* New York: Guilford Press.

Webster-Stratton, C., Reid, M. J., & Hammond, M. (2004). Treating children with early-onset conduct problems: Intervention outcomes for parent, child, and teacher training. *Journal of Clinical Child and Adolescent Psychology, 33,* 105–124.

Wechsler, D. (1997). *Wechsler Adult Intelligence Scale–Third Edition.* San Antonio, TX: Psychological Corporation.

Wechsler, D. (2001). *Wechsler Individual Achievement Test–Second Edition.* San Antonio, TX: Psychological Corporation

Wechsler, D. (2002). *The Wechsler Preschool and Primary Scale of Intelligence–Third Edition.* San Antonio, TX: Psychological Corporation.

Wechsler, D. (2003). *The Wechsler Intelligence Scale for Children–Fourth Edition.* San Antonio, TX: PsychCorp.

Welfel, E. R. (2002). *Ethics in counseling and psychotherapy: Standards, research, and emerging issues* (2nd ed.). Pacific Grove, CA: Brooks/Cole.

White, M. A., & Harris, M. W. (1961). *The school psychologist.* New York: Harper & Brothers.

Wickman, E. K. (1928). *Children's behavior and teachers' attitudes.* New York: Commonwealth Fund Division of Publications.

Wiederholt, J. L., & Bryant, B. R. (2001). *Gray Oral Reading Tests–Fourth Edition.* Austin, TX: Pro-Ed.

Wilkinson, G. S. (1993). *Wide Range Achievement Test* (3rd ed.). Wilmington, DE: Wide Range.

Williams, C. L., & Berry, J. W. (1991). Primary prevention of acculturative stress among refugees. *American Psychologist, 46,* 632–641.

Wilson, M. S., & Reschly, D. J. (1995). Gender and school psychology: Issues, questions, and answers. *School Psychology Review, 24,* 45–61.

Wilson, M. S., & Reschly, D. J. (1996). Assessment in school psychology training and practice. *School Psychology Review, 25,* 9–23.

Witt, J. C., Daly, E. M., & Noell, G. (2000). *Functional assessments: A step by step guide to solving academic and behavior problems.* Longmont, CO: Sopris West.

Witt, J. C., Elliott, S. N., Daly, E. J., Gresham, F. M., & Kramer, J. J. (1997). *Assessment of at-risk and special needs children* (2nd ed.). New York: McGraw Hill.

Wolery, M., Bailey, D. B., & Sugai, G. M. (1989). *Effective teaching: Applied behavior analysis with exceptional students.* Boston: Allyn & Bacon.

Woodcock, R. W. (1987). *Woodcock Reading Mastery Tests–Revised.* Circle Pines, MN: American Guidance Service.

Woodcock, R. W. (1998). *Woodcock Reading Mastery Tests–Revised–Normative update.* Circle Pines, MN: American Guidance Service.

Woodcock, R. W., McGrew, K. S., & Mather, N. (2001a). *The Woodcock–Johnson III–Tests of Achievement*. Itasca, IL: Riverside.

Woodcock, R. W., McGrew, K. S., & Mather, N. (2001b). *The Woodcock–Johnson III–Tests of Cognitive Abilities*. Itasca, IL: Riverside.

Woodcock, R. W., & Munoz-Sandoval, A. F. (1995). *Woodcock Language Proficiency Battery–Revised, Spanish form*. Itasca, IL: Riverside Publishing.

World Health Organization. (1992). *The ICD-10 classification of mental disorders*. Geneva: Author.

Worthen, B. R., Sanders, J. R., & Fitzpatrick, J. L. (1997). *Program evaluation: Alternative approaches and practical guidelines* (2nd ed.). New York: Longman.

Yansen, E. A., & Shulman, E. L. (1996). Language assessment: Multicultural considerations. In L. A. Suzuki, P. J. Meller, & J. G. Ponterotto (Eds.), *Handbook of multicultural assessment* (pp. 353–393). San Francisco: Jossey-Bass.

Yell, M. (1998). *The law and special education*. Upper Sdalle River, NJ: Prentice-Hall.

Ysseldyke, J. (2000). Commentary: Déjà vu all over again: What will it take to solve big instructional problems? *School Psychology Review, 29*, 575–576.

Ysseldyke, J., Dawson, P., Lehr, C., Reschly, D., Reynolds, M., & Telzrow, C. (1997). *School psychology: A blueprint for training and practice–II*. Bethesda, MD: National Association of School Psychologists.

Ysseldyke, J. E., Algozzine, B., & Epps, S. (1983). A logical and empirical analysis of current practice in classifying students as handicapped. *Exceptional Children, 50*, 160–166.

Ysseldyke, J. E., Christenson, S. L., Thurlow, M. L., & Bakewell, D. (1989). Are different kinds of instructional tasks used by different categories of students in different settings? *School Psychology Review, 18*, 98–111.

Ysseldyke, J. E., & Thurlow, M. L. (1984). Assessment practices in special education: Adequacy and appropriateness. *Educational Psychologist, 19*, 123–136.

Zhang, D., & Katsiyannis, A. (2002). Minority representation in special education: A persistent challenge. *Remedial and Special Education, 25*, 180–187.

# Index

*f* indicates figure, *t* indicates table

ABAB design, 253–254*f*, 257. *See also* Research
Accountability stage of program evaluation, 258–259. *See also* Program evaluation
Accreditation of doctoral programs, 34, 63–64, 65*t*–72*t*. *See also* Doctoral level of training
Acculturation, 49. *See also* Cultural diversity; Linguistic diversity
Achievement testing, 169–170. *See also* Assessments
ADA. *See* Americans with Disabilities Act (ADA)
Adaptive development, 25, 118, 228
ADHD. *See* Attention-deficit/hyperactivity disorder (ADHD)
Administrators, school, 130, 135, 148–149, 252
Advertising, 135, 295–297, 326–327
African Americans/blacks, 43, 46, 51, 57. *See also* Cultural diversity; Minority students
American Board of Professional Psychology (ABPP), 91
American Indian/Alaskan Natives, 43, 46, 57. *See also* Cultural diversity; Minority students
American Psychological Association (APA). *See also* Division of School

Psychology (Division 16) of the APA
accreditation and, 63–64, 82
continuing professional development and, 92–93
ethical issues and, 130–135
Ethical Principles of Psychologists and Code of Conduct (Revised 2002), 281–307
job postings by, 97
lack of diversity among school psychologists, 47–48
practicum and internships, 84, 85–87
questions regarding, 41
tensions experienced between NASP and, 37–39
timeline, 40*t*
training and, 63–64, 73, 76–77, 82, 92–93
American School Counselor Association, 16
Americans with Disabilities Act (ADA), 115*t*, 126–128. *See also* Legislation
Analysis of problems
assessment and, 182–183
evidence-based instruction and, 194–195
mental health services and, 213
overview, 152*f*, 153–154
prevention and intervention and, 203
Anxiety, 218–220, 243

APA. *See* American Psychological Association (APA)
APA Division of School Psychology. *See* Division of School Psychology (Division 16) of the APA
APA's Ethical Principles of Psychologists and Code of Conduct (Revised 2002), 281–307
Applied research. *See also* Research
conducting in the schools, 251–255, 254*f*, 256*f*, 257
evaluation of programs and, 240, 257–260
Aristotle, 22
Asian Americans/Pacific Islanders, 43, 46. *See also* Cultural diversity; Minority students
Assessing program utility stage of program evaluation, 259–260. *See also* Program evaluation
Assessments. *See also* Functional behavioral assessment (FBA); Intellectual assessment; IQ testing; Problem-solving assessment
of academic skills, 168–172
of acculturation, 49
balancing with other roles of school psychologists, 105–107
bias in, 52–53, 58*t*, 176–177
case example regarding, 7–8

359